T0309122

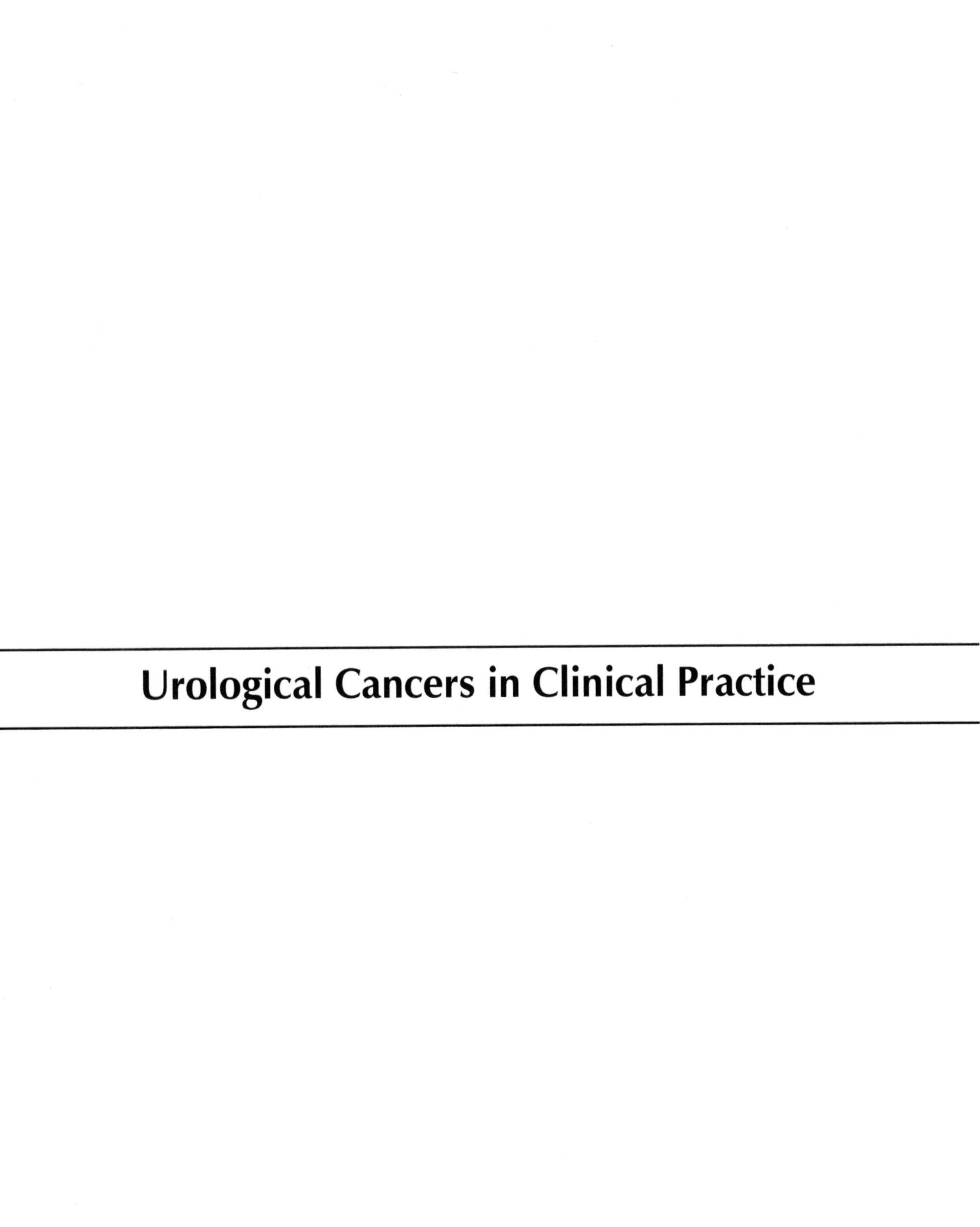

Urological Cancers in Clinical Practice

Urological Cancers in Clinical Practice

Editor: Klara Walker

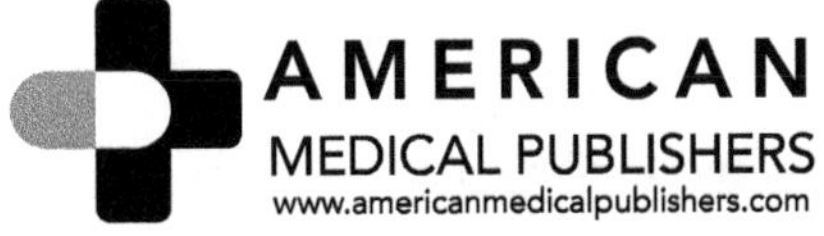

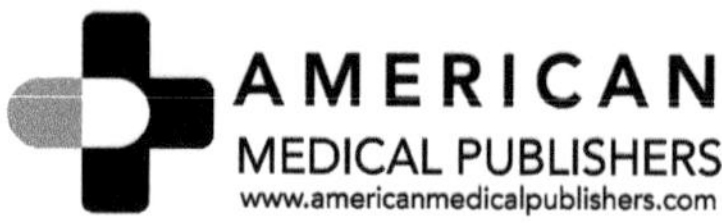

Cataloging-in-Publication Data

Urological cancers in clinical practice / edited by Klara Walker.
p. cm.
Includes bibliographical references and index.
ISBN 978-1-63927-821-3
1. Urinary organs--Cancer. 2. Urinary organs--Cancer--Treatment. 3. Oncology. 4. Genitourinary organs--Cancer.
5. Genitourinary organs--Cancer--Treatment. I. Walker, Klara.
RC280.U74 U763 2023
616.994 6--dc23

American Medical Publishers,
41 Flatbush Avenue,
1st Floor, New York,
NY 11217, USA

ISBN 978-1-63927-821-3 (Hardback)

Contents

Preface

This book has been a concerted effort by a group of academicians, researchers and scientists, who have contributed their research works for the realization of the book. This book has materialized in the wake of emerging advancements and innovations in this field. Therefore, the need of the hour was to compile all the required researches and disseminate the knowledge to a broad spectrum of people comprising of students, researchers and specialists of the field.

Urological cancers refer to a group of diseases that develop in the organs of the urinary tract and the male reproductive tract as a result of aberrant cell development. These can affect the urethra, kidneys, bladder and ureter, as well as the testicles, penis and prostate in males. Cancers in these organs cause symptoms like a lump, pain, blood in the urine and urinary tract infections (UTIs). Urological cancers can be caused by a variety of factors, including the environment, genetics, lifestyle or other factors. Many of these cancers are treatable if detected early. Majority of these cancers are treated surgically in an attempt to eliminate the tumor. In certain cases, radiation therapy like cyberknife is preferred after surgery or in its place. This method employs high-energy beams, such as X-rays, to regulate or stop the development of cancer cells. Some patients may receive chemotherapy to kill cancer cells or slow their growth. This book is a compilation of chapters that discuss the most vital concepts and emerging studies on urological cancers. It aims to understand the clinical perspectives of these cancers. This book is appropriate for students seeking detailed information in this area as well as for experts.

At the end of the preface, I would like to thank the authors for their brilliant chapters and the publisher for guiding us all-through the making of the book till its final stage. Also, I would like to thank my family for providing the support and encouragement throughout my academic career and research projects.

Editor

A Mini-Review of Reactive Oxygen Species in Urological Cancer: Correlation with NADPH Oxidases, Angiogenesis and Apoptosis

Yasuyoshi Miyata [1,*], Tomohiro Matsuo [1], Yuji Sagara [1], Kojiro Ohba [1], Kaname Ohyama [2] and Hideki Sakai [1]

1 Department of Urology, Nagasaki University Graduate School of Biomedical Sciences, 1-7-1 Sakamoto, Nagasaki 852-8501, Japan; tomo1228@nagasaki-u.ac.jp (T.M.); gaasara3@gmail.com (Y.S.); ohba-k@nagasaki-u.ac.jp (K.O.); hsakai@nagasaki-u.ac.jp (H.S.)

2 Department of Pharmaceutical Science, Nagasaki University Graduate School of Biomedical Sciences, 1-7-1 Sakamoto, Nagasaki 852-8501, Japan; k-ohyama@nagasaki-u.ac.jp

* Correspondence: yasu-myt@nagasaki-u.ac.jp

Abstract: Oxidative stress refers to elevated reactive oxygen species (ROS) levels, and NADPH oxidases (NOXs), which are one of the most important sources of ROS. Oxidative stress plays important roles in the etiologies, pathological mechanisms, and treatment strategies of vascular diseases. Additionally, oxidative stress affects mechanisms of carcinogenesis, tumor growth, and prognosis in malignancies. Nearly all solid tumors show stimulation of neo-vascularity, termed angiogenesis, which is closely associated with malignant aggressiveness. Thus, cancers can be seen as a type of vascular disease. Oxidative stress-induced functions are regulated by complex endogenous mechanisms and exogenous factors, such as medication and diet. Although understanding these regulatory mechanisms is important for improving the prognosis of urothelial cancer, it is not sufficient, because there are controversial and conflicting opinions. Therefore, we believe that this knowledge is essential to discuss observations and treatment strategies in urothelial cancer. In this review, we describe the relationships between members of the NOX family and tumorigenesis, tumor growth, and pathological mechanisms in urological cancers including prostate cancer, renal cell carcinoma, and urothelial cancer. In addition, we introduce natural compounds and chemical agents that are associated with ROS-induced angiogenesis or apoptosis.

Keywords: reactive oxygen species; NADPH oxidases; angiogenesis; apoptosis; urological cancers

---

1. Introduction

Oxidative stress is defined as the imbalance between the production of pro-oxidants, such as free radicals and reactive metabolites, and their elimination by protective mechanisms, referred to as antioxidants (Figure 1) [1]. The oxide balance is maintained by an endogenous enzymatic mechanism, but it is also affected by exogenous factors, such as lifestyle, medications, and diet [2,3]. There is a general agreement that oxidative stress is closely associated with various complex physiological and pathological mechanisms [3,4]. In addition, there is growing support for the concept that oxidative stress plays important roles in carcinogenesis, malignant behavior, and prognosis, in various types of cancer [4,5]. Thus, understanding the pathological roles and regulatory mechanisms of oxidative stress in malignant cells and tissues is essential to discuss the observations and treatment strategies in patients with malignancies.

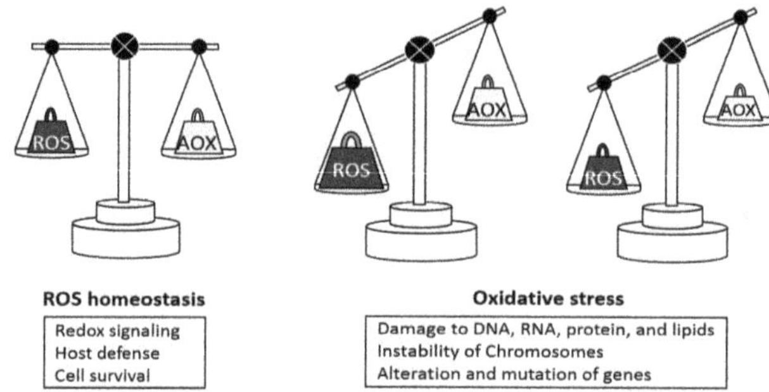

Figure 1. Oxidative stress is defined as an imbalance between the cellular production of reactive oxygen species (ROS) and antioxidants (AOX). Under natural conditions, the production of pro- and antioxidants is in a stable equilibrium. Excessive ROS production or depletion of antioxidants can cause oxidative stress, which may damage cellular lipids, proteins, and DNA, with the latter leading to chromosomal instability and gene mutations.

Oxidative stress refers to elevated intracellular levels of reactive oxygen species (ROS). ROS are a heterogeneous group of highly reactive ions and molecules derived from molecular oxygen (O_2), including superoxide anions, hydroxyl radicals, hydrogen peroxide, HOCl, and singlet oxygen [6]. Although ROS were initially believed to be toxic and associated with various pathological mechanisms, subsequent studies have shown that ROS also play crucial roles in physiological processes [7]. In fact, ROS can act as an antioxidant system to maintain redox homeostasis, even though they are recognized as strong pro-oxidants themselves [8]. Thus, various evidence supports the fact that the biological roles of ROS are complex and paradoxical [7,9]. The degree of ROS production is speculated to be the determinant factor in such dual roles. In short, a low or moderate increase in ROS promotes cell proliferation, apoptosis, angiogenesis, and migration in physiological conditions, and ROS act to maintain cellular homeostasis [10]. In contrast, excessive production of ROS can cause oxidative stress, which may damage cellular lipids, proteins, and DNA [6,11]. Thus, balancing the ROS level is important for regulating cell proliferation, apoptosis, migration, and angiogenesis, and under normal conditions, the production and elimination of ROS are tightly controlled through the help of ROS scavengers (endogenous antioxidants) of an enzymatic (e.g., catalase, glutathione peroxidase system) or a non-enzymatic (e.g., ascorbic acid, lipoic acid, α-tocopherol) nature.

As mentioned above, excessive ROS production causes DNA damage and promotes the activities of oncogenes and/or inhibits tumor-suppressor genes. For example, H_2O_2 has been shown to stimulate an activating mutation of the proto-oncogene, c-Ha-ras-1, whereas it inhibits the function of the tumor-suppressor gene, p53 [12]. In addition to such genetic changes, ROS are known to stimulate carcinogenesis via various epigenetic alterations. The methylation of tumor-suppressor genes is the most representative epigenetic alteration in oxidative stress-induced carcinogenesis. For example, H_2O_2 has been reported to hypermethylate tumor-suppressor genes, such as retinoblastoma, Von Hippel–Lindau, and breast cancer 1 [13,14]. Furthermore, the activities of various proteins and signaling molecules, such as mitogen-activated protein kinase (MAPK) and extracellular regulated kinase (Erk)1/2 (associated with cell proliferation [15,16]), nuclear factor κB (NFκB) (involved in cell proliferation and the cell cycle [17]), and 3-phosphoinositide-dependent kinase (PDK)-1 (involved in cell proliferation and apoptosis [16]), are affected by ROS. Phosphoinositide 3-kinase (PI3K)/Akt (protein kinase B) signaling, implicated in cancer cell proliferation, is also modulated by ROS [18]. Interestingly, ROS can suppress the activity of phosphatase and tensin homolog (PTEN), recognized as inhibitor of PI3K/Akt signaling [19]. PI3K/Akt signaling is also associated with various malignant behaviors, including apoptosis, angiogenesis, and chemotherapy resistance [18]. Thus, ROS can regulate the activities of cancer-related pathways, via direct and indirect mechanisms.

The mitochondrial electron transport chain is suggested to be the major endogenous source of ROS [20]. Other important sources of ROS are enzymes, such as NADPH oxidase (NOX), xanthine oxidase (XO), and lipoxygenase (LOX) [21]. Among these, special attention has been paid to NOX because it is the best-known source of cellular ROS and because of its cross-talk with mitochondria [22,23]. Furthermore, increased ROS lead to the upregulation of cyclooxygenase (COX)-2 activity [24]. ROS also activate matrix metalloproteinases (MMPs), which can degrade basement membranes and the extracellular matrix [25]. Interestingly, tissue inhibitors of metalloproteinases (TIMPs), endogenous inhibitors of MMPs, are downregulated by ROS [26]. In addition to the MMP/ TIMP system, urokinase-type plasminogen activator (uPA) is well known to degrade extracellular compounds, and ROS have been reported to induce uPA expression via regulation of MAPK [15]. Furthermore, ROS directly regulate the activity of β-actin, a regulator of cell adhesion [27]. Previous reports have shown that such ROS-related molecules play crucial roles in carcinogenesis and malignant aggressiveness, via the regulation of cell differentiation, proliferation, invasion, and angiogenesis in several types of cancer [11,16,21,28]. Based on these facts, ROS are speculated to be closely associated with pathological mechanisms as well as with outcomes in cancer patients. In fact, elevated oxidative signaling because of excessive production of ROS has been reported to be associated with carcinogenesis and malignant behavior [28–31], and cancer cells have higher ROS levels than their normal counterparts [32].

Thus, information on ROS-related molecules and pathways is important to understand the pathological mechanisms and to discuss the treatment strategies in several types of malignancies, including urological cancers. Several investigators are of the opinion that ROS are crucial for cell survival, angiogenesis, invasion, and extravasation [33,34]. Among these biological phenomena, angiogenesis plays crucial roles in cell survival, via the supply of oxygen and nutrients, and cell dissemination in solid tumors. In other words, solid malignant tumors are regarded as "vascular diseases". In fact, increased levels of ROS have been reported in several cancer cells, and play important roles in tumor development, cell survival, and progression [34–36]. Therefore, in this review, we present a simplified outline of the proposed mechanisms of oxidative stress under normal and pathological conditions, including malignancies. Further, we summarize the pathological significance of NOXs in urological cancers, such as prostate cancer, renal cell carcinoma (RCC), and urothelial cancer. Finally, we show the relationships between ROS and apoptosis in pathological conditions, including malignancies, and natural products and chemical agents that influence ROS-related apoptosis in urological cancers are introduced.

2. NOX and Urological Cancer

2.1. Pathological Significance of NOX1–5 in Malignancies

NOX was first described in the context of leukemia. The NOX family comprises seven isoforms: NOX 1–5 and dual oxidases (DUOX) 1 and 2. NOX 1–5 generate superoxide anions, whereas DUOX1 and 2 generate H_2O_2 [37]. As mentioned above, the NOX family is one of the major sources of ROS and one of the key regulators in ROS-related mechanisms expressed in various epithelial cells. In regard to stimuli of mammalian NOXs, chemicals, inflammatory factors, and changed cellular environments are the best known [38,39]. NOX-mediated ROS are reported to stimulate various pro-oncogenes, such as Src and Ras, and to inhibit tumor suppressors, such as p53 and PTEN [40]. In addition, NOXs and NOX-mediated ROS can mediate cellular transformation and genetic programming related to cell growth [40–42]. Furthermore, malignant cells generate NOX-dependent extracellular superoxide anions, which contribute to the control of cell proliferation and intracellular ROS/reactive nitrogen species-dependent signaling pathways that cause apoptosis [43,44]. Consequently, during tumor progression, tumor cells establish resistance towards intracellular signaling, though the expression of membrane-associated catalase [45]. Thus, information about the pathological significance of NOXs is essential for understanding the relationship between oxidative stress and tumorigenesis, cell survival and death, cell dissemination, and the prognosis of malignancies.

NOX1 is most highly expressed in the colon epithelium and to a lesser extent in endothelial cells, vascular smooth muscle, and the prostate [41,46,47]. NOX1 has been reported to be closely associated with malignant potential, apoptosis, and angiogenesis, under various conditions [47,48]. The overexpression of NOX1 in NIH3T3 fibroblasts has induced malignant transformation, rendering them slightly tumorigenic in athymic mice [41]. Because of these facts, the function of NOX1 in human cancer has been focused on among the NOX family members [49]. In fact, NOX1 is associated with cell proliferation in colon cancer [50] and carcinogenesis in skin cancer [51].

NOX2 was first described in phagocytic leukocytes and recognized as a mediator of inflammation. NOX2 has also been widely studied in humans. Similar to NOX1, NOX2 is suggested to play important roles in carcinogenesis. Actually, NOX1- and NOX2-induced ROS production is a cause of DNA damage by acidic bile reflux in esophageal cells [52]. From this finding, it has been suggested that inhibition of ROS, induced by reflux, could be a useful strategy for preventing DNA damage and decreasing the risk of tumorigenic transformation caused by gastroesophageal reflux disease, which is the greatest risk factor for esophageal adenocarcinoma. Investigators have also reported pathological roles of NOX2 in malignancies. For example, NOX2-derived ROS facilitate the metastasis of melanoma cells, by downmodulation of NK-cell function [53], immunosuppression by chronic myelomonocytic leukemia (which depends on NOX2 [54]), and cell proliferation—which is associated with NOX2 in gastric cancer [55].

NOX3 is expressed in the inner ear [56]. Increased NOX3 protein expression has been detected after heavy ion irradiation, which also induces other NOXs (NOX 1, 2, 4, and 5) [57]. In non-small cell lung cancer, NOX3 has been linked to tumor growth [58]. The mechanism of NOX3 regulation is less well known than those of other isoforms.

NOX4 is highly expressed in the kidneys [59]. Various growth factors and their receptors, such as insulin-like growth factor (IGF)-1, transforming growth factor β (TGF-β), and toll-like receptor 4 (TLR4), have been reported to stimulate NOX4 activity [60–62]. Interestingly, stimulation of the IGF-1 receptor was positively associated with cell survival via induction of NOX4-generated ROS in a variety of cancers [60]. Furthermore, NOX4 is associated with tumor growth and the prevention of apoptosis in the presence of growth factors in several malignancies [63,64]. In addition, NOX4 stimulates angiogenesis through the upregulation of vascular endothelial growth factor (VEGF)-A and hypoxia-inducible factor (HIF)-1α in a variety of cancers [65], and siRNA-mediated knockdown of NOX4 inhibited VEGF-induced endothelial cell migration and proliferation [66]. In a mouse model, NOX4 expression was upregulated in new capillaries in brain ischemia-induced angiogenesis [67]. Thus, NOX4 is suggested to play crucial roles in aggressive malignancy.

NOX5 is detected in various normal tissues, including the fetal tissues, as well as in the adult spleen and uterus [59]. Increased mRNA expression of NOX5 has been detected in cell lines and tumor tissues of various malignancies, including melanoma and breast cancer, but not in colorectal, hepatic, and ovarian cancer and Ewing's sarcoma [68]. In contrast, NOX5 mRNA expression in testicular tumor tissues was significantly lower than that in the adjacent normal ones [68]. On the other hand, NOX5 is reportedly associated with pathological significance in esophageal carcinoma [69], and plays important roles in angiogenesis via the stimulation of endothelial cells and vascular muscle cells in malignancies [70]. Thus, the pathological functions of NOX5 in malignancies have widely been investigated in both in vivo and in vitro studies.

2.2. Pathological Significance of DUOX1 and 2 in Malignancies

In contrast to the quite well elucidated roles of NOXs, the functions of the two DUOX isoforms remain unclear. DUOX1 expression was not detected in lung cancer cells [71]. In addition, the DUOX1 mRNA expression level in hepatocellular carcinoma tissues is lower than that in non-cancerous tissues [72]. Similar results have been found in various other cancers, including esophagus cancer, lung cancer, and thyroid cancer [73]. Thus, DUOX1 expression is suppressed in various malignancies. In contrast, in one report, the reintroduction of functional DUOX1 into lung cancer cell lines increased cell migration and wound repair, without affecting cell growth [71]. In addition, DUOX1 has been identified as a risk factor for the prognosis of hepatocellular carcinoma patients after surgery [74].

DUOX2 mRNA and protein are reportedly expressed in several malignancies, including lung, breast, colorectal, gastric, and pancreatic cancers [75,76]. In contrast, lung cancer cells show losses of DUOX2 expression [71]. In another report, no significant differences in DUOX2 expression were found in carcinomas originating from the breast, lung, skin, stomach, or thyroid [73]. Thus, there is no general agreement on the pathological significance of DUOXs in malignant tumors.

3. Pathological Significance of the NOX Family in Urological Cancers

3.1. NOX 1–5 in Prostate Cancer

In an in vivo study, the overexpression of NOX1 mRNA was not detected in three prostate cancer cell lines (DU145, LNCaP, and PC-3) [77]. In addition, DU145 cells do not express NOX1 mRNA [78]. On the other hand, one study reported that NOX1 m-RNA is expressed at a low level in DU145 cells and at higher levels in LNCaP and VCaP cells [79]. Thus, while there is controversy regarding NOX1 expression in prostate cancer cells, NOX1 expression seems to be absent or low in DU145 cells.

In animal experiments using nude mice, NOX1 overexpression increased tumorigenesis and tumor growth in DU145 human prostate cancer cells [80]. A similar result in an animal model has been reported by other investigators [81]. In the transgenic adenocarcinoma of the mouse prostate (TRAMP) mice, NOX1 expression was significantly higher in high-grade prostatic intraepithelial neoplasia (PIN) and cancer cells, than in low-grade PIN and normal prostate epithelial cells [82]. However, NOX1 acted as a potent trigger of angiogenesis via the upregulation of VEGF in a DU145 xenograft model [80]. Thus, animal experiments have shown that NOX1 is positively associated with tumorigenesis and malignant behavior in prostate cancer. Furthermore, in recent years, in vitro models using adenovirus vectors have shown that NOX1 plays a role in the cell death of prostate cancer cells [83], and NOX1 has been associated with metastatic potential in a series of cell lines developed from LNCaP [81].

In humans, NOX1 mRNA and protein are overexpressed in prostate cancer as compared to non-tumor prostate tissues [81,84]. However, according to the Human Protein Atlas repository version 12 (www.proteinatlas.org), high protein expression has been detected in both tumor cells and non-tumoral epithelium, and several studies in humans have reported that the NOX1 mRNA level did not significantly differ between benign and malignant prostate tissues [68,79]. Unfortunately, there are few reports on the relationship between NOX1 expression and pathological features in patients with prostate cancer. In the report by Arnold et al. [84], the high protein expression of NOX1 was not associated with any clinicopathological features, biochemical failure, or survival.

In contrast to NOX1, NOX2 mRNA expression has been detected in DU145, PC-3, and LNCaP cells, but not in normal cell lines [78]. mRNA levels of NOX2 were reported to be higher in PC-3, DU145, and VCaP cells than in the benign prostate cell lines, EP156T and RWPE1 [79]. However, other investigators have shown that mRNA expression of NOX2 was low or undetectable in three of these cancer cell lines (LNCaP, DU145, and PC-3) [68]. A similar observation has been reported in 17 patients with moderately to poorly differentiated prostate adenocarcinoma tissues [68]. According to the Human Protein Atlas repository version 12 (www.proteinatlas.org), NOX2 shows low protein expression in both tumor cells and non-tumoral epithelium, while it is prominently expressed in stromal tissues. As for mRNA expression, the NOX2 status in malignant prostate tissues is similar to that in benign tissues [79]. Thus, although several studies have shown that NOX2 expression is increased in prostate cancer as compared to non-tumoral tissues, opposite results have been shown by in vivo studies. Unfortunately, there is little information on the pathological significance of NOX2 expression in prostate cancer.

As mentioned above, the pathological significance of NOX3 in malignancies is not yet fully understood. NOX3 mRNA and protein expression was not observed in the prostate cancer cell lines, DU145, LNCaP, and PC-3 [68,77,78]. Protein expressions of NOX 1, 2, 4, and 5 have been detected in PC-3 cells, while NOX3 expression was absent [85]. Furthermore, no significant difference in NOX3 mRNA expression was detected between human prostate cancer tissues and non-tumoral tissues [68,79]. Although the information on NOX3 expression in prostate cancer is scarce, studies have shown that NOX3 has limited or no pathological significance in prostate cancer.

NOX4 is reportedly expressed in DU145, PC-3, and LNCaP cells, but not in a normal prostate cell line [78]. In addition, NOX4 mRNA levels in prostate cancer are significantly higher than those in benign prostate tissues [79]. In contrast, in a study by Juhasz et al., overexpression of NOX4 mRNA was not detected in the above three cell lines and human prostate cancer tissues [68]. According to the Human Protein Atlas repository version 12 (Available online: www.proteinatlas.org), tumor cells and non-tumoral epithelium show low NOX4 protein expression. Regarding its pathological roles, NOX4 is reported to contribute to angiogenesis via the upregulation of VEGF [65]. Interestingly, in rat prostate cancer, castration results in dramatic increases in NOX1, NOX2, and NOX4 [86]. Regarding the relationship between hormonal conditions and NOXs, NOX2 and NOX4 mRNA levels were upregulated by androgens and downregulated in the absence of androgens in the human androgen-responsive but not dependent prostate cell line, 22Rv1 [87]. This NOX-related mechanism, which involves ROS production, is associated with radiosensitivity in prostate cancer cells [87]. On the other hand, no significant change in NOX5 mRNA levels was observed upon castration in rats with prostate cancer [86]. In addition to androgens, adiponectin has induced a strong increase in NOX2 and NOX4 mRNA expression in DU145 and 22Rv1 human prostate cancer cells, which were NOX2-dominated and NOX4-dominated, respectively [88].

Kumar et al. reported NOX5 expression in prostate cancer cell lines (DU145, PC-3, and LNCaP cells), while it was not detected in a normal prostate cell line [78]. Other investigators detected NOX5 mRNA in benign prostate cancer cells (RWPE1) and cancer cell lines (LNCaP, VCaP, DU145, and PC-3), with the highest levels being observed in LNCaP and PC-3 cells [77,79]. From these results, it can be said that NOX5 mRNA is widely expressed in prostate cancer cell lines. Actually, NOX5 is held to be the most consistently expressed member of the NOX family in prostate cancer cell lines [79]. However, Juhasz et al. observed overexpression of NOX5 mRNA in PC-3, but not in DU145 cells [68]. Thus, there is a possibility that NOX5 mRNA expression may rely on androgens. Furthermore, a comparative analysis of NOX5 gene expression in tumor samples vs. adjacent non-malignant tissue showed no significant differences [68]. Brar et al. reported that, in human prostate tissues, NOX5 mRNA is widely expressed in both cancer and normal glands, based on which, the authors concluded that NOX5 mRNA expression is not a marker of malignant transformation [77]. Similar results have been reported for NOX5 protein expression in human tissues; NOX5 protein was expressed in 50 out of 62 human prostate cancer tissues (80.6%) in a study by Antony et al. [89]. Based on data in the Human Protein Atlas repository version 12 (Available online: www.proteinatlas.org), both tumor cells and non-tumoral epithelium highly express NOX5 protein. In addition, it has been reported that protein expression levels of NOX-5 are not significantly different between cancer and benign tissues [79]. On the other hand, decreased mRNA expression of NOX5 in prostate cancer, as compared to benign tissues, has been reported [79]. This finding suggested that NOX5 acts as a tumor suppressor in the carcinogenesis of prostate cancer. However, the relationship between NOX5 expression and carcinogenesis is not entirely clear, and more detailed and wider studies are necessary. Regarding the pathological roles of NOX5, several reports have shown that downregulation of NOX5 expression inhibits cell proliferation and tumor growth and induces apoptosis in PC cells [77–79,90]. In addition, in PC-3 cells, NOX5 silencing led to a significant increase in apoptosis via the stimulation of caspase-3 and -7 [79]. From these facts, NOX5 is thought to stimulate the cell survival of prostate cancer cells.

3.2. DUOX1 and 2 in Prostate Cancer

Overexpression of DUOX1 mRNA was not detected in the three prostate cancer cell lines, LNCaP, DU145, and PC-3 [63]. Other investigators reported that DUOX1 mRNA was detected at high levels in DU145 cells; however, such high expression was also detected in the benign prostate cell lines, EP156T and RWPE1 [79]. PC-3 cells express DUOX1 protein, but at a level similar to that in HeLa cells [85]. In humans, DUOX1 is highly expressed in both normal and prostate tumor tissues, and while some patients showed higher DUOX1 expression in tumoral tissues than in normal ones, the authors did not judge that the difference was significant [68]. According to the Human Protein Atlas repository version 12 (Available online: www.proteinatlas.org), DUOX1 protein expression is not detected in tumor cells and non-tumoral epithelium. On the other hand, it has been reported that DUOX1 mRNA expression in prostate cancer tissues is significantly lower than that in non-tumor tissues [79]. Thus, although DUOX1 expression has been detected in prostate cancer cells, its pathological significance is not fully understood.

DUOX2 mRNA expression has been reported to be low or undetectable in prostate cancer cell lines [68]. Other investigators detected high expression of DUOX2 mRNA in DU145 cells, but not in PC-3 cells [79]. Although DUOX2 expression has been observed in human cancer tissues, it is also highly expressed in normal tissues, indicating that DUOX2 is not overexpressed in human cancer tissues [68]. In addition, DUOX2 mRNA expression in prostate cancer tissues did not differ from that in non-tumoral tissues [68].

Several reports have shown pathological roles of DUOXs in prostate cancer. For example, BxPC-3 cells responded to interferon-γ treatment by upregulating DUOX2 protein [75]. There is a report that ROS levels in prostate cancer (PC-3 cells) are constitutively maintained by DUOX1 and 2, and these ROS lead to increased apoptosis resistance via positive regulation of Akt signaling [85].

3.3. NOXs and DUOXs in RCC

In contrast to prostate cancer, there is very limited information on the expression of NOXs in RCC. In an in vitro study, the activation of NOX1 and NOX4 maintained HIF-2α protein expression and thereby contributed to the tumorigenesis of RCC [91]. NOX4 expression in RCC cell lines was higher than that in a normal renal tubular cell line [91]. In vivo, inhibition of NOX4 expression by siRNA, abrogated tumorigenesis, cell invasion, and tumor growth in a murine xenograft model of RCC [92]. In a study by Chang et al., NOX4 contributed to the chemoresistance of RCC, by regulating apoptotic signaling, including anti-apoptotic B-cell lymphoma (Bcl)-XL and Bcl-2 and pro-apoptotic Bax [93]. Unfortunately, there are only a few reports on the expression and pathological roles of NOX2, 3, and 5 in RCC.

DUOX1 and 2 were reported to be highly expressed in both normal and RCC tissues [68]. However, there is no report with detailed information on the pathological significance of DUOXs in RCC. There is a general agreement that ROS-mediated mechanisms of oxidative stress play important roles in carcinogenesis, tumor development, and progression in RCC [94]. Specifically, angiogenesis is one of the important processes for tumor growth, cell dissemination, and prognosis in RCC. Unfortunately, there is no report on the angiogenic roles of NOXs. Therefore, more detailed and wider studies are necessary to discuss the pathological characteristics of this disease.

3.4. NOXs and DUOXs in Urothelial Cancer

Similar to RCC, the information on NOXs in urothelial cancer is insufficient to discuss their pathological roles in tumorigenesis and malignant aggressiveness. NOX1 protein expression is higher in high-grade and invasive disease than in low-grade and non-invasive disease, in human bladder cancer tissues [49]. Unfortunately, additional results on NOX1 expression in urothelial cancer have not yet been reported. However, several reports suggest that NOX1 is associated with tumor development and apoptosis in urothelial cancer. For example, the silencing of ALKBH8, a member of the human AlkB family of DNA repair molecules [95], leads to a decrease in ROS production, via the downregulation of NOX1 in urothelial cancer and to apoptosis resistance, resulting in bladder cancer development [49]. In addition, other reports have shown that the knockdown of NOX1 reduces ROS production and apoptosis by FK228, a histone deacetylase inhibitor, in a human bladder cancer cell line (J82 cells) [96].

Overexpression of NOX2 has been detected in urothelial cancer cells, whereas expression in normal urothelial cells is low, suggesting that NOX2 may play a crucial role in the carcinogenesis of urothelial cancer [97]. However, this study also showed that NOX2 expression was not significantly associated with grade or pT stage in 93 patients with urothelial cancer [97]. In another report, the

DNA repair molecule, ALKBH3, was positively associated with urothelial cancer cell survival, through NOX2-dependent ROS production [97]. Thus, NOX2 is speculated to be required for tumor growth in urothelial cancer.

NOX4 is highly expressed in the urothelial cancer cell lines, T24, UMUC6, and KK47 [93]. In addition, NOX4 overexpression was detected in the cancer tissues of patients with low- or high-grade and non-invasive or invasive urothelial cancers, including carcinoma in situ, as compared to normal urothelium [98]. However, its level was not significantly correlated with the grade, pT stage, or tumor growth in 82 patients with urothelial cancer [98]. Although pathological roles of NOX4 expression were not speculated to be important, the authors observed significantly higher NOX4 immunostaining in the percutaneous lesion dysplasia than in normal urothelium [98]. Regarding apoptosis, NOX4 gene silencing did induce a change in the apoptotic activity of urothelial cancer cells [49]. Conversely, leukotriene B4 receptor 2 regulates cell invasion and metastasis by ROS production in urothelial cancer, and NOX1 and NO4 are associated with the mechanism of this phenomenon [99].

To our knowledge, there are no reports on the expression of NOX3 and NOX5 in urothelial cancer. We emphasize the importance for further investigation into the expression and pathological roles of NOX3 and NOX5 in urothelial cancer. Furthermore, we should note that the discussion of the biological activities and pathological significances of NOX family members was based on mRNA expression in cell culture. In other words, there is less information on the protein expression of the NOX family in human cancer tissues because of the lack of reliable antibodies. In recent years, specific antibodies for NOX family members have been developed. Wider and more detailed studies are expected to clarify the pathological significance and prognostic roles of these enzymes in urological cancers. We summarized pathological roles of NOX family in prostate cancer, renal cell cancer, and urothelial cancer in Table 1.

Table 1. Summary of pathological roles of NOXs in urological cancers.

Characteristics as Malignant Cells	Types	NOX					DUOX		References
		1	2	3	4	5	1	2	
Overexpression in cancer cells	PCa	Y/N	Y/N	N	Y/N	Y/N	N	N	[68,77–82,84,85,89]
	RCC	N	N	N	Y/N	N	N	N	[68,91]
	UC	–	Y	–	Y	–	–	–	[97,98]
Tumorigenesis	PCa	Y	–	–	–	–	–	–	[80,81]
	RCC	Y	–	–	Y	–	–	–	[91,92]
	UC	–	–	–	–	–	–	–	–
Cell death/Apoptosis	PCa	Y	–	–	–	Y	Y	Y	[77,79,83,85]
	RCC	–	–	–	Y	–	–	–	[93]
	UC	Y	–	–	N	–	–	–	[49,96]
Angiogenesis/ Angiogenesis-related factors	PCa	Y	–	–	Y	–	–	–	[65,80]
	RCC	–	–	–	–	–	–	–	–
	UC	–	N	–	–	–	–	–	[97]
Gleason score/Grade	PCa	N	–	–	–	–	–	–	[84]
	RCC	–	–	–	–	–	–	–	–
	UC	Y	N	–	N	–	–	–	[49,97,98]
T stage/Tumor growth/Invasion	PCa	Y/N	Y	–	Y	Y	–	–	[65,77–80,82,84]
	RCC	–	–	–	Y	–	–	–	[92]
	UC	Y	Y/N	–	Y/N	–	–	–	[49,97–99]
N stage/M stage/Metastasis	PCa	Y/N	–	–	–	–	–	–	[81,84]
	RCC	–	–	–	–	–	–	–	–
	UC	Y	–	–	Y	–	–	–	[99]
Outcome/Survival	PCa	N	–	–	–	–	–	–	[84]
	RCC	–	–	–	–	–	–	–	–
	UC	–	–	–	–	–	–	–	

NOX; NADPH oxidases, DUOX; dual oxidases, Y; Yes, N; No, PCa; prostate cancer, RCC; renal cell carcinoma, UC; urothelial cancer.

4. Angiogenesis and ROS

Proliferation, migration, and tube formation of endothelial cells are well known to be important steps of cancer-related angiogenesis. ROS can modulate tumor angiogenesis via the regulation of these steps [28]. VEGF-A is well known as one of the strongest pro-angiogenic factors under physiological and pathological conditions. Numerous studies have reported a positive correlation between VEGF-A expression and angiogenesis in cancer tissues evaluated by micro-vessel density [100,101]. Although various pathways have been reported to be regulators of VEGF-A expression, ROS are also known to be a representative VEGF-A-related factor under pathological conditions, including malignancies [102–104]. In addition to VEGF-A, information on hypoxia-induced changes is essential for a discussion of the pathological roles of tumor angiogenesis in urological cancers, especially in RCC. Hypoxia can also affect ROS production and this is recognized as a regulator of angiogenesis in these cancers [105–107]. Therefore, several investigators have paid special attention to the relationship between angiogenesis and ROS production in malignant tumors. In fact, detailed molecular regulatory mechanisms of angiogenesis, induced by ROS under pathological conditions, including malignancies, have been described in previous excellent reviews [28,108,109]. In this review, we demonstrate the factors modulating angiogenesis by ROS production in urological cancers.

4.1. Angiogenesis and ROS in Prostate Cancer

Various types of chemical agents, chemokines, and natural compounds can mediate carcinogenesis, malignant behavior, and treatment response, via the regulation of tumor angiogenesis. In addition, ROS are often associated with angiogenesis-related mechanisms in prostate cancer. In this section, we describe representative examples of factors that produce ROS and thus affect angiogenesis in prostate cancer.

Arsenite, an environmental toxicant, widely distributed in water, food, and air, acts as a carcinogen for prostate cancer, via the activation of PI3K/Akt signaling and the expression of VEGF and HIF-1α. ROS have been associated with this mechanism in DU145 cells [110]. In addition, Ampelopsin (dihydromyricetin), a natural flavonoid, is suggested to be a useful agent for the prevention and treatment of prostate cancer, and suppression of ROS and angiogenesis is thought to underlie its anti-cancer effects [111]. Similar effects of other flavonoids have been reported in the androgen-independent prostate cancer cell line, PC-3 [112].

Regarding chemical agents, vanadate, known as sodium orthovanadate, is associated with carcinogenesis for prostate cancer, via angiogenesis- and ROS-related mechanisms [105]. Conversely, when the anti-cancer effects of a combination therapy with paclitaxel and S13 (a tyrosine kinase inhibitor with a prevalent specificity for Src) were analyzed in a hormone-insensible prostate cancer cell model, tumor growth and angiogenesis were suppressed by the concomitant impairment of endothelial migration and VEGF production [113]. Interestingly, significant effects were observed in combination therapy versus control and single treatments, and a reduction in ROS production was similarly found only in combination therapy [113]. In brief, the combination of paclitaxel and S13 may strongly inhibit tumor angiogenesis, via the reduction of ROS production. In addition to anti-cancer agents, ROS are associated with interleukin-6-related radio-sensitivity and tumor angiogenesis in animal models [114]. However, angiogenesis is suppressed by exosomes derived from menstrual stem cells through a reduction in the secretion/activity of pro-angiogenic molecules, such as VEGF and NF-κB, and ROS inhibition is associated with this mechanism in prostate cancer [115]. Thus, ROS plays important roles in angiogenesis, caused by various stimuli, in prostate cancer.

4.2. Angiogenesis and ROS in RCC and Urothelial Cancer

As mentioned above, as angiogenesis is the most important step in tumor growth and progression in RCC, anti-angiogenetic agents are useful for angiogenesis treatment. In fact, hypoxia induces ROS production, and subsequently activates RhoA, which leads to angiogenesis through HIF-1α induction and VEGF production in RCC [106]. Unfortunately, the information about ROS-induced angiogenesis in RCC is very limited. In regard to natural compounds, piperlongumine—an alkaloid present in the fruit of the long pepper (*Piper longum*)—and its analogs, rapidly reduced protein and mRNA levels of c-Met, a regulator of angiogenesis, via a ROS-dependent mechanism in the RCC cell lines, 786-0 and PNX0010 [116]. However, the combination of quercetin (a flavonoid) and hyperoside (an organic compound) was reported to decrease ROS production by up to 2.25-fold, which correlated with angiogenesis in 786-0 cells [117].

Similar to RCC, there are few reports on ROS-induced angiogenesis in urothelial cancer. Platinum agents, such as cisplatin and carboplatin, are key drugs for the treatment of patients with advanced urothelial cancer. Cis-dichlorodiammineplatinum has been reported to increase ROS production in the urothelial cancer cell lines, T24, KU-1, and KU-19-19. In addition, it upregulates angiotensin II type 1 receptor (AT1R) expression though ROS production and enhances VEGF production [118]. Conversely, AT1R expression has been reported to be significantly associated with microvessel density in non-muscle-invasive bladder cancer [119]. The same research group showed that AT1R signaling was upregulated when tumors progressed after cisplatin-based regimens, and there was increased ROS production related to this phenomenon in bladder cancer [118]. The knockdown of ALKBH3 led to the downregulation of angiogenesis, ROS production, and VEGF expression in bladder cancer, in vitro and in vivo, in an orthotopic mouse model [97]. In addition to ALKBH3, ALKB8 is reported to be significantly associated with tumor grade, cancer cell invasion, and prognosis, via the regulation of angiogenesis and ROS production in urothelial cancer [49]. Other investigators have reported that MMP-1, which is associated with cell invasion and metastasis, is upregulated under hypoxic conditions. Such hypoxia-induced changes in MMP-1 expression are accompanied by the stabilization of HIF-1α and -2α and a rise in intracellular ROS in metastatic 253J-BV cells [107]. The authors concluded that ROS play important roles in hypoxia-mediated MMP-1 expression, and that HIF stabilization under hypoxia is dependent on increases in intracellular ROS levels.

5. Apoptosis and ROS

Apoptosis or programmed cell death is executed via two major pathways: the extrinsic (death receptor-dependent) and the intrinsic (mitochondrial) pathway. In the extrinsic pathway, apoptosis is regulated by the binding of death-inducing ligand. For example, the interaction between Fas ligand (FasL) and its receptor, Fas receptor (FasR), leads to the activation of the caspase cascade and the induction of apoptosis. Apoptosis via the caspase cascade can be also stimulated by the ligation of tumor necrosis factor (TNF)-α and TNF-related apoptosis-inducing ligand (TRAIL) to their respective receptors, such as TNF receptor and death receptors. The intrinsic pathway is not necessarily initiated by intracellular effects, but may be initiated by outside triggers as well [120,121]. However, apoptosis by the intrinsic pathway is often initiated by increased mitochondrial membrane permeability. In short, pro-apoptotic factors, such as cytochrome-c and apoptosis-inducing factor, are released from the mitochondria though the mitochondrial permeability transition pore. The intrinsic pathway of apoptosis is tightly regulated by the balance of the B-cell lymphoma 2 (Bcl-2) family, composed of pro- and anti-apoptotic Bcl-2 proteins. As pro-apoptotic members, Bax, Bad, and Bid, are well known. Bcl-2, Bcl-cl, and Mcl-1 are representative anti-apoptotic factors. These members of the Bcl-2 family are regulated by ROS, via direct and indirect mechanisms [122,123]. Detailed apoptotic mechanisms induced by ROS under pathological conditions have been described in previous reviews [124,125]. Therefore, we here pay special attention to natural products and chemical agents that produce ROS and consequently modulate apoptosis in urothelial cancers.

5.1. *ROS and Apoptosis in Prostate Cancer*

Total flavonoids extracted from persimmon leaves, which are used as a herbal medicine in Asia, have been recently reported to induce mitochondrial apoptosis, via the inactivation of Bcl-2, upregulation of Bax, and release of cytochrome c in the androgen-independent prostate cancer cell line,

PC-3 [125,126]. In addition to these mitochondria-related pathways, flavonoids induced apoptosis by ROS production [126]. Anethole, which is a major constituent of *Foeniculum vulgare* (fennel) essential oil and is widely used in folk medicine, inhibited cell proliferation, migration, and colony formation and induced apoptosis and cell arrest by ROS production [127]. Actually, numerous studies have shown that the induction of apoptosis by natural products reduced ROS production in prostate cancer cells. Because of space constraints, we introduce only the most recent reports published in 2017; *Punica granatum* (pomegranate) peel in mouse prostate cancer cells (TRAMP-C1) [128]; a new nanoemulsion system of rutin in PC-3 [129]; benzyl isothiocyanate in cruciferous plants in CRW-22Rv1 and PC-3 [130]; curcumin and resveratrol in LNCaP and PC-3 cells [131]; Chikusetsu saponin Iva, isolated from *Aralia taibaiensis* in PC-3 [132]; chrysin, a natural flavone found in numerous plant extracts, honey, and propolis, in DU145 and PC-3 cells [133]; lasalocid, an antibiotic from the group of carboxylic ionophores produced by *Streptomyces lasaliensis*, in PC-3 [134]; naringenin, an anti-oxidant flavonoid derived from citrus, in PC-3 [135]; and coumestrol, a major phytoestrogen abundant in soybeans, legumes, Brussels sprouts, and spinach, in LNCaP and PC-3 cells [136]. Furthermore, treatment with WZ35, a chemical analog of curcumin, induced apoptosis in two prostate cancer cell lines (RM-1 and DU145), and this anti-cancer effect depended on ROS production [137].

In addition to natural products, various chemicals have been reported to modulate apoptosis via ROS production. For example, salinomycin, a promising anti-cancer drug, induced apoptosis via ROS production, and this mechanism was related to ROS-mediated autophagy through the regulation of the PI3K/Akt/ mechanistic target of rapamycin (mTOR) and ERK/p38 MAPK signaling pathways [138]. In addition, toyocamycin, an antibiotic agent isolated from *Streptomyces* species, enhanced the apoptosis of PC-3 cells by the ROS-mediated signaling pathway, ERK/p38 MAPKs [139]. Conversely, there are several reports on the relationship between ROS production and treatment efficacy in prostate cancer. For example, treatment with JS-K, a glutathione S transferase-activated nitric oxide donor prodrug, for 24 h, increased the proportion of apoptotic cells, by inducing ROS production in prostate cancer cells (22RV1, C4-2, LNCaP, and PC-3) [140]. Interestingly, these authors also showed that the pro-apoptotic effect of JS-K is dose-dependent, and 22RV1 and C4-2 cells were more sensitive than LNCaP and PC-3 cells [141]. Furthermore, although selenite had a partial pro-apoptotic effect and carmustine showed no apoptosis induction in EGF-stimulated PC-3 cells, combination treatment with carmustine and selenite dramatically induced apoptosis in EGF-stimulated PC-3 cells [141]. This combination treatment increased ROS production, which triggered apoptosis in 22RV1 and PC-3 cells [141,142]. Based on these facts, this combination treatment was speculated to induce apoptosis via ROS production in prostate cancer cells. Similar findings have reported for the combination of orlistat, an anti-obesity drug, and 5-aminoimidazole-4-carboxamide ribonucleotide, an analog of adenosine monophosphate (AMP) that is capable of stimulating AMP-dependent protein kinase (AMPK) activity [143].

5.2. Apoptosis and ROS in RCC

Similar to prostate cancer, various substances and agents are associated with apoptosis via ROS production in RCC. Various chemical compounds have been shown to induce ROS production and to modulate apoptosis in RCC cells. Galangin, a flavonoid extracted from the root of *Alpinia officinarum*, induced apoptosis by increasing the intracellular concentration of ROS [144]. Eupatilin, a pharmacologically active component found in *Artemisia asiatica*, induced apoptosis in 786-O cells by ROS-mediated activation of the MAPK signaling pathway and inhibition of the PI3K/Akt signaling pathway [145]. Additionally, carnosic acid, the major bioactive compound of *Rosmarinus officinalis* L., is reported to induce apoptosis via a ROS-related mechanism in RCC cells (Caki cells) [146]. Thus, several natural compounds have been reported to be associated with ROS-induced apoptosis in RCC cells. We suggest that further studies are necessary because the number of studies on RCC are lower than those on prostate cancer.

A variety of chemical agents have been reported to induce apoptosis via ROS-related mechanisms. For example, the anti-hepatitis drug, bicyclol (4,4′-dimethoxy-5,6,5′,6′-bis(methylenedioxy)-

2-hydroxymethy-L-2′-methoxy-carbonyl biphenyl, reportedly induces apoptosis and cell-cycle arrest, which depended on ROS production in RCC cells [147]. Furthermore, niclosamide, an anthelmintic drug, especially used for the treatment of tapeworm infection, can inhibit cell proliferation and induce apoptosis in RCC cell lines, and Wnt/β-catenin activities are associated with these anti-cancer effects [148]. The study also showed that niclosamide induces mitochondrial dysfunction, resulting in increased ROS levels [148]. These results support the possibility that existing therapeutic drugs for other diseases may be useful as new treatment strategies in patients with RCC. In fact, the combination of chloroquine and ABT-737, a small-molecule BH3 mimetic with very high affinity to Bcl-2, Bcl-xL, and Bcl-w, which induces apoptosis by inhibiting pro-survival Bcl-2 proteins and activating caspases, synergistically decreased RCC cell viability as compared to treatment with a single reagent, and the level of ROS was increased after treatment with ABT-737 and chloroquine [149]. On the other hand, sorafenib, a multikinase inhibitor approved for the treatment of advanced RCC, induces apoptosis by ROS production, and such ROS-dependent apoptotic processes are independent of caspase activities and Bcl-2 family proteins, including bax and bak; however, sorafenib-induced ROS accumulation mediates increased caspase-8 activation [150]. These findings may help to improve the anti-cancer effects of sorafenib-based therapy.

ROS negatively regulates cellular FLICE-inhibitory protein (c-FLIP) via proteasomal degradation, leading to the induction of apoptosis via the extrinsic pathway [151]. In RCC cells, the anti-cancer alkaloid, berberine, sensitized TRAIL-induced apoptosis, through the downregulation of c-FLIP in renal cancer cells [152]. Similarly, 6-shogaol, a potent bioactive compound in ginger, enhanced TRAIL-mediated apoptosis in Caki RCC cells, via ROS-mediated cytochrome c release and downregulation of c-FLIP expression [153]. Similar effects in Caki cells have been reported for thymoquinones—phytochemical compounds found in the plant Nigella sativa [154]. Thus, ROS can modulate apoptosis, through direct and indirect mechanisms, in RCC cells.

5.3. *Apoptosis and ROS in Urothelial Cancer*

Compared to prostate cancer and RCC, less information is available on regulators of ROS-induced apoptosis in urothelial cancer. Guizhi Fuling Wan, a traditional Chinese medicine, suppressed cell proliferation and induced apoptosis in bladder cancer cells, and the authors speculated that one possible mechanism underlying these effects is an increase in intracellular ROS, leading to the activation of the ATM/CHK2 and ATM/P53 pathways [155]. Furthermore, a high concentration of aristolochic acid, extracted from species of *Aristolochia*, induced cell death, partly via apoptosis, activated via increased ROS production [156]. In addition, dioscin, a natural steroid saponin, and thymol, a phenolic compound, triggered ROS-induced apoptosis in T24 bladder cancer cells [157].

Regarding chemical agents, *O*2-(2,4-dinitrophenyl) 1-[(4-ethoxycarbonyl)piperazin-1-yl]diazen-1-ium-1,2-diolate (JS-K) suppressed cell proliferation and induced the apoptosis of bladder cancer cells, in a concentration-dependent manner, by increasing ROS levels [158]. Furthermore, 5-bromo-3-(3-hydroxyprop-1-ynyl)-2*H*-pyran-2-one has been reported to induce apoptosis, via the activation of caspases and increased ROS production [159]. Conversely, chloroquine reportedly induced ROS production and affected cell death in prostate cancer cells, but not in bladder cancer cells [160,161]. Thus, the activity for ROS-induced apoptosis depends on the type of cancer.

6. Conclusions

This review mainly discussed the relationships between ROS and malignant potential in urological cancers. In particular, we paid special attention to the NOX family, angiogenesis, and apoptosis, which are key factors for carcinogenesis, tumor growth, and the cell dissemination of prostate cancer, renal cell carcinoma, and urothelial cancer. There is no general agreement on the overexpression of NOX family members in prostate cancer. On the other hand, the information on expression of NOXs in RCC and urothelial cancer is insufficient to draw definitive conclusions. However, NOX3 does not seem to play an important role in malignant aggressiveness in all urological cancers. Thus, readers may notice that the information on the pathological significance of oxidative stress is insufficient to discuss observations and treatment strategies based on ROS in urological cancers, especially in RCC and urothelial cancer. We emphasize that further investigations are necessary to understand the biological and pathological characteristics of urological cancers as vascular diseases. Once such detailed information is available, there is a possibility that the NOX family may provide useful predictive factors and/or potential therapeutic targets for patients with these types of cancer.

Acknowledgments: This study was supported by ISPS KAKENHI Grant Number 16K15690. No private funding was received for this study.

Author Contributions: Yasuyoshi Miyata designed and wrote the paper; Tomohiro Matsuo, Yuji Sagara, and Kojiro Ohba wrote the paper; Kaname Ohyama and Hideki Sakai designed the paper.

References

1. Sies, H. Oxidative stress: Oxidants and antioxidants. *Exp. Physiol.* **1997**, *82*, 291–295. [CrossRef] [PubMed]
2. Goodman, M.; Bostick, R.M.; Dash, C.; Terry, P.; Flanders, W.D.; Mandel, J. A summary measure of pro- and anti-oxidant exposures and risk of incident, sporadic, colorectal adenomas. *Cancer Causes Control* **2008**, *19*, 1051–1064. [CrossRef] [PubMed]
3. Pizzino, G.; Irrera, N.; Cucinotta, M.; Pallio, G.; Mannino, F.; Arcoraci, V.; Squadrito, F.; Altavilla, D.; Bitto, A. Oxidative Stress: Harms and Benefits for Human Health. *Oxid. Med. Cell. Longev.* **2017**, *2017*, 8416763. [CrossRef] [PubMed]
4. Andrisic, L.; Dudzik, D.; Barbas, C.; Milkovic, L.; Grune, T.; Zarkovic, N. Short overview on metabolomics approach to study pathophysiology of oxidative stress in cancer. *Redox Biol.* **2017**, *14*, 47–58. [CrossRef] [PubMed]
5. Carini, F.; Mazzola, M.; Rappa, F.; Jurjus, A.; Geagea, A.G.; Al Kattar, S.; Bou-Assi, T.; Jurjus, R.; Damiani, P.; Leone, A.; et al. Colorectal carcinogenesis: Role of oxidative stress and antioxidants. *Anticancer Res.* **2017**, *37*, 4759–4766. [PubMed]
6. Schieber, M.; Chandel, N.S. ROS function in redox signaling and oxidative stress. *Curr. Biol.* **2014**, *24*, R453–R462. [CrossRef] [PubMed]
7. D'Autréaux, B.; Toledano, M.B. ROS as signaling molecules: Mechanisms that generate specificity in ROS homeostasis. *Nat. Rev. Mol. Cell Biol.* **2007**, *8*, 813–824. [CrossRef] [PubMed]
8. Valko, M.; Leibfritz, D.; Moncol, J.; Cronin, M.T.; Mazur, M.; Telser, J. Free radicals and antioxidants in normal physiological functions and human disease. *Int. J. Biochem. Cell Biol.* **2007**, *39*, 44–84. [CrossRef] [PubMed]
9. Halliwell, B. The antioxidant paradox: Less paradoxical now? *Br. J. Clin. Pharmacol.* **2013**, *75*, 637–644. [CrossRef] [PubMed]
10. Brown, D.I.; Griendling, K.K. Regulation of signal transduction by reactive oxygen species in the cardiovascular system. *Circ. Res.* **2015**, *116*, 531–549. [CrossRef] [PubMed]
11. Trachootham, D.; Alexandre, J.; Huang, P. Targeting cancer cells by ROS-mediated mechanisms: A radical therapeutic approach? *Nat. Rev. Drug Discov.* **2009**, *8*, 579–591. [CrossRef] [PubMed]
12. Du, M.Q.; Carmichael, P.I.; Phillips, D.H. Induction of activating mutations in the human c-Ha-ras-a proto-oncogene by oxygen free radicals. *Mol. Carcinog.* **1994**, *11*, 170–175. [CrossRef] [PubMed]
13. Ushijima, T. detection and interpretation of altered methylation patterns in cancer cells. *Nat. Rev. Cancer.* **2005**, *5*, 223–231. [CrossRef] [PubMed]
14. Toyokuni, S. Molecular mechanisms of oxidative stress-induced carcinogenesis: From epidemiology to oxygenomics. *IUBMB Life* **2008**, *60*, 441–447. [CrossRef] [PubMed]
15. Lee, K.H.; Kim, S.W.; Kim, J.R. Reactive oxygen species regulate urokinase plasminogen activator expression and cell invasion via mitogen-activated protein kinase pathways after treatment with hepatocyte growth factor in stomach cancer cells. *J. Exp. Clin. Cancer Res.* **2009**, *28*, 73. [CrossRef] [PubMed]
16. Liou, G.Y.; Storz, P. Reactive oxygen species in cancer. *Free Radic. Res.* **2010**, *44*, 479–496. [CrossRef] [PubMed]
17. Li, Q.; Engelhardt, J.F. Interleukin-1β induction of NFκB is partially regulated by H_2O_2-mediated activation of NFκB-inducing kinase. *J. Biol. Chem.* **2006**, *281*, 1495–1505. [CrossRef] [PubMed]

18. Fresno Vara, J.A.; Casado, E.; de Castro, J.; Cejas, P.; Belda-Iniesta, C.; González-Barón, M. PI3K/Akt signaling pathway and cancer. *Cancer Treat. Rev.* **2004**, *30*, 193–204. [CrossRef] [PubMed]
19. Kwon, J.; Lee, S.R.; Yang, K.S.; Ahn, Y.; Kim, Y.J.; Stadtman, E.R.; Rhee, S.G. Reversible oxidation and inactivation of the tumor suppressor PTEN in cells stimulated with peptide growth factor. *Proc. Natl. Acad. Sci. USA* **2004**, *101*, 16419–16424. [CrossRef] [PubMed]
20. Saybasilli, H.; Yülsel, M.; Haklar, G.; Yalçin, A.S. Effect of mitochondrial electron transport chain inhibitors on superoxide radical generation in rat hippocampal and striatal slices. *Antioxid. Redox Signal.* **2001**, *3*, 1099–1104. [CrossRef] [PubMed]
21. Li, X.; Fang, P.; Mai, J.; Choi, E.T.; Wang, H.; Yang, X.F. Targeting mitochondrial reactive oxygen species as novel therapy for inflammatory diseases and cancers. *J. Hematol. Oncol.* **2013**, *6*, 19. [CrossRef] [PubMed]
22. Segal, A.W.; Shatwell, K.P. The NAPDH oxidase of phagocytic leukemia. *Ann. N. Y. Acad. Sci.* **1997**, *832*, 215–222. [CrossRef] [PubMed]
23. Kröller-Schön, S.; Steven, S.; Kossmann, S.; Scholz, A.; Daub, S.; Oelze, M.; Xia, N.; Hausding, M.; Mikhed, Y.; Zinssius, E.; et al. Molecular mechanisms of the crosstalk between mitochondria and NADPH oxidase through reactive oxygen species-studies in white blood cells and in animal models. *Antioxid. Redox Signal.* **2015**, *20*, 247–266. [CrossRef] [PubMed]
24. Korbecki, J.; Baranowska-Bosiacka, I.; Gutowska, I.; Chlubek, D. The effect of reactive oxygen species on the synthesis of prostanoids from arachidonic acid. *J. Physiol. Pharmacol.* **2013**, *64*, 409–421. [PubMed]
25. Nelson, K.K.; Melendez, J.A. Mitochondrial redox control of matrix metalloproteinases. *Free Radic. Biol. Med.* **2004**, *37*, 768–784. [CrossRef] [PubMed]
26. Siwik, D.A.; Colucci, W.S. Regulation of matrix metalloproteinases by cytokines and reactive oxygen/nitrogen species in the myocardium. *Heart Fail. Rev.* **2004**, *9*, 43–51. [CrossRef] [PubMed]
27. Fiaschi, T.; Cozzi, G.; Raugei, G.; Formigli, L.; Ramponi, G.; Chiarugi, P. Redox regulation of β-actin during integrin-mediated cell adhesion. *J. Biol. Chem.* **2006**, *281*, 22983–22991. [CrossRef] [PubMed]
28. Galadari, S.; Rahman, A.; Pallichankandy, S.; Thayyullathil, F. Reactive oxygen species and cancer paradox: To promote or to suppress? *Free Radic. Biol. Med.* **2017**, *104*, 144–164. [CrossRef] [PubMed]
29. Leufkens, A.M.; van Duijnhoven, F.J.; Woudt, S.H.; Siersema, P.D.; Jenab, M.; Jansen, E.H.; Pischon, T.; Tjønneland, A.; Olsen, A.; Overvad, K.; et al. Biomarkers of oxidative stress and risk of developing colorectal cancer: A cohort-nested case-control study in the European Prospective Investigation Into Cancer and Nutrition. *Am. J. Epidemiol.* **2012**, *175*, 653–663. [CrossRef] [PubMed]
30. Tochhawng, L.; Deng, S.; Pervaiz, S.; Yap, C.T. Redox regulation of cancer cell migration and invasion. *Mitochondrion* **2013**, *13*, 246–253. [CrossRef] [PubMed]
31. Prasad, S.; Gupta, S.C.; Tyagi, A.K. Reactive oxygen species (ROS) and cancer: Role of antioxidative nutraceuticals. *Cancer Lett.* **2017**, *387*, 95–105. [CrossRef] [PubMed]
32. Toyokuni, S.; Okamoto, K.; Yodoi, J.; Hiai, H. Persistent oxidative stress in cancer. *FEBS Lett.* **1995**, *358*, 1–3. [CrossRef]
33. Schumacker, P.T. Reactive oxygen species in cancer: A dance with the devil. *Cancer Cell.* **2015**, *27*, 156–157. [CrossRef] [PubMed]
34. Morry, J.; Ngamcherdtrakul, W.; Yantasee, W. Oxidative stress in cancer and fibrosis: Opportunity for therapeutic intervention with antioxidant compounds, enzymes, and nanoparticles. *Redox Biol.* **2017**, *11*, 240–253. [CrossRef] [PubMed]
35. Szatrowski, T.P.; Nathan, C.F. Production of large amounts of hydrogen peroxide by human tumor cells. *Cancer Res.* **1991**, *51*, 794–798. [PubMed]
36. Panieri, E.; Santoro, M.M. ROS homeostasis and metabolism: A dangerous liason in cancer cells. *Cell Death Dis.* **2016**, *7*, e2253. [CrossRef] [PubMed]
37. Lambeth, J.D.; Kawahara, T.; Diebold, B. Regulation of Nox and Duox enzymatic activity and expression. *Free Radic. Biol. Med.* **2007**, *43*, 319–331. [CrossRef] [PubMed]
38. Jiang, F.; Zhang, Y.; Dusting, G.J. NADPH oxidase-mediated redox signaling: Roles in cellular stress response, stress tolerance, and tissue repair. *Pharmacol. Rev.* **2011**, *63*, 218–242. [CrossRef] [PubMed]
39. Gào, X.; Schöttker, B. Reduction-oxidation pathways involved in cancer development: A systematic review of literature reviews. *Oncotarget* **2017**, *8*, 51888–51906. [CrossRef] [PubMed]
40. Block, K.; Gorin, Y. Aiding and abetting roles of NOX oxidases in cellular transformation. *Nat. Rev. Cancer* **2012**, *12*, 627–637. [CrossRef] [PubMed]

41. Suh, Y.A.; Arnold, R.S.; Lassegue, B.; Shi, J.; Xu, X.; Sorescu, D.; Chung, A.B.; Griendling, K.K.; Lambeth, J.D. Cell transformation by the superoxide-generating oxidase MOX1. *Nature* **1999**, *13*, 16–22.
42. Arnold, R.S.; Shi, J.; Murad, E.; Whalen, A.M.; Sun, C.Q.; Polavarapu, R.; Parthasarathy, S.; Petros, J.A.; Lambeth, J.D. Hydrogen peroxide mediates the cell growth and transformation caused by the mitogenic oxidase Nox1. *Proc. Natl. Acad. Sci. USA* **2001**, *98*, 5550–5555. [CrossRef] [PubMed]
43. Böhm, B.; Heinzelmann, S.; Motz, M.; Bauer, G. Extracellular localization of catalase is associated with the transformed state of malignant cells. *Biol. Chem.* **2015**, *396*, 1339–1356. [CrossRef] [PubMed]
44. Heinzelmann, S.; Bauer, G. Multiple protective functions of catalase against intercellular apoptosis inducing ROS signaling of human tumor cells. *Biol. Chem.* **2010**, *391*, 675–693. [CrossRef] [PubMed]
45. Bauer, G. Increasing the endogenous NO level causes catalase inactivation and reactivation of intercellular apoptosis signaling specifically in tumor cells. *Redox Biol.* **2015**, *6*, 353–371. [CrossRef] [PubMed]
46. Bánfi, B.; Muturana, A.; Jaconi, S.; Arnaudeau, S.; Laforge, T.; Sinha, B.; Ligeti, E.; Demaurex, N.; Krause, K.H. A mammalian H^+ channel generated trough alternative splicing of the NADPH oxidase homolog NOH-1. *Science* **2000**, *287*, 138–142. [PubMed]
47. Kobayashi, S.; Nojima, Y.; Shibuya, M.; Maru, Y. Nox1 regulates apoptosis and potentially stimulates branching morphogenesis in sinusoidal endothelial cells. *Exp. Cell Res.* **2004**, *300*, 455–462. [CrossRef] [PubMed]
48. Shinihara, M.; Shang, W.H.; Kubodera, M.; Harada, S.; Mitsushita, J.; Kato, M.; Miyazaki, H.; Sumimoto, H.; Kamata, T. Nox1 redox signaling mediates oncogenic Ras-induced disruption of stress fibers and focal adhesion by down-regulating Rho. *J. Biol. Chem.* **2007**, *282*, 17640–17648. [CrossRef] [PubMed]
49. Shimada, K.; Nakamura, M.; Anai, S.; De Velasco, M.; Tanaka, M.; Tsujikawa, K.; Ouji, Y.; Konishi, N. A novel human AlkB homologue, ALKBH8, contributes to human bladder cancer progression. *Cancer Res.* **2009**, *69*, 3157–3164. [CrossRef] [PubMed]
50. De Carvalbo, D.D.; Sadok, A.; Bourgarel-Rey, V.; Gattacceca, F.; Penel, C.; Lehmann, M.; Kovacic, H. Nox1 downstream of 12-lipoxygenase controls cell proliferation but not cell spreading of colon cancer. *Int. J. Cancer* **2008**, *122*, 1757–1764. [CrossRef] [PubMed]
51. Raad, H.; Serrano-Sanchez, M.; Harfouche, G.; Mahfouf, W.; Bortolotto, D.; Bergeron, V.; Kasraian, Z.; Dousset, L.; Hosseini, M.; Taieb, A.; et al. NADPH oxidase-1 plays a key role in keratinocyte responses to UV radiation and UVB-induced skin carcinogenesis. *J. Investig. Dermatol.* **2017**, *137*, 1311–1321. [CrossRef] [PubMed]
52. Bhardwaj, V.; Gokulan, R.C.; Horvat, A.; Yermalitskaya, L.; Korolkova, O.; Washington, K.M.; El-Rifai, W.; Dikalov, S.I.; Zaika, A.I. Activation of NADPH oxidases leads to DNA damage in esophageal cells. *Sci. Rep.* **2017**, *7*, 9956. [CrossRef] [PubMed]
53. Aydin, E.; Johansson, J.; Nazir, F.H.; Hellstrand, K.; Martner, A. Role of NOX2-derived reactive oxygen species in NK cell-mediated control of murine melanoma metastasis. *Cancer Immunol. Res.* **2017**, *5*, 804–811. [CrossRef] [PubMed]
54. Aurelius, J.; Hallner, A.; Werlenius, O.; Riise, R.; Möllgård, L.; Brune, M.; Hansson, M.; Martner, A.; Thorén, F.B.; Hellstrand, K. NOX2-dependent immunosuppression in chronic myelomonocytic leukemia. *J. Leukoc. Biol.* **2017**, *102*, 459–466. [CrossRef] [PubMed]
55. Montalvo-Javé, E.E.; Olguín-Martínez, M.; Hernández-Espinosa, D.R.; Sánchez-Sevilla, L.; Mendieta-Condado, E.; Contreras-Zentella, M.L.; Oñate-Ocaña, L.F.; Escalante-Tatersfield, T.; Echegaray-Donde, A.; Ruiz-Molina, J.M.; et al. Role of NADPH oxidases in inducing a selective increase of oxidant stress and cyclin D1 and checkpoint 1 over-expression during progression to human gastric adenocarcinoma. *Eur. J. Cancer.* **2016**, *57*, 50–57. [CrossRef] [PubMed]
56. Bánfi, B.; Malgrange, B.; Knisz, J.; Steger, K.; Steger, K.; Dubois-Dauphin, M.; Krause, K.H. NOX3, a superoxide-generating NADPH oxidase of the inner ear. *J. Biol. Chem.* **2004**, *279*, 46065–46072. [CrossRef] [PubMed]
57. Wang, Y.; Liu, Q.; Zhao, W.; Zhou, X.; Miao, G.; Sun, C.; Zhang, H. NADPH oxidase activation contributes to heavy ion irradiation-induced cell death. *Dose Response* **2017**, *15*, 1559325817699697. [CrossRef] [PubMed]
58. Leung, E.L.; Fan, X.X.; Wong, M.P.; Jiang, Z.H.; Liu, Z.Q.; Yao, X.J.; Lu, L.L.; Zhou, Y.L.; Yau, L.F.; Tin, V.P.; et al. Targeting tyrosine kinase inhibitor-resistant non-small cell lung cancer by inducing epidermal growth factor receptor degradation via methionine 790 oxidation. *Antioxid. Redox Signal.* **2016**, *24*, 263–279. [CrossRef] [PubMed]

59. Cheng, G.; Cao, Z.; Xu, X.; van Meir, E.G.; Lambeth, J.D. Homologs of gp91phox: Cloning and tissue expression of Nox3, Nox4, and Nox5. *Gene* **2001**, *269*, 131–140. [CrossRef]
60. Lee, J.K.; Edderkaoui, M.; Truong, P.; Ohno, I.; Jang, K.T.; Berti, A.; Pandol, S.J.; Gukovskaya, A.S. NADPH oxidase promotes pancreatic cancer cell survival via inhibiting JAK2 dephosphorylation by tyrosine phosphatases. *Gastroenterology* **2007**, *133*, 1637–1648. [CrossRef] [PubMed]
61. Maloney, E.; Sweet, I.R.; Hockenbery, D.M.; Pharm, M.; Rizzo, N.O.; Tateya, S.; Handa, P.; Schwartz, M.W.; Kim, F. Activation of NF-κB by palmitate in endothelial cells, a key role for NADPH oxidase-derived superoxide in response to TLR4. *Activation* **2009**, *29*, 1370–1375.
62. Liu, R.-M.; Choi, J.; Wu, J.-H.; Gaston Pravia, K.A.; Lewis, K.M.; Brand, J.D.; Mochel, N.S.; Krzywanski, D.M.; Lambeth, J.D.; Hagood, J.S.; et al. Oxidative modification of nuclear mitogen-activated protein kinase phosphatase 1 is involved in transforming growth factor β1-induced expression of plasminogen activator inhibitor 1 in fibroblasts. *J. Biol. Chem.* **2010**, *285*, 16239–16247. [CrossRef] [PubMed]
63. Brar, S.S.; Kennedy, T.P.; Whorton, A.R.; Sturrock, A.B.; Huecksteadt, T.P.; Ghio, A.J.; Hoidal, J.R. Reactive oxygen species from NAD(P)H: Quinone oxidoreductase constitutively activate NF-κB in malignant melanoma cells. *Am. J. Physiol.* **2001**, *280*, C659–C676.
64. Vaquero, E.C.; Edderkaoui, M.; Pandol, S.; Gukovsky, I.; Gukovskaya, A.S. Reactive oxygen species produced by NAD(P)H oxidase inhibit apoptosis in pancreatic cancer cells. *J. Biol. Chem.* **2004**, *279*, 34643–34654. [CrossRef] [PubMed]
65. Xia, C.; Meng, Q.; Liu, L.Z.; Rojanasakul, Y.; Wang, X.R.; Jiang, B.H. Reactive oxygen species regulate angiogenesis and tumor growth through vascular endothelial growth factor. *Cancer Res.* **2007**, *67*, 10823–10830. [CrossRef] [PubMed]
66. Datla, S.R.; Peshavariya, H.; Dusting, G.J.; Mahadev, K.; Goldstein, B.J.; Jiang, F. Important role of Nox4 type NADPH oxidase in angiogenic responses in human microvascular endothelial cells in vitro. *Arterioscler. Thromb. Vasc. Biol.* **2007**, *27*, 2319–2324. [CrossRef] [PubMed]
67. Vallet, P.; Charnay, Y.; Steger, K.; Ogier-Denis, E.; Kovari, E.; Herrmann, F.; Michel, J.P.; Szanto, I. Neuronal expression of the NADPH oxidase NOX4, and its regulation in mouse experimental brain ischemia. *Neuroscience* **2005**, *132*, 233–238. [CrossRef] [PubMed]
68. Juhasz, A.; Ge, Y.; Markel, S.; Chiu, A.; Matsumoto, L.; Van, B.J.; Roy, K.; Doroshow, J.H. Expression of NADPH oxidase homologues and accessory genes in human cancer cell lines, tumours and adjacent normal tissues. *Free Radic. Res.* **2009**, *43*, 523–532. [CrossRef] [PubMed]
69. Si, J.; Fu, X.; Behar, J.; Wands, J.; Beer, D.G.; Souza, R.F.; Spechler, S.J.; Lambeth, D.; Cao, W. NADPH oxidase NOX5-S mediates acid-induced cyclooxygenase-2 expression via activation of NF-κB in Barrett's esophageal adenocarcinoma cells. *J. Biol. Chem.* **2007**, *282*, 16244–16255. [CrossRef] [PubMed]
70. Ushio-Fukai, M.; Nakamura, Y. Reactive oxygen species and angiogenesis: NADPH oxidase as target for cancer therapy. *Cancer Lett.* **2008**, *266*, 37–52. [CrossRef] [PubMed]
71. Luxen, S.; Belinsky, S.A.; Knaus, U.G. Silencing of DUOX NADPH oxidases by promoter hypermethylation in lung cancer. *Cancer Res.* **2008**, *68*, 1037–1045. [CrossRef] [PubMed]
72. Chen, S.; Ling, Q.; Yu, K.; Huang, C.; Li, N.; Zheng, J.; Bao, S.; Cheng, Q.; Zhu, M.; Chen, M. Dual oxidase 1: A predictive tool for the prognosis of hepatocellular carcinoma patients. *Oncol. Rep.* **2016**, *35*, 3198–3208. [CrossRef] [PubMed]
73. Little, A.C.; Sulovari, A.; Danyal, K.; Heppner, D.E.; Seward, D.J.; van der Vliet, A. Paradoxical roles of dual oxidases in cancer biology. *Free Radic. Biol. Med.* **2017**, *110*, 117–132. [CrossRef] [PubMed]
74. Chen, S.S.; Yu, K.K.; Ling, Q.X.; Huang, C.; Li, N.; Zheng, J.M.; Bao, S.X.; Cheng, Q.; Zhu, M.Q.; Chen, M.Q. The combination of three molecular markers can be a valuable predictive tool for the prognosis of hepatocellular carcinoma patients. *Sci. Rep.* **2016**, *6*, 24582. [CrossRef] [PubMed]
75. Wu, Y.; Antony, S.; Hewitt, S.M.; Jiang, G.; Yang, S.X.; Meitzler, J.L.; Juhasz, A.; Lu, J.; Liu, H.; Doroshow, J.H.; Roy, K. Functional activity and tumor-specific expression of dual oxidase 2 in pancreatic cancer cells and human malignancies characterized with a novel monoclonal antibody. *Int. J. Oncol.* **2013**, *42*, 1229–1238. [CrossRef] [PubMed]
76. Qi, R.; Zhou, Y.; Li, X.; Guo, H.; Gao, L.; Wu, L.; Wang, Y.; Gao, Q. DUOX2 expression is increased in Barrett esophagus and cancerous tissues of stomach and colon. *Gastroenterol. Res. Pract.* **2016**, *2016*, 1835684. [CrossRef] [PubMed]

77. Brar, S.S.; Corbib, Z.; Kennedy, T.P.; Hemendinger, R.; Thornton, L.; Bommarius, B.; Arnold, R.S.; Whorton, A.R.; Sturrock, A.B.; Huecksteadt, T.P.; et al. NOX5 NAD(P)H oxidase regulates growth and apoptosis in DU145 prostate cancer cells. *Am. J. Physiol. Cell Physiol.* **2003**, *285*, C353–C369. [CrossRef] [PubMed]
78. Kumar, B.; Koul, S.; Khandrika, L.; Meacham, R.B.; Koul, H.K. Oxidative stress in inherent in prostate cancer cells and is required for aggressive phenotype. *Cancer Res.* **2008**, *68*, 1777–1785. [CrossRef] [PubMed]
79. Höll, M.; Koziel, R.; Schäfer, G.; Pircher, H.; Pauck, A.; Hermann, M.; Klocker, H.; Jansen-Dürr, P.; Sampson, N. ROS signaling by NADPH oxidase 5 modulates the proliferation and survival of prostate carcinoma cells. *Mol. Carcinog.* **2016**, *55*, 27–39. [CrossRef] [PubMed]
80. Arbiser, J.L.; Petros, J.; Klafter, R.; Govindajaran, B.; McLaughlin, E.R.; Brown, L.F.; Cohen, C.; Moses, M.; Kilroy, S.; Arnold, R.S.; et al. Reactive oxygen generated by Nox1 triggers the angiogenic switch. *Proc. Natl. Acad. Sci. USA* **2001**, *99*, 715–720. [CrossRef] [PubMed]
81. Lim, S.D.; Sun, C.Q.; Lambeth, J.D.; Marshall, F.; Amin, M.; Chung, L.; Petros, J.A.; Arnold, R.S. Increased Nox1 and hydrogen peroxide in prostate cancer. *Prostate* **2005**, *62*, 200–207. [CrossRef] [PubMed]
82. Deep, G.; Kumar, R.; Jain, A.K.; Dhar, D.; Panigrahi, G.K.; Hussain, A.; Agarwal, C.; El-Elimat, T.; Sica, V.P.; Oberlies, N.H.; et al. Graviola inhibits hypoxia-induced NADPH oxidase activity in prostate cancer cells reducing their proliferation and clonogenicity. *Sci. Rep.* **2016**, *6*, 23135. [CrossRef] [PubMed]
83. Tamura, R.E.; Hunger, A.; Fernandes, D.C.; Laurindo, F.R.; Costanzi-Strauss, E.; Strauss, B.E. Induction of oxidants distinguishes susceptibility of prostate carcinoma cell lines to p53 gene transfer mediated by an improved adenoviral vector. *Hum. Gene Ther.* **2017**, *28*, 639–653. [CrossRef] [PubMed]
84. Arnold, R.S.; He, J.; Remo, A.; Ritsick, D.; Yin-Goen, Q.; Lambeth, J.D.; Datta, M.W.; Young, A.N.; Petros, J.A. Nox1 expression determines cellular reactive oxygen and modulates c-fos-induced growth factor, interleukin-8 and cav-1. *Am. J. Pahol.* **2007**, *171*, 2021–2032. [CrossRef] [PubMed]
85. Pettigrew, C.A.; Clerkin, J.S.; Cotter, T.G. DUOX enzyme activity promotes AKT signalling in prostate cancer cells. *Anticancer Res.* **2012**, *32*, 5175–5181. [PubMed]
86. Tam, N.; Gao, Y.; Leung, Y.; Ho, S.M. Androgenic regulation of oxidative stress in the rat prostate: Involvement of NAD(P)H oxidase and antioxidant defense machinery during prostatic involution and regrowth. *Am. J. Pathol.* **2003**, *163*, 2513–2522. [CrossRef]
87. Lu, J.P.; Monardo, L.; Bryskin, I.; Hou, Z.F.; Trachtenberg, J.; Wilson, B.C.; Pinthus, J.H. Androgens induce oxidative stress and radiation resistance in prostate cancer cells though NADPH oxidase. *Prostate Cancer Prostatic Dis.* **2010**, *13*, 39–46. [CrossRef] [PubMed]
88. Lu, J.P.; Hou, Z.F.; Duivenvoorden, W.C.; Whelan, K.; Honig, A.; Pinthus, J.H. Adiponectin inhibits oxidative stress in human prostate carcinoma cells. *Prostate Cancer Prostatic Dis.* **2012**, *15*, 28–35. [CrossRef] [PubMed]
89. Antony, S.; Wu, Y.; Hewitt, S.M.; Anver, M.R.; Butcher, D.; Jiang, G.; Meitzler, J.L.; Liu, H.; Juhasz, A.; Lu, J.; et al. Characterization of NADPH oxidase 5 expression in human tumors and tumor cell lines with a novel mouse monoclonal antibody. *Free Radic. Biol. Med.* **2013**, *65*, 497–508. [CrossRef] [PubMed]
90. Huang, W.C.; Li, X.; Liu, J.; Lin, J.; Chung, L.W. Activation of androgen receptor, lipogenesis, and oxidative stress converged by SREBP-1 is responsible for regulating growth and progression of prostate cancer cells. *Mol. Cancer Res.* **2012**, *10*, 133–142. [CrossRef] [PubMed]
91. Block, K.; Gorin, Y.; Hoover, P.; Williams, P.; Chelmicki, T.; Clark, R.A.; Yoneda, T.; Abboud, H.E. NAD(P)H oxidases regulate HIF-2α protein expression. *J. Biol. Chem.* **2007**, *282*, 8019–8026. [CrossRef] [PubMed]
92. Gregg, J.L.; Turner, R.M., 2nd; Chang, G.; Joshi, D.; Zhan, Y.; Chen, L.; Maranchie, J.K. NADPH oxidase NOX4 supports renal tumorigenesis by promoting the expression and nuclear accumulation of HIF2α. *Cancer Res.* **2014**, *74*, 3501–3511. [CrossRef] [PubMed]
93. Chang, G.; Chen, L.; Lin, H.M.; Lin, Y.; Maranchie, J.K. Nox4 inhibition enhances the cytotoxicity of cisplatin in human renal cancer cells. *J. Exp. Ther. Oncol.* **2012**, *10*, 9–18. [PubMed]
94. Shanmugasundaram, K.; Block, K. Renal carcinogenesis, tumor heterogeneity, and reactive oxygen species: Tactics evolved. *Antioxid. Redox Signal.* **2016**, *25*, 685–701. [CrossRef] [PubMed]
95. Tsujikawa, K.; Koike, K.; Kitae, K.; Shinkawa, A.; Arima, H.; Suzuki, T.; Tsuchiya, M.; Makino, Y.; Furukawa, T.; Konishi, N.; et al. Expression and sub-cellular localization of human ABH family molecules. *J. Cell. Mol. Med.* **2007**, *11*, 1105–1116. [CrossRef] [PubMed]

96. Choudhary, S.; Rathore, K.; Wang, H.C. Differential induction of reactive oxygen species through Erk1/1 and Nox-1 by FK228 for selective apoptosis of oncogenic H-Ras-expressing human urinary bladder cancer J82 cells. *J. Cancer Res. Clin. Oncol.* **2011**, *137*, 471–480. [CrossRef] [PubMed]
97. Shimada, K.; Fujii, T.; Tsujikawa, K.; Anai, S.; Fujimoto, K.; Konishi, N. ALKBH3 contributes to survival and angiogenesis of human urothelial carcinoma cells through NADPH oxidase and Tweak/Fn14/VEGF signals. *Clin. Cancer Res.* **2012**, *18*, 5247–5255. [CrossRef] [PubMed]
98. Shimada, K.; Fujii, T.; Anai, S. ROS generation via NOX4 and its utility in the cytological diagnosis of urothelial carcinoma of the urinary bladder. *BMC Cancer* **2011**, *11*, 22. [CrossRef] [PubMed]
99. Kim, E.Y.; Seo, J.M.; Kim, C.; Lee, J.E.; Lee, K.M.; Kim, J.H. BLT2 promotes the invasion and metastasis of aggressive bladder cancer cells through a reactive oxygen species-linked pathway. *Free Radic. Biol. Med.* **2010**, *49*, 1072–1081. [CrossRef] [PubMed]
100. Matsuo, T.; Miyata, Y.; Asai, A.; Sagara, Y.; Furusato, B.; Fukuoka, J.; Sakai, H. Green tea polyphenol induces changes in cancer-related factors in an animal model of bladder cancer. *PLoS ONE* **2017**, *12*, e0171091. [CrossRef] [PubMed]
101. Miyata, Y.; Mitsunari, K.; Asai, A.; Takehara, K.; Mochizuki, Y.; Sakai, H. Pathological significance and prognostic role of microvessel density, evaluated using CD31, CD34, and CD105 in prostate cancer patients after radical prostatectomy with neoadjuvant therapy. *Prostate* **2015**, *75*, 84–91. [CrossRef] [PubMed]
102. Abid, M.R.; Spokes, S.C.; Shih, W.C.; Aird, W.C. NAPDH oxidase activity selectively modulates vascular endothelial growth factor signaling pathway. *J. Biol. Chem.* **2007**, *282*, 35373–35385. [CrossRef] [PubMed]
103. Kilmova, T.; Chandel, N.S. Mitochondrial complex III regulates hypoxic activation of HIF. *Cell Death Differ.* **2008**, *15*, 660–666. [CrossRef] [PubMed]
104. Jing, Y.; Liu, L.Z.; Jiang, Y.; Zhu, Y.; Guo, N.L.; Barnett, J.; Rojanasakul, Y.; Agani, F.; Jiang, B.H. Cadmium increases HIF-1 and VEGF expression through ROS, ERK, and Akt signaling pathways and induces malignant transformation of human bronchial epithelial cells. *Toxicol. Sci.* **2012**, *125*, 10–19. [CrossRef] [PubMed]
105. Gao, N.; Ding, M.; Zheng, J.Z.; Zhang, Z.; Leonard, S.S.; Liu, K.J.; Shi, X.; Jiang, B.H. Vanadate-induced expression of hypoxia-inducible factor 1 alpha and vascular endothelial growth factor through phosphatidylinositol 3-kinase/Akt pathway and reactive oxygen species. *J. Biol. Chem.* **2002**, *277*, 31963–31971. [CrossRef] [PubMed]
106. Turcotte, S.; Desrosiers, R.R.; Béliveau, R. HIF-1α mRNA and protein upregulation involves Rho GTPase expression during hypoxia in renal cell carcinoma. *J. Cell Sci.* **2003**, *116*, 2247–2260. [CrossRef] [PubMed]
107. Shin, D.H.; Dier, U.; Melendez, J.A.; Hempel, N. Regulation of MMP-1 expression in response to hypoxia is dependent on the intracellular redox status of metastatic bladder cancer cells. *Biochim. Biophys. Acta* **2015**, *1852*, 2593–2602. [CrossRef] [PubMed]
108. Coso, S.; Harrison, I.; Harrison, C.B.; Vinh, A.; Sobey, C.G.; Drummond, G.R.; Williams, E.D.; Selemidis, S. NADPH oxidases as regulators of tumor angiogenesis: Current and emerging concepts. *Antioxid. Redox Signal.* **2012**, *16*, 1229–1247. [CrossRef] [PubMed]
109. Prieto-Bermejo, R.; Hernández-Hernández, A. The Importance of NADPH Oxidases and Redox Signaling in Angiogenesis. *Antioxidants (Basel)* **2017**, *6*, 32. [CrossRef] [PubMed]
110. Gao, N.; Shen, L.; Zhang, Z.; Leonard, S.S.; He, H.; Zhang, X.G.; Shi, X.; Jiang, B.H. Arsenite induces HIF-1α and VEGF through PI3K, Akt and reactive oxygen species in DU145 human prostate carcinoma cells. *Mol. Cell. Biochem.* **2004**, *255*, 33–45. [CrossRef] [PubMed]
111. Kou, X.; Fan, J.; Chen, N. Potential molecular targets of ampelopsin in prevention and treatment of cancers. *Anticancer Agents Med. Chem.* **2017**. [CrossRef]
112. Zhang, M.; Liu, C.; Zhang, Z.; Yang, S.; Zhang, B.; Yin, L.; Swarts, S.; Vidyasagar, S.; Zhang, L.; Okunieff, P. A new flavonoid regulates angiogenesis and reactive oxygen species production. *Adv. Exp. Med. Biol.* **2014**, *812*, 149–155. [PubMed]
113. Delle, M.S.; Sanità, P.; Calgani, A.; Schenone, S.; Botta, L.; Angelucci, A. Src inhibition potentiates antitumoral effect of paclitaxel by blocking tumor-induced angiogenesis. *Exp. Cell Res.* **2014**, *328*, 20–31. [CrossRef] [PubMed]
114. Wu, C.T.; Chen, M.F.; Chen, W.C.; Hsieh, C.C. The role of IL-6 in the radiation response of prostate cancer. *Radiat. Oncol.* **2013**, *8*, 159. [CrossRef] [PubMed]

115. Alcayaga-Miranda, F.; González, P.; Lopez-Verrilli, A.; Varas-Godoy, M.; Aguila-Diaz, C.; Contreras, L.; Khoury, M. Prostate tumor-induced angiogenesis is blocked by exosomes derived from menstrual stem cells through the inhibition of reactive oxygen species. *Oncotarget* **2016**, *7*, 44462–44477. [CrossRef] [PubMed]
116. Golovine, K.; Makhov, P.; Naito, S.; Raiyani, H.; Tomaszewski, J.; Mehrazin, R.; Tulin, A.; Kutikov, A.; Uzzo, R.G.; Kolenko, V.M. Piperlongumine and its analogs down-regulate expression of c-Met in renal cell carcinoma. *Cancer Biol. Ther.* **2015**, *16*, 743–749. [CrossRef] [PubMed]
117. Li, W.; Liu, M.; Xu, Y.F.; Feng, Y.; Che, J.P.; Wang, G.C.; Zheng, J.H. Combination of quercetin and hyperoside has anticancer effects on renal cancer cells through inhibition of oncogenic microRNA-27a. *Oncol. Rep.* **2014**, *31*, 117–124. [CrossRef] [PubMed]
118. Tanaka, N.; Miyajima, A.; Kosaka, T.; Shirotake, S.; Hasegawa, M.; Kikuchi, E.; Oya, M. Cis-dichlorodiammineplatinum upregulates angiotensin II type 1 receptors through reactive oxygen species generation and enhances VEGF production in bladder cancer. *Mol. Cancer Ther.* **2010**, *9*, 2982–2992. [CrossRef] [PubMed]
119. Shirotake, S.; Miyajima, A.; Kosaka, T.; Tanaka, N.; Maeda, T.; Kikuchi, E.; Oya, M. Angiotensin II type 1 receptor expression and microvessel density in human bladder cancer. *Urology* **2011**, *77*, e19–e25. [CrossRef] [PubMed]
120. Li, D.; Urta, E.; Kimura, T.; Yamamoto, Y.; Osaki, T. Reactive oxygen species (ROS) control the expression of Bcl-2 family proteins by regulating their phosphorylation and ubiquitination. *Cancer Sci.* **2004**, *95*, 644–650. [CrossRef] [PubMed]
121. Scheit, K.; Bauer, G. Direct and indirect inactivation of tumor cell protective catalase by salicylic acid and anthocyanidins reactivates intercellular ROS signaling and allows for synergistic effects. *Carcinogenesis* **2015**, *36*, 400–411. [CrossRef] [PubMed]
122. Bauer, G. Central signaling elements of intercellular reactive oxygen/nitrogen species-dependent induction of apoptosis in malignant cells. *Anticancer Res.* **2017**, *37*, 499–513. [CrossRef] [PubMed]
123. Luanpitpong, S.; Chanvorachote, P.; Stehlik, C.; Tse, W.; Callery, P.S.; Wang, L.; Rojanasakul, Y. Regulation of apoptosis by Bcl-2 cysteine oxidation in human lung epithelial cells. *Mol. Biol. Cell* **2013**, *24*, 858–869. [CrossRef] [PubMed]
124. Moloney, J.N.; Cotter, T.G. ROS signalling in the biology of cancer. *Semin. Cell Dev. Biol.* **2017**. [CrossRef] [PubMed]
125. Zhao, Y.; Hu, X.; Liu, Y.; Dong, S.; Wen, Z.; He, W.; Zhang, S.; Huang, Q.; Shi, M. ROS signaling under metabolic stress: Cross-talk between AMPK and AKT pathway. *Mol. Cancer* **2017**, *16*, 79. [CrossRef] [PubMed]
126. Ding, Y.; Ren, K.; Dong, H.; Song, F.; Chen, J.; Guo, Y.; Liu, Y.; Tao, W.; Zhang, Y. Flavonoids from persimmon (*Diospyros kaki* L.) leaves inhibit proliferation and induce apoptosis in PC-3 cells by activation of oxidative stress and mitochondrial apoptosis. *Chem. Biol. Interact.* **2017**, *275*, 210–217. [CrossRef] [PubMed]
127. Elkady, A.I. Anethole inhibits the proliferation of human prostate cancer cells via induction of cell cycle arrest and apoptosis. *Anticancer Agents Med. Chem.* **2017**. [CrossRef] [PubMed]
128. Deng, Y.; Li, Y.; Yang, F.; Zeng, A.; Yang, S.; Luo, Y.; Zhang, Y.; Xie, Y.; Ye, T.; Xia, Y.; et al. The extract from Punica granatum (pomegranate) peel induces apoptosis and impairs metastasis in prostate cancer cells. *Biomed. Pharmacother.* **2017**, *93*, 976–984. [CrossRef] [PubMed]
129. Ahmad, M.; Sahabjada; Akhtar, J.; Hussain, A.; Badaruddeen; Arshad, M.; Mishra, A. Development of a new rutin nanoemulsion and its application on prostate carcinoma PC3 cell line. *EXCLI J.* **2017**, *16*, 810–823. [PubMed]
130. Lin, J.F.; Tsai, T.F.; Yang, S.C.; Lin, Y.C.; Chen, H.E.; Chou, K.Y.; Hwang, T.I. Benzyl isothiocyanate induces reactive oxygen species-initiated autophagy and apoptosis in human prostate cancer cells. *Oncotarget* **2017**, *8*, 20220–20234. [CrossRef] [PubMed]
131. Rodriguez-Garcia, A.; Hevia, D.; Mayo, J.C.; Gonzalez-Menendez, P.; Coppo, L.; Lu, J.; Holmgren, A.; Sainz, R.M. Thioredoxin 1 modulates apoptosis induced by bioactive compounds in prostate cancer cells. *Redox Biol.* **2017**, *12*, 634–647. [CrossRef] [PubMed]
132. Zhu, W.B.; Tian, F.J.; Liu, L.Q. Chikusetsu (CHI) triggers mitochondria-regulated apoptosis in human prostate cancer via reactive oxygen species (ROS) production. *Biomed. Pharmacother.* **2017**, *90*, 446–454. [CrossRef] [PubMed]

133. Ryu, S.; Lim, W.; Bazer, F.W.; Song, G. Chrysin induces death of prostate cancer cells by inducing ROS and ER stress. *J. Cell. Physiol.* **2017**, *232*, 3786–3797. [CrossRef] [PubMed]
134. Kim, K.Y.; Kim, S.H.; Yu, S.N.; Park, S.G.; Kim, Y.W.; Nam, H.W.; An, H.H.; Yu, H.S.; Kim, Y.W.; Ji, J.H.; et al. Lasalocid induces cytotoxic apoptosis and cytoprotective autophagy through reactive oxygen species in human prostate cancer PC-3 cells. *Biomed. Pharmacother.* **2017**, *8*, 1016–1024. [CrossRef] [PubMed]
135. Lim, W.; Park, S.; Bazer, F.W.; Song, G. Naringenin-induced apoptotic cell death in prostate cancer cells Is mediated via the PI3K/AKT and MAPK signaling pathways. *J. Cell. Biochem.* **2017**, *118*, 1118–1131. [CrossRef] [PubMed]
136. Lim, W.; Jeong, M.; Bazer, F.W.; Song, G. Coumestrol inhibits proliferation and migration of prostate cancer cells by regulating AKT, ERK1/2, and JNK MAPK cell signaling cascades. *J. Cell. Physiol.* **2017**, *232*, 862–871. [CrossRef] [PubMed]
137. Chen, M.; Zhou, B.; Zhong, P.; Rajamanickam, V.; Dai, X.; Karvannan, K.; Zhou, H.; Zhang, X.; Liang, G. Increased intracellular reactive oxygen species mediates the anti-cancer effects of WZ35 via activating mitochondrial apoptosis pathway in prostate cancer cells. *Prostate* **2017**, *77*, 489–504. [CrossRef] [PubMed]
138. Kim, K.Y.; Park, K.I.; Kim, S.H.; Yu, S.N.; Park, S.G.; Kim, Y.W.; Seo, Y.K.; Ma, J.Y.; Ahn, S.C. Inhibition of autophagy promotes salinomycin-induced apoptosis via reactive oxygen species-mediated PI3K/AKT/mTOR and ERK/p38 MAPK-dependent signaling in human prostate cancer. *Int. J. Mol. Sci.* **2017**, *18*, 1088. [CrossRef] [PubMed]
139. Park, S.G.; Kim, S.H.; Kim, K.Y.; Yu, S.N.; Choi, H.D.; Kim, Y.W.; Nam, H.W.; Seo, Y.K.; Ahn, S.C. Toyocamycin induces apoptosis via the crosstalk between reactive oxygen species and p38/ERK MAPKs signaling pathway in human prostate cancer PC-3 cells. *Pharmacol. Rep.* **2017**, *69*, 90–96. [CrossRef] [PubMed]
140. Qiu, M.; Chen, L.; Tan, G.; Ke, L.; Zhang, S.; Chen, H.; Liu, J. JS-K promotes apoptosis by inducing ROS production in human prostate cancer cells. *Oncol. Lett.* **2017**, *13*, 1137–1142. [CrossRef] [PubMed]
141. Thamilselvan, V.; Menon, M.; Stein, G.S.; Valeriote, F.; Thamilselvan, S. Combination of carmustine and selenite inhibits EGFR mediated growth signaling in androgen-independent prostate cancer cells. *J. Cell. Biochem.* **2017**. [CrossRef] [PubMed]
142. Thamilselvan, V.; Menon, M.; Thamilselvan, S. Combination of carmustine and selenite effectively inhibits tumor growth by targeting androgen receptor, androgen receptor-variants, and Akt in preclinical models: New hope for patients with castration resistant prostate cancer. *Int. J. Cancer* **2016**, *139*, 1632–1647. [CrossRef] [PubMed]
143. Wright, C.; Iyer, A.K.V.; Kaushik, V.; Azad, N. Anti-tumorigenic potential of a novel orlistat-AICAR combination in prostate cancer cells. *J. Cell. Biochem.* **2017**. [CrossRef] [PubMed]
144. Cao, J.; Wang, H.; Chen, F.; Fang, J.; Xu, A.; Xi, W.; Zhang, S.; Wu, G.; Wang, Z. Galangin inhibits cell invasion by suppressing the epithelial-mesenchymal transition and inducing apoptosis in renal cell carcinoma. *Mol. Med. Rep.* **2016**, *13*, 4238–4244. [CrossRef] [PubMed]
145. Zhong, W.F.; Wang, X.H.; Pan, B.; Li, F.; Kuang, L.; Su, Z.X. Eupatilin induces human renal cancer cell apoptosis via ROS-mediated MAPK and PI3K/AKT signaling pathways. *Oncol. Lett.* **2016**, *12*, 2894–2899. [CrossRef] [PubMed]
146. Park, J.E.; Park, B.; Chae, I.G.; Kim, D.H.; Kundu, J.; Kundu, J.K.; Chun, K.S. Carnosic acid induces apoptosis through inactivation of Src/STAT3 signaling pathway in human renal carcinoma Caki cells. *Oncol. Rep.* **2016**, *35*, 2723–2732. [CrossRef] [PubMed]
147. Wu, J.; Zheng, W.; Rong, L.; Xing, Y.; Hu, D. Bicyclol exerts an anti-tumor effect via ROS-mediated endoplasmic reticulum stress in human renal cell carcinoma cells. *Biomed. Pharmacother.* **2017**, *91*, 1184–1192. [CrossRef] [PubMed]
148. Zhao, J.; He, Q.; Gong, Z.; Chen, S.; Cui, L. Niclosamide suppresses renal cell carcinoma by inhibiting Wnt/β-catenin and inducing mitochondrial dysfunctions. *Springerplus* **2016**, *5*, 1436. [CrossRef] [PubMed]
149. Yin, P.; Jia, J.; Li, J.; Song, Y.; Zhang, Y.; Chen, F. ABT-737, a Bcl-2 selective inhibitor, and chloroquine synergistically kill renal cancer cells. *Oncol. Res.* **2016**, *24*, 65–72. [CrossRef] [PubMed]
150. Gillissen, B.; Richter, A.; Richter, A.; Preissner, R.; Schulze-Osthoff, K.; Essmann, F.; Daniel, P.T. Bax/Bak-independent mitochondrial depolarization and reactive oxygen species induction by sorafenib overcome resistance to apoptosis in renal cell carcinoma. *J. Biol. Chem.* **2017**, *292*, 6478–6492. [CrossRef] [PubMed]

151. Wang, L.; Azad, N.; Kongkaneramit, L.; Chen, F.; Lu, Y.; Jiang, B.H.; Rojanasakul, Y. The Fas death signaling pathway connecting reactive oxygen species generation and FLICE inhibitory protein down-regulation. *J. Immunol.* **2008**, *180*, 3072–3080. [CrossRef] [PubMed]
152. Lee, S.J.; Noh, H.J.; Sung, E.G.; Song, I.H.; Kim, J.Y.; Kwon, T.K.; Lee, T.J. Berberine sensitizes TRAIL-induced apoptosis through proteasome-mediated downregulation of c-FLIP and Mcl-1 proteins. *Int. J. Oncol.* **2011**, *38*, 485–492. [CrossRef] [PubMed]
153. Han, M.A.; Woo, S.M.; Min, K.J.; Kim, S.; Park, J.W.; Kim, D.E.; Kim, S.H.; Choi, Y.H.; Kwon, T.K. 6-Shogaol enhances renal carcinoma Caki cells to TRAIL-induced apoptosis through reactive oxygen species-mediated cytochrome c release and down-regulation of c-FLIP(L) expression. *Chem. Biol. Interact.* **2015**, *228*, 69–78. [CrossRef] [PubMed]
154. Park, E.J.; Chauhan, A.K.; Min, K.J.; Park, D.C.; Kwon, T.K. Thymoquinone induces apoptosis through downregulation of c-FLIP and Bcl-2 in renal carcinoma Caki cells. *Oncol. Rep.* **2016**, *36*, 2261–2267. [CrossRef] [PubMed]
155. Lu, C.C.; Shen, C.H.; Chang, C.B.; Hsieh, H.Y.; Wu, J.D.; Tseng, L.H.; Hwang, D.W.; Chen, S.Y.; Wu, S.F.; Chan, M.W.; et al. Guizhi Fuling Wan as a novel agent for intravesical treatment for bladder cancer in mouse model. *Mol. Med.* **2017**. [CrossRef] [PubMed]
156. Romanov, V.; Whyard, T.C.; Waltzer, W.C.; Grollman, A.P.; Rosenquist, T. Aristolochic acid-induced apoptosis and G2 cell cycle arrest depends on ROS generation and MAP kinases activation. *Arch. Toxicol.* **2015**, *89*, 47–56. [CrossRef] [PubMed]
157. Li, Y.; Wen, J.M.; Du, C.J.; Hu, S.M.; Chen, J.X.; Zhang, S.G.; Zhang, N.; Gao, F.; Li, S.J.; Mao, X.W.; et al. Thymol inhibits bladder cancer cell proliferation via inducing cell cycle arrest and apoptosis. *Biochem. Biophys. Res. Commun.* **2017**. [CrossRef] [PubMed]
158. Qiu, M.; Chen, L.; Tan, G.; Ke, L.; Zhang, S.; Chen, H.; Liu, J. A reactive oxygen species activation mechanism contributes to JS-K-induced apoptosis in human bladder cancer cells. *Sci. Rep.* **2015**, *5*, 15104. [CrossRef] [PubMed]
159. Yu, G.Q.; Dou, Z.L.; Jia, Z.H. 5-bromo-3-(3-hydroxyprop-1-ynyl)-2*H*-pyran-2-one induces apoptosis in T24 human bladder cancer cells through mitochondria-dependent signaling pathways. *Mol. Med. Rep.* **2017**, *15*, 153–159. [CrossRef] [PubMed]
160. Saleem, A.; Dvorzhinski, D.; Santanam, U.; Mathew, R.; Bray, K.; Stein, M.; White, E.; DiPaola, R.S. Effect of dual inhibition of apoptosis and autophagy in prostate cancer. *Prostate* **2012**, *72*, 1374–1381. [CrossRef] [PubMed]
161. Hsin, I.L.; Wang, S.C.; Li, J.R.; Ciou, T.C.; Wu, C.H.; Wu, H.M.; Ko, J.L. Immunomodulatory proteins FIP-gts and chloroquine induce caspase-independent cell death via autophagy for resensitizing cisplatin-resistant urothelial cancer cells. *Phytomedicine* **2016**, *23*, 1566–1573. [CrossRef] [PubMed]

2

Dual-Time Point [^{68}Ga]Ga-PSMA-11 PET/CT Hybrid Imaging for Staging and Restaging of Prostate Cancer

Manuela A. Hoffmann [1,2,*], Hans-Georg Buchholz [2], Helmut J. Wieler [3], Florian Rosar [2,4], Matthias Miederer [2], Nicolas Fischer [5] and Mathias Schreckenberger [2]

1 Department of Occupational Health & Safety, Federal Ministry of Defense, 53123 Bonn, Germany
2 Clinic of Nuclear Medicine, Johannes Gutenberg-University, 55101 Mainz, Germany; hans-georg.buchholz@unimedizin-mainz.de (H.-G.B.); florian.rosar@uks.eu (F.R.); matthias.miederer@unimedizin-mainz.de (M.M.); mathias.schreckenberger@unimedizin-mainz.de (M.S.)
3 Clinic of Nuclear Medicine, Bundeswehr Central Hospital, 56072 Koblenz, Germany; helmut.wieler@web.de
4 Department of Nuclear Medicine, Saarland University Medical Center, 66421 Homburg, Germany
5 Department of Urology, University of Cologne, 50937 Cologne, Germany; nicolas.fischer@uk-koeln.de
* Correspondence: manuhoffmann@web.de

Simple Summary: Early diagnosis and tumor characterization of prostate cancer (PCa) are important for accurate treatment. [^{68}Ga]Ga-PSMA-11 PET/CT turns out to constitute a major step toward improved diagnostic procedures to detect primary, recurrent, and metastatic PCa. The aim of our study is to evaluate the effect of a second imaging modality for the staging and restaging of PCa by possibly detecting additional PCa lesions due to the well-known increase of PSMA uptake over time. There was a significant increase in tracer uptake on delayed images in comparison to early [^{68}Ga]Ga-PSMA-11 PET/CT in our study, but the lesion positivity rate was comparable. However, in a few individual cases, additional delayed scans provided an information advantage in PCa lesion detection. The findings of our study are likely to be of major interest to clinicians as well as to researchers defining the algorithms that are necessary to implement this promising method with its specific tracer into clinical routine.

Abstract: Routine [^{68}Ga]Ga-PSMA-11 PET/CT (one hour post-injection) has been shown to accurately detect prostate cancer (PCa) lesions. The goal of this study is to evaluate the benefit of a dual-time point imaging modality for the staging and restaging of PCa patients. Biphasic [^{68}Ga]Ga-PSMA-11 PET/CT of 233 patients, who underwent early and late scans (one/three hours post-injection), were retrospectively studied. Tumor uptake and biphasic lesion detection for 215 biochemically recurrent patients previously treated for localized PCa (prostatectomized patients (P-P)/irradiated patients (P-I) and 18 patients suspected of having primary PCa (P-T) were separately evaluated. Late [^{68}Ga]Ga-PSMA-11 PET/CT imaging detected 554 PCa lesions in 114 P-P patients, 187 PCa lesions in 33 P-I patients, and 47 PCa lesions in 13 P-T patients. Most patients (106+32 P-P/P-I, 13 P-T) showed no additional PCa lesions. However, 11 PSMA-avid lesions were only detected in delayed images, and 33 lesions were confirmed as malignant by a SUVmax increase. The mean SUVmax of pelvic lymph node metastases was 25% higher ($p < 0.001$) comparing early and late PET/CT. High positivity rates from routine [^{68}Ga]Ga-PSMA-11 PET/CT for the staging and restaging of PCa patients were demonstrated. There was no decisive influence of additional late imaging with PCa lesion detection on therapeutic decisions. However, in a few individual cases, additional delayed scans provided an information advantage in PCa lesion detection due to higher tracer uptake and improved contrast.

Keywords: [^{68}Ga]Ga-PSMA PET/CT; prostate cancer; dual-time point imaging; delayed imaging; biphasic imaging; lesion positivity rate

1. Introduction

Prostate cancer (PCa) is the most commonly diagnosed cancer with an incidence of 1.276 million worldwide in 2018 [1]. Early diagnosis, accurate staging, and tumor characterization are critical for selection of optimal therapy. Molecular imaging with positron-emission tomography (PET) is regarded as a relevant diagnostic approach and has found its way into the guidelines of the European Association of Urology (EAU guidelines) on PCa [2,3]. The prostate-specific membrane antigen (PSMA) is a transmembrane glycoprotein that is significantly overexpressed in most prostate adenocarcinomas, compared with other PSMA-expressing tissues [4]. After many years of preclinical research on PSMA ligands, a breakthrough was achieved in 2011 with the clinical introduction of Glu-NH-CO-NH-Lys(Ahx)-{^{68}Ga-(N,N′-bis-[2-hydroxy-5-(carboxyethyl)benzyl]ethylen-ediamine-N,N′-diacetic-acid)}([^{68}Ga]Ga-HBED-CC-PSMA or [^{68}Ga]Ga-PSMA-11) as a ^{68}Gallium (^{68}Ga)-labeled PSMA-targeted radioligand for PET/computed tomography (CT) [5,6]. PSMA PET/CT offers an appealing combination of PCa specificity and high sensitivity at low tumor volumes [7]. Sensitive and specific imaging is a fundamental requirement for the definition of the target volume in radiotherapy planning. One of the main limitations of both CT and magnetic resonance imaging (MRI) for lymph node (LN) staging is their limited capability to detect metastatic clusters in normal sized nodes; and microscopic LNM are often not enlarged [8,9]. The accurate assessment of locoregional LN metastases (LNM) is much more sensitive with PSMA PET/CT than with MRI [9]. Whereas PSMA PET/CT can detect an LNM of diameter of 3 mm, MRI can generally only identify pathological LN when they show aberrant anatomical characteristics such as a short-axis diameter >1 cm and/or non-oval shape. However, up to 80% of metastasis-involved nodes are smaller than this threshold limit that is typically used in clinical practice [10]. Meta-analytical data for the traditional CT and MRI imaging approaches suggest sensitivity of only 39–42% and specificity of 82% [10]. Since normal lymphatic or retroperitoneal fatty tissue does not demonstrate PSMA expression, metastatic LNs can be detected with a favorable lesion-to-background ratio. [^{68}Ga]Ga-PSMA PET/CT imaging has been shown to accurately detect PCa lesions for LNM [11,12]. These characteristics have led to the evolution of PSMA PET/CT as an important diagnostic tool in nuclear medicine [7,9,13]. In 130 patients with intermediate to high-risk PCa, a sensitivity of 65.9% and a specificity of 98.9% for LN staging using [^{68}Ga]Ga-PSMA-11 PET/CT was reported by Maurer et al. [12].

It has been described that PCa metastases demonstrate an increase of PSMA ligand uptake over time [5,14]. According to the Heidelberg group [5], 70% of PCa lesions have increased uptake and contrast three hours (h) post-injectionem (p.i.) compared to one h p.i. Clarification of the special situation of pelvic LNM and the possible impact of additional delayed imaging for salvage or primary therapy would be important for improved clinical decision making.

The goal of our study is to evaluate the effect of a second (late) imaging modality for the restaging and initial staging of patients with recurrent PCa, using additional findings in the abdominopelvic area based on the well-known increase of PSMA uptake over time.

2. Results

2.1. Overall Lesion Positivity Rate

A positivity rate in 147 out of 215 restaging patients (68%) (mean prostate-specific antigen (PSA) serum level 19.2 ± 82.5 ng/mL) and in 13 out of 18 primary staging patients (72%) (mean PSA 39.1 ± 67.5 ng/mL) was shown by [^{68}Ga]Ga-PSMA-11 PET/CT. At least one lesion suspect for malignancy was detected in these patients. This retrospective study includes 147 restaging patients (prostatectomized patients (P-P) and irradiated patients (P-I)) and 13 staging patients (patients suspected of having primary PCa (P-T)), both with PSMA-positive findings (Table 1). To ensure accurate statistical analysis and a homogenous patient population, the biochemically recurrent (BC)-patients, previously treated by radical prostatectomy (patient group P-P) and those previously treated by irradiation (patient group P-I) were separately evaluated according to the definition protocol of BC patients [15].

Table 1. Patient characteristics.

Characteristics (*n*)	**Parameters**
Number of patients	233
Age (y) (233)	
Median	72
Range	47–85
Mean ± SD	70.3 ± 7.3
Primary Gleason score (228)	
≤6 (low risk + grade group 1)	16
7a, 7b (intermediate risk + grade group 2 + 3)	96
8 (high risk + grade group 4)	33
>8 (high risk + grade group 5)	83
PSA (ng/mL) (233)	
Median	2.32
Range	0.2–960
Mean ± SD	15.1 ± 71.9
Prior treatment of primary tumor (233)	
Surgery (radical prostatectomy)	178
Radiotherapy and other	37
Primary staging (pre-therapy)	18
Further treatment	
Anti-androgen therapy (x/233)	101
Lesion positivity rate (160/233)	68.7%
Restaging (PET/CT-positive/total)	147/215
Primary staging (PET/CT-positive/total)	13/18

Abbreviations: PSA, prostate-specific antigen; SD, standard deviation; *n*, number of patients; y, year.

2.1.1. Lesion Positivity Rate Post-Prostatectomized (P-P)

- Baseline: 551 lesions in 114 patients

In this subgroup (P-P and baseline PET/CT), the detection efficacy was 27% (33) for PSA levels of 0.2 to <0.5 ng/mL and 32% (25), 70% (27), 77% (43), and 90% (50) for PSA levels of 0.5 to <1 ng/mL, 1 to <2 ng/mL, 2 to <5 ng/mL, and ≥5 ng/mL, respectively ($p < 0.001$) (Table 2).

Patients with a PSMA-positive scan showed local recurrence in 24% (27/114) and metastases in 90%. Of the patients with metastases, 39% exhibited local metastases and 30% exhibited distant metastases, and 31% showed both. In 70% of the patients, LNM were detected, 78% of which were pelvic LNM (Table 2).

- Delayed: 554 lesions in 114 patients

Late imaging (3 h after intravenous injection (p.i.)) showed no difference in the detection efficacy when considering the patients without separate division of the number of lesions (Table 2).

Table 2. PET/CT findings: Lesion positivity rate (LPR) post-prostatectomized (P-P) related to different PSA values.

PSA (ng/mL)	0.2–<0.5	0.5–<1.0	1.0–<2.0	2.0–<5.0	≥5.0	Chi², p
Number (x/178) post-prostatectomized patients	33	25	27	43	50	
PET/CT-positive (x/114)	9	8	19	33	45	$r = 0.507; p < 0.001$
Lesion positivity rate	27.3%	32.0%	70.4%	76.6%	90.0%	
Regions:						
Local recurrence	2	0	5	6	14	$r = 0.236; p = 0.01$
Metastases	7	8	16	31	41	$r = 0.471; p < 0.001$
Site of metastases:						$r = 0.459; p < 0.001$
Local metastases	4	4	9	11	12	
Distant metastases	0	4	4	10	13	
Local + distant metastases	3	0	3	10	16	
Number of metastases:						$r = 0.536; p < 0.001$
Single metastases	3	6	7	7	2	
Multiple metastases	4	2	9	24	39	
Lymph node metastases (LNM)	7	4	12	21	28	$r = 0.296; p = 0.001$
Site of LNM:						$r = 0.297; p < 0.042$
Pelvic LNM	6	4	10	17	19	
Extra-pelvic LNM	0	0	1	1	2	
Pelvic + extra-pelvic LNM	1	0	1	3	7	
Bone metastases	2	4	5	18	24	$r = 0.355; p < 0.001$
Visceral metastases	0	0	1	1	4	$r = 0.153; p = 0.352$ *

* Fisher's exact test. Abbreviations: PSA, prostate-specific antigen; LNM, lymph node metastases; $p < 0.05$ is considered significant; r, Pearson correlation coefficient.

2.1.2. Lesion Positivity Rate Post-Irradiated (P-I)

- Baseline: 186 lesions in 33 patients

This subgroup (P-I and baseline PET/CT) showed a detection efficacy rate of 100% for PSA levels of 2 to <5 ng/mL and 94% for PSA levels of ≥5 ng/mL, respectively. Local recurrence was detected in 79% and metastases were detected in 67%. A total of 42% of the patients showed LNM, while 80% of them showed pelvic LNM. Due to the small number of patients, a statistical analysis would not have given meaningful results.

- Delayed: 187 lesions in 33 patients

The detection efficacy rates 3 h p.i. showed the same results as baseline images.

2.1.3. Lesion Positivity Rate Pre-Therapy (P-T)

All patients (13) with PSMA-positive lesions showed histopathologically (biopsy-proven) adenocarcinoma PCa.

- Baseline: 47 lesions in 13 patients

In this subgroup (P-T and baseline PET/CT), the detection efficacy was shown in 69% for PSA levels of >4 to <50 ng/mL and in 100% for PSA levels of ≥50 ng/mL. Primary tumor lesions in the prostate were detected in 100%, metastases were detected in 38%, and LNM were detected in 31%, of which pelvic LNM were shown in 75%. Statistical analysis was not done due to the small patient number.

- Delayed: 47 lesions in 13 patients

No difference in the detection efficacy was shown in late compared to baseline imaging.

2.2. *Impact of Delayed Imaging on Lesion Positivity Rate*

A combination of results from both scans (baseline and delayed [^{68}Ga]Ga-PSMA-11 PET/CT) revealed a total of 788 lesions (554 P-P, 187 P-I, 47 P-T) (Figures 1 and 2).

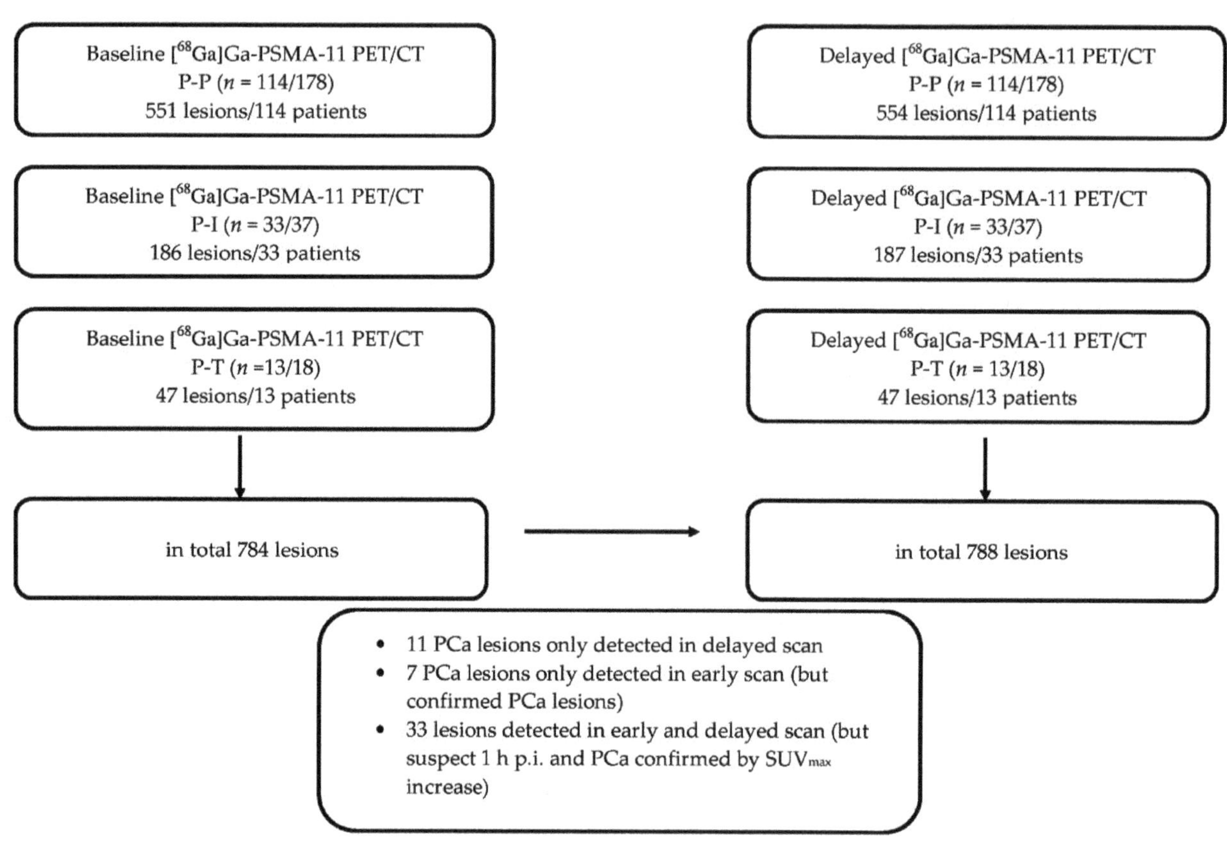

Figure 1. Flow chart showing baseline and delayed [^{68}Ga]Ga-PSMA-11 PET/CT results regarding LPR in patients.

2.2.1. Impact of Delayed Imaging on Lesion Positivity Rate P-P

A total of 551 lesions in 114 patients were detected on early scans. Twenty-nine of these lesions were local recurrent findings, and 326 were LNM (262 pelvic LNM and 64 extra-pelvic LNM). In delayed images, 328 LNM (262 pelvic LNM and 66 extra-pelvic LNM) were found. A total of 106 patients showed no additional malignant lesions in late images. Three lesions were only found in the late imaging (two extra-pelvic LNM and one bone metastasis). Comparison of tracer accumulation in pathologic lesions between baseline and delayed scans was statistically significant ($p < 0.001$ pelvic LNM, bone metastases), but this increase in maximum standardized uptake value (SUVmax) did not correspond to a significant influence of late images on the lesion positivity rates (LPR) (Table 3, Figure 1).

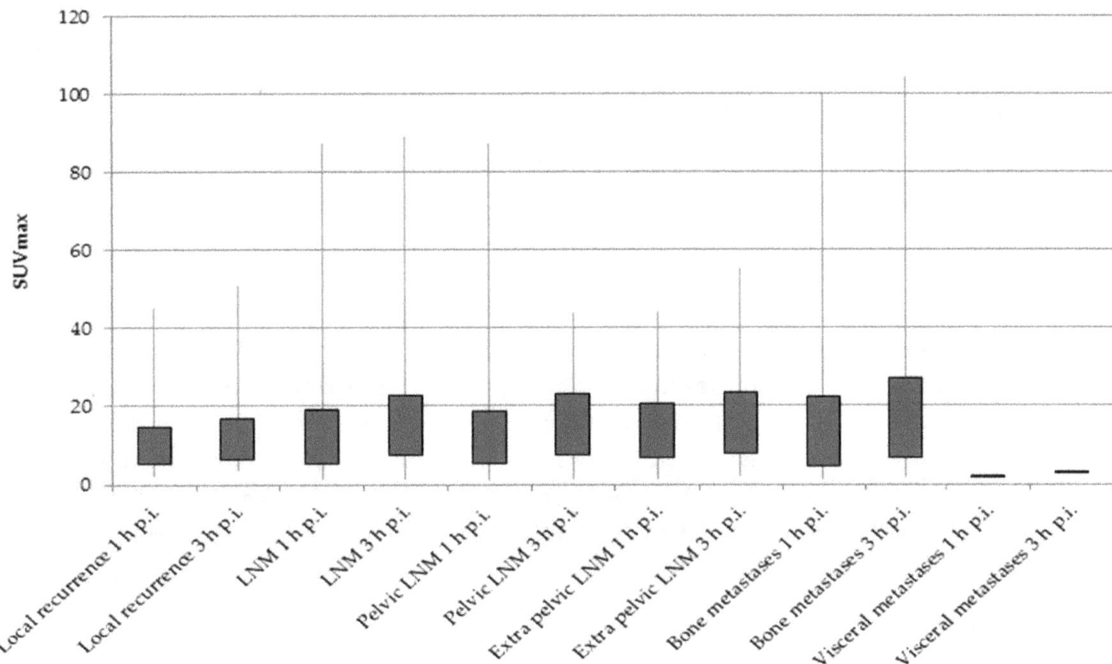

Figure 2. Comparison of baseline and delayed [^{68}Ga]Ga-PSMA-11 positron-emission tomography/computed tomography (PET/CT) regarding tracer uptake of prostate-specific membrane antigen (PSMA)-positive lesions (P-P).

Table 3. Comparison of baseline and delayed PET/CT P-P related to tracer uptake of PSMA-positive lesions.

Tumor Location	Number of Patients (x/178)	PET/CT-Positive Patients (x/114)	Number of PSMA-Positive Lesions	SUV_{max} Mean ± SD Range	Wilcoxon p
Local recurrence 1 h p.i.	27	27	29	10.1 ± 9.5/2.1–45.2	
Local recurrence 3 h p.i.	27	27	29	11.7 ± 10.7/3.6–50.9	$p < 0.001$
LNM 1 h p.i.	72	72	326	12.2 ± 13.6/1.1–87.2	
LNM 3 h p.i.	72	72	328	15.0 ± 15.1/1.2–89.2	$p < 0.001$
Pelvic LNM 1 h p.i.	68	68	262	12.0 ± 13.7/0.9–87.2	
Pelvic LNM 3 h p.i.	68	68	262	15.2 ± 15.5/1.2–89.2	$p < 0.001$
Extra-pelvic LNM 1 h p.i.	16	16	64	13.8 ± 13.8/1.2–44.2	
Extra-pelvic LNM 3 h p.i.	16	16	66	15.6 ± 15.6/2.0–55.5	$p < 0.005$
Bone metastases 1 h p.i.	53	53	195	13.5 ± 18.0/1.3–100.1	
Bone metastases 3 h p.i.	53	53	196	17.0 ± 20.2/1.8–104.5	$p < 0.001$
Visceral metastases 1 h p.i.	1	1	1	2.1	
Visceral metastases 3 h p.i.	1	1	1	3.2	

Abbreviations: LNM, lymph node metastases; SUVmax, maximum standardized uptake value; $p < 0.05$ is considered significant.

2.2.2. Impact of Delayed Imaging on Lesion Positivity Rate P-I

In 33 patients, 186 lesions were found in baseline PET/CT (Figure 1). By comparison, the 33 patients showed 187 findings in late imaging. No additional PCa lesions were shown in 32 patients. In total, a single lesion in one patient was noted 3 h p.i. (one local recurrent PCa lesion in the prostate bed). The comparison of SUVmax in pathologic lesions between early and late images was statistically significant ($p = 0.008$ pelvic LNM). However, there was no significant impact of delayed imaging on LPR.

2.2.3. Impact of Delayed Imaging on Lesion Positivity Rate P-T

All 13 [^{68}Ga]Ga-PSMA-11 PET/CT-positive patients showed 47 lesions (Figure 1). No additional PCa lesions were identified by late imaging.

2.2.4. Total Comparison of Biphasic Lesion Detection

Eleven patients with discordant results showed 51 discordant lesions. All unclear lesions (33 lesions moderately suspicious of malignancy) detected by [^{68}Ga]Ga-PSMA-11 PET/CT on standard imaging (1 h p.i.) could be clarified by additional late images (3 h p.i.). The decision to classify the lesions as malignant was made on the basis of various criteria such as a higher tracer uptake with increased SUVmax in the late images compared to the early images (Table 3), and an improved contrast as well as presentation of the lesions with a more focal character. The assessment was carried out by nuclear medicine and radiological specialists with several years of diagnostic experience with regard to the analysis of oncologic PET/CT imaging of PCa foci.

- LPR on PET, but not on CT:

By comparison of PET and CT imaging separately, nine LNM with high PSMA avidity were detected on PET, but these were not suspect of malignancy on CT alone.

- Lesions only detected on early imaging:

Seven PSMA-avid lesions (five LNM and two bone metastases) were only shown on early imaging (two P-P and zero P-I). These findings could not be confirmed as PCa lesions on delayed images.

- Lesions only detected on delayed imaging:

In this study, 11 lesions suspicious of malignancy were detected exclusively by delayed imaging (eight P-P and one P-I).

- Additional impact of delayed imaging:

A total of 33 PSMA-avid lesions (of which 15 were LNM, eight were bone metastases, and five were lesions in the prostate bed) suspected of being malignant were confirmed as malignant by increased tracer uptake in the delayed scans.

- No additional impact of delayed imaging/concordant lesions:

In 222 of 233 evaluable patients (95%), the baseline PET/CT and the delayed PET/CT were concordant.

- Time dependency of LPR:

PSMA avidity in pelvic LNM was related more often to scan time than in other metastases (e.g., extra-pelvic LNM, bone metastases, visceral metastases) ($p < 0.001$). Comparing early and late PET/CT imaging, the mean SUVmax of pelvic LNM was 25% higher ($p < 0.001$) and the mean SUVmax of extra-pelvic LNM was 14% higher ($p = 0.003$), respectively.

2.3. SUVmax

An increase of tracer accumulation over time was observed in patient groups P-P, P-I, and P-T. The SUV_{max} values of the detected sites of PCa lesions of the late scans were higher than those of the baseline scans. Overall, the SUV_{max} values of tumor lesions in the late PET/CT scans was higher in 22.1% (P-P), 22.5% (P-I), and 17.8% (P-T) than the SUV_{max} values in the baseline scans (each $p < 0.001$) (Table 3).

2.3.1. SUV_{max} of Malignant Lesions (P-P)

The Wilcoxon test showed a statistically significant difference in SUVmax between baseline and delayed scans. SUVmax was the highest in bone metastases (mean + standard deviation/SD: 17.0 ± 20.2 3 h p.i.; $p < 0.001$) and lowest in local recurrence in the prostate bed (10.1 ± 9.5 1 h p.i./11.7 ± 10.7 3 h p.i.; $p < 0.001$). The SUVmax of LNM showed high values of 15.2 ± 15.5 3 h p.i. for pelvic LNM ($p < 0.001$) and 15.6 ± 15.6 3 h p.i. for extra-pelvic LNM ($p < 0.005$) (Table 3, Figure 2).

2.3.2. SUV_{max} of Malignant Lesions (P-I)

The greatest increase of tracer uptake over time was seen in bone metastases: at 1 h p.i. SUVmax 24.3 ± 44.6 vs. at 3 h p.i. SUVmax 29.3 ± 48.6 ($p = 0.002$).

2.3.3. SUV_{max} of Malignant Lesions (P-T)

In P-T patients, an increase of tracer accumulation was also observed in bone metastases, but these data were not statistically significant ($p = 0.068$).

2.4. *Gleason Score*

The LPR showed a clear differentiation depending on the primary histological starting situation, which is expressed by the evaluation system for determining the aggressiveness of PCa. According to previous studies, PCa with a Gleason score (GS) of 7b (4 + 3) has a significantly worse prognosis than PCa with a GS of 7a (3 + 4). For this reason, 7a is classified as grade group 2 and 7b is classified as grade group 3, although they belong to the same group of intermediate-risk PCa. In our study, 11% of the PSMA-positive subgroup P-P was previously categorized as low-risk PCa (GS < 7) with grade 1 according to the International Society of Urological Pathology (ISUP) and intermediate-risk with grade 2 (GS 7a), whereas a categorization of PCa grade 3 to grade 5 (GS 7b, 8 and >8; intermediate up to high-risk) was found in 89% (Table 4) [3,16,17]. By comparison of the LNM-LPR of grade group 1 to 2 PCa-patients (GS ≤ 7a) with that of grade group 3 to 5 (GS ≥7b), a statistically significant difference ($p = 0.029$) was noted (12% vs. 88% respectively) (Table 4).

Table 4. Gleason score in relation to [^{68}Ga]Ga-PSMA-11 PET/CT LPR P-P.

$n = 178$	GS < 7 (11)	GS 7a (33)	GS 7b (51)	GS 8 (26)	GS > 8 (57)	Chi^2 r, p Value
PSMA-positive (xx/114)	1	11	38	25	39	0.326; $p < 0.001$
Local recurrence (xx/27)	1	4	5	6	11	0.112; $p = 0.446$
Metastases (xx/103)	0	9	34	23	37	0.346; $p < 0.001$
LNM (xx/68)	0	8	22	17	21	0.186; $p = 0.029$

Abbreviations: GS, Gleason score; n, number of patients; $p < 0.05$ is considered significant; r, Pearson correlation coefficient.

When comparing grade 1 to 2 PCa patients (GS ≤ 7a) with grade 3 to 5 PCa patients (GS ≥ 7b) in the subgroup P-I, we evaluated an LNM-LPR in 10% for grade 1 to 2 and in 80% for grade 3 to 5. In the subgroup P-T, all PSMA-avid LNM belong to grade group 3 to 5 (GS ≥ 7b). However, these results were not statistically significant.

2.5. *Subpopulation*

Based on EAU guidelines, which suggest the examination of PSMA PET/CT in patients with PSA serum values of ≥1 ng/mL and based on the definition of BC (PSA is >0.2 ng/mL in prostatectomized patients), we highlighted and examined the patient collective of restaging patients (P-P) in the range from 0.2 to <1 ng/mL as particularly assessable [3,15]. In baseline PET/CT, 33% (58/178) of patients (P-P) showed PSA values in the range of 0.2 to <1 ng/mL, of which 29% were PSMA-positive and 14%

showed local metastases ($p < 0.001$) (Table 5). There was no difference in the results determined by delayed PET/CT images.

In one of our previous studies, we determined an optimal PSA cutoff level of 1.24 ng/mL for distinguishing between positive and negative PSMA PET/CT results for BC patients after primary prostatectomy (P-P) [13]. In this study, P-P patients in baseline shots, with PSA < 1.24 ng/mL, showed an overall positivity in 34% (24/71), PSMA-avid local metastases in 13% (9/71), and distant metastases in 10% (7/71), compared to 84% (90/107), 29% (31/107), and 22% (24/107) in patients with PSA ≥ 1.24 ng/mL ($p < 0.001$) (Table 5). The results were comparable in delayed images.

Table 5. Baseline PET/CT: LPR P-P of different subgroups related to PSA subgroups.

PSA Range (ng/mL)	Overall Positivity	Chi² *p*/*r* Value	Single Metastases		Multiple Metastases	Chi² *p*/*r* Value
0.2 to <1 (58)	17 (29.3%)		9 (15.5%)		6 (10.3%)	
<1.24 (71)	24 (33.8%)		12 (16.9%)		9 (12.7%)	
≥1.24 (107)	90 (84.1%)		13 (12.1%)		69 (64.5%)	
Total (178)	114 (64%)	$p < 0.001$ r 0.513	25		78	$p < 0.001$ r 0.522
PSA Range (ng/mL)	**Local Recurrence**	***p*/*r* Value**	**Local Metastases**	**Distant Metastases**	**Local + Distant Metastases**	***p*/*r* Value**
0.2 to <1 (58)	2 (3.4%)		8 (13.8%)	4 (6.9%)	3 (5.2%)	
<1.24 (71)	3 (4.2%)		9 (12.7%)	7 (9.9%)	5 (7.0%)	
≥1.24 (107)	24 (22.4%)		31 (29.0%)	24 (22.4%)	27 (25.2%)	
Total (178)	27	$p = 0.001$ r 0.249	40	31	32	$p < 0.001$ r 0.412

Abbreviations: PSA, prostate-specific-antigen; $p < 0.05$ is considered significant; r, Pearson correlation coefficient.

3. Discussion

In this study, the biphasic [^{68}Ga]Ga-PSMA-11 PET/CT of 233 patients was retrospectively studied. A total of 178 prostatectomized patients and 37 irradiated patients as well as 18 pre-therapy patients were assessed, and their data (e.g. tumor uptake, biphasic LPR) were separately evaluated. As reported in other studies, we also found high LPR from baseline [^{68}Ga]Ga-PSMA-11 PET/CT for the staging (72%) and restaging (68%) of PCa patients [11,13,18].

A recently published prospective, randomized, multi-center study from Australia [9] including 300 men with biopsy-proven PCa found that [^{68}Ga]Ga-PSMA PET/CT yielded 92% accuracy in identifying those with distant metastatic or pelvic nodal disease compared with 65% accuracy from traditional imaging (CT, bone scan). Furthermore, conventional imaging had more equivocal findings, fewer management changes, and higher radiation doses (19.2 mSv vs. 8.4 mSv; $p < 0.001$) [9]. In addition to improving detection, PSMA PET/CT will have a significant impact on a patient's treatment plan and disease management in future guidelines [9,11].

Several acquisition protocols with different acquisition times, including early dynamic to 3 h p.i. imaging, have been proposed for [^{68}Ga]Ga-PSMA PET/CT studies [18–22]. Time activity curves acquired from PCa lesions showed a continuously increasing tracer accumulation during early dynamic PET acquisition, which also supports the essential role of additional late imaging [22]. The addition of delayed scans has been considered to offer substantial advantages for the discrimination of PCa versus non-PCa lesions, as the malignant foci usually show a further increase in tracer accumulation on the late scans. Benign lesions, on the other hand, usually show a decrease in SUV [18–22]. The optimal time point for the various currently available tracers for PSMA PET/CT imaging and the potential of additional late images have been and are currently being investigated. In the present study, we evaluated the incremental value of [^{68}Ga]Ga-PSMA-11 PET delayed imaging, especially abdominopelvic imaging.

As described by previous studies, there is a significant increase in SUVmax of PCa lesions on delayed images when evaluating dual time point [^{68}Ga]Ga-PSMA-11 PET/CT imaging [18,21,23,24]. Beheshti et al. reported that this increase relates to suspicious lesions ($p < 0.001$) in the prostate bed (11.6 ± 8.2 to 14.8 ± 1.0) as well as to LNs (9.7 ± 5.9 to 12.3 ± 8.8) [23]. Nevertheless, lesions' tracer accumulation on early imaging has been sufficient for diagnosis [23], which is consistent with our results.

Afshar-Oromieh et al. reported a mixed pattern of tracer behavior (increase/decrease of SUVmax in metastases) in the same patient in 11.6% (8/69 patients), whereas six of 69 patients (8.7%) showed a consistent decrease in metastatic uptake [20]. We did not find similar results in our patient group. Another study showed a SUVmax decrease in 26 out of 157 lesions [23]. Beheshti et al. reported [23] an increase of SUVmax over time in most lesions, which was also in agreement with our findings. Delayed images could confirm malignancy of 33 moderately PSMA-avid lesions, which were suspicious of being malignant on early scans, due to the increase of tracer uptake. However, some of the findings were ambiguous (11 lesions only detected in delayed scan, seven lesions only detected in early scan), but all of them were characteristic for PCa in follow-up (such as PSMA PET/CT, PSMA PET/MRI, CT, MRI), which support the results of a previous study that demonstrated [^{68}Ga]Ga-PSMA PET/CT to be a helpful tool to determine malignancy in ambiguous lesions [24]. These different results might be explained by various tumor cell biologies. Afshar et al. suspect that individual lesions may have a decreased rate of internalization of the PSMA ligand [20]. We speculate that miscellaneous and mixed patient populations may also account for at least some of the different findings that have been reported in the literature. In the large patient group with recurrent PCa, the role of primary treatment (e.g., prostatectomy, radiation therapy) could be an important factor as well.

In our study, the clinically most important group (P-P) of recurrent PCa-patients ($n = 114/178$) showed no significant difference in LPR (551 lesions early vs. 554 late). However, a statistically significant increase of tumor uptake in PCa lesions detected by baseline PET/CT compared with delayed PET/CT was shown. As described by previous PSMA PET studies, the standardized uptake values (SUVs) of LNs are significantly higher 3 h p.i. than 1 h p.i., and nearly all LNM of PCa show high PSMA expression [18,25]. The increase of SUVmax values between baseline and delayed scan in our study also did not significantly raise the number of pathological findings in the P-I and in the P-T-groups, especially for LN lesions, which are of important clinical interest for therapy planning. Due to the fact that microscopic LNs uploaded with metastatic tumor cells are frequently non-enlarged, LN staging and restaging by CT and MRI alone is limited [8], and PSMA PET/CT or PET/MRI is preferred [9,11,12,26]. In a series of PCa patients, the authors found 72% [25] of [^{68}Ga]Ga-PSMA-avid LNs to be metastatic in normal-sized LNs (<1 cm) [25,26]. Our data demonstrated nine LNM with high PSMA avidity on PET, which showed no signs of malignancy on CT alone. Aside from the overexpressed PSMA avidity in prostate tumor cells, the LPR of microscopic LNs could improve in the near future as the next generation of scanners (including time-of-flight technique) results in increased spatial resolution, which—compared to the older scanner systems—leads to a higher contrast as well as a higher intrinsic sensitivity [24,27].

A just published comprehensive literature search [28], including nine retrospective and two prospective studies, reported detection rates of [^{68}Ga]Ga-PSMA-PET in recurrent patients for PSA <0.2 ng/mL, for 0.2–0.49 ng/mL, and for PSA 0.5 to <1.0 ng/mL ranged from 11% to 50%, 20% to 73%, and 25% to 88%. Our results match those of Luiting et al. We had LPR values of 27% for 0.2 to <0.5 ng/mL and 32% for 0.5 to <1.0 ng/mL. The subgroup of patients with PSA < 0.2 ng/mL was excluded in our study, because they do not belong to BC patients per definition [15]. The authors [28] observed high specificity rates of [^{68}Ga]Ga-PSMA-PET imaging for pelvic LNM detection in primary staging as well as in restaging, while sensitivity was modest, and they concluded that [^{68}Ga]Ga-PSMA PET has a high impact in patient management concerning the salvage setting [11,28,29]. In our study, we found LNM in 70% of the PSMA-avid metastases, 78% of which were pelvic LNM in restaging patients (P-P). In primary tumor staging, LNM were detected in 31%, of which pelvic LNM were shown in 75%. Previous studies report the dynamic uptake of PSMA in ganglia (e.g., celiac ganglia) [18,30]. However, none of the patients in the present study showed PSMA-positive celiac ganglia, neither 1 h p.i. nor 3 h p.i.

The impact of delayed imaging in our patient groups (P-P, P-I, P-T) was limited due to the lack of significantly increased rates of pathological findings 3 h p.i. Our findings were consistent with the results of a study by Derlin et al. [31] using [^{68}Ga]Ga-THP-PSMA, who also found that delayed imaging did not increase the number of detected metastases significantly (two out of 99 patients). In contrast, Afshar-Oromieh et al. [32], using [^{68}Ga]Ga-PSMA-11, found a 3-h delay as an optimal time point for imaging, as the majority of cancer lesions could be detected then. However, their patient cohort was very small ($n = 4$). It is known from early pharmacokinetic studies that the background activity decreases significantly between 1 and 3 h p.i., resulting in an improved tumor/background (T/B) ratio [5]. However, in the present study, these higher T/B ratios or contrasts to lesions' tracer accumulation did not result in significantly higher LPR on delayed images, compared to other authors [21]. It must be taken into account here that due to the ^{68}Ga's relatively short half-life of 68 minutes, the count statistics in the 3-hour measurement are significantly lower. Most PC lesions (97%) in our study were already detected early in the imaging process, which sheds some doubt on the need for a second late examination in clinical routine. However, sometimes, it can also be useful to perform late images, e.g., if the effect of urinary activity in assessing pelvic PCa lesions remains unclear in baseline scans [26,33]. In this setting, imaging with ^{18}F-labeled compounds (PSMA-based radiopharmaceuticals such as [^{18}F]PSMA-1007) should be considered [34], since it offers advantages in late imaging due to the longer half-life of 110 minutes and the significantly lower positron range with improved resolution and the detection of small LNs. However, with regard to a theranostic approach, therapies with [^{177}Lu]Lu-PSMA make a pre-therapeutic PET/CT with [^{68}Ga]Ga-PSMA appear more meaningful [6,35]. From our theranostic point of view, dual-time point imaging definitely has an important teaching value. The results of our study do not really support a routine performance of supplementary late images for every PSMA PET/CT examination. However, delayed imaging is useful to confirm or rule out a suspicious abnormality seen in early images in individual cases. An important point to emphasize is that additional late images are useful for clearing up unclear lesions whose signs of malignancy would lead to a change in the therapeutic approach.

4. Materials and Methods

4.1. Patient Characteristics

The clinical characteristics of the 233 included patients are summarized in Table 1. From 2015 to 2018, 233 patients for staging and restaging were retrospectively evaluated. [^{68}Ga]Ga-PSMA-11 PET/CT of 215 BC patients who had previously undergone either radical prostatectomy (178, patient group P-P, PSA elevation to >0.2 ng/mL by definition) or radiation therapy (37, patient group P-I, PSA elevation to >2 ng/mL above nadir by definition) and 18 patients with elevated PSA serum level of >4.0 ng/mL, highly suspicious of having primary PCa (group P-T) were separately assessed [15]. All PSMA-positive lesions of P-T were histopathologically confirmed as PCa by biopsy. In case of BC (P-P, P-I), when the biopsy or surgery of PSMA-avid lesions was not possible or considered too invasive for the patients (e.g., bone metastases), we rated the increase of PSA before therapy and decrease after therapy as a tumor confirmation and marker. Additionally, we have included the findings of follow-up examinations (such as PSMA PET/CT, PSMA PET/MRI, CT, MRI).

This retrospective study was done in accordance with the Declaration of Helsinki. All reported investigations were conducted according to the national regulations (German Medical Products Act, AMG § 13.2b). The protocol was approved by the Ethics Committee of Laek Rlp (2018-13390).

All patients signed an informed consent (including participation in the study and for evaluation and publication of their anonymized data).

4.2. Imaging Protocol and Analysis

^{68}Ga-labeled PSMA ligand, Glu-urea-Lys(Ahx)-HBED-CC ([^{68}Ga]Ga-PSMA-11), was synthesized using sterile methods as previously described by Eder et al. [36]. The included patients underwent imaging on a Biograph 64 TruePoint (True V HD) PET/CT scanner (Siemens/Erlangen/Germany) 60 ± 10 min (whole body; baseline scan) p.i. of 195.5 ± 48.3 MBq (median activity: 193 MBq, range: 97–299 MBq) and 180 ± 10 min. p.i. (pelvic, abdominal, and suspicious regions; delayed scan). The following parameters were used: three-dimensional acquisition mode (168 × 168); acquisition time of three min. per bed position; axial field of view (FOV): 21.8 cm; random, scatter, and decay correction; ordered-subsets expectation maximization method (OSEM) for PET image reconstruction (two iterations, 14 subsets, Gaussian filtering, 4.2 mm transaxial resolution, full-width at half-maximum). Attenuation corrections were performed using the low-dose non-enhanced CT data (120 kV, 20–60 mAs, CT transverse scan-field 50 cm, 70 cm extended FOV, resolution 1.0 s, 0.6 mm) or the contrast-enhanced CT data (140 kV, 100–400 mAs, dose modulation). The images were assessed by nuclear medicine clinicians and radiologists (each with more than 5 years experience in PET/CT imaging) and reviewed visually in consensus by two board-certified nuclear medicine clinicians and one board-certified radiologist. The term "lesion positivity rate" is used based on the imaging result and its interpretation by the nuclear medicine and radiological expert team in relation to the PSMA-positive tumor lesions. Any lesion with an increased radiotracer uptake (measured with SUV_{max}) above physiological uptake was considered suspicious of malignancy, and biphasic lesion detection (baseline and delayed images) was taken into account. If no consensus could be found between the board-certified nuclear medicine clinicians and the board-certified radiologist, these lesions were classified as moderately suspicious of malignancy. However, in this case, all the experts classified the lesions as abnormal and probably malignant. SUV_{max} of PSMA-avid lesions detected by baseline and by delayed scan were compared. There have been extensive efforts to develop quantitative criteria for the analysis of oncologic PET images. The measures proposed are based on the SUV in a certain volume of interest (VOI) enclosing the lesion. The principle of the SUV was introduced by Strauss and Conti [37]. For a defined VOI, the mean SUV value (SUV_{mean}) of all included pixels is usually calculated as a representative measure of tracer uptake. As a result of the VOI definition dependence, the SUV_{mean} suffers from a limited reproducibility. To overcome this problem, the SUV_{max} has been introduced, which is the maximal SUV value in the lesion. Thus, we have only used the SUV_{max} in the present study. LNM were divided into two groups based on their location (pelvic LNM: iliac and/or pararectal) and extra-pelvic distant LNM (retroperitoneal and/or above the iliac bifurcation).

4.3. Statistical Analysis

Data were analyzed using IPM SPSS Statistics version 23.0 (IBM Corporation, Ehningen, Germany). First, variables were tested for normal distribution using the Shapiro–Wilk test. To compare normally distributed values of two patient groups, Student's-*t*-test was used. The Mann–Whitney U-test was used for non-normally distributed continuous variables. For further analysis, we evaluated PSA-stratified LPR and evaluated categorical differences by Chi-square test and Pearson correlation. For comparing values of baseline and delayed imaging, i.e., SUV_{max} of PET-positive lesions, the Wilcoxon-signed-rank-test was used. Mean and SD are given if normality was observed. Additionally, for non-normal distributed variables, median and range were evaluated. p values < 0.05 were considered statistically significant.

5. Conclusions

Although there was a significant increase in SUVmax on delayed images in pelvic and extra-pelvic LNM in comparison to early [^{68}Ga]Ga-PSMA PET/CT in our study, the LPR was comparable, especially in the assessment of small subcentimeter pelvic PCa lesions in patients with multiple metastases.

The few additional findings, respectively, the confirmed lesions in the late images, had no effect on staging or restaging of PCa, as they did not lead to any modification of the final interpretation or TNM classification and did not change patient management. However, in a few individual cases, additional late scans provided an information advantage in PCa lesion detection due to a higher tracer uptake and an improved contrast.

Author Contributions: Conceptualization, M.A.H., H.-G.B., H.J.W., M.M. and M.S.; methodology, M.A.H., H.-G.B., H.J.W., M.M., F.R. and M.S.; software, M.A.H., H.-G.B. and N.F.; validation, M.A.H., H.-G.B., H.J.W., M.M., F.R., N.F. and M.S.; formal analysis, M.A.H., H.-G.B., H.J.W., M.M., F.R. and N.F.; investigation, M.A.H., H.J.W. and M.M.; resources, M.A.H., H.-G.B., H.J.W. and M.M.; data curation, H.J.W., M.M. and M.S.; writing—original draft preparation, M.A.H., H.-G.B., H.J.W., M.M. and M.S.; writing—review and editing, H.J.W., M.M., F.R., N.F. and M.S.; visualization, M.A.H., H.-G.B. and M.S.; supervision, M.M. and M.S.; project administration, H.J.W., M.M. and M.S. All authors have read and agreed to the published version of the manuscript.

Acknowledgments: The authors wish to express their gratitude to Ed Michaelson, MD, Fort Lauderdale, Florida, USA for language revision and to Rainer Arenz, Wolken, Germany, for technical support.

References

1. Ferlay, J.; Colombet, M.; Soerjomataram, I.; Mathers, C.; Parkin, D.M.; Piñeros, M.; Znaor, A.; Bray, F. Estimating the global cancer incidence and mortality in 2018: GLOBOCAN sources and methods. *Int. J. Cancer* **2019**, *144*, 1941–1953. [CrossRef] [PubMed]
2. Wibmer, A.G.; Burger, I.A.; Sala, E.; Hricak, H.; Weber, W.A.; Vargas, H.A. Molecular Imaging of Prostate Cancer. *Radiographics* **2016**, *36*, 142–159. [CrossRef] [PubMed]
3. Mottet, N.; Bellmunt, J.; Bolla, M.; Briers, E.; Cumberbatch, M.G.; De Santis, M.; Fossati, N.; Gross, T.; Henry, A.M.; Joniau, S.; et al. EAU-ESTRO-SIOG Guidelines on Prostate Cancer. Part 1: Screening, Diagnosis, and Local Treatment with Curative Intent. *Eur Urol.* **2017**, *71*, 618–629. [CrossRef] [PubMed]
4. Ghosh, A.; Heston, W.D. Tumor target prostate specific membrane antigen (PSMA) and its regulation in prostate cancer. *J. Cell. Biochem.* **2004**, *91*, 528–539. [CrossRef]
5. Afshar-Oromieh, A.; Malcher, A.; Eder, M.; Eisenhut, M.; Linhart, H.G.; Hadaschik, B.A.; Holland-Letz, T.; Giesel, F.L.; Kratochwil, C.; Haufe, S.; et al. PET imaging with a [^{68}Ga]gallium-labelled PSMA ligand for the diagnosis of prostate cancer: Biodistribution in humans and first evaluation of tumour lesions. *Eur. J. Nucl. Med. Mol. Imaging* **2013**, *40*, 486–495. [CrossRef]
6. Coenen, H.H.; Gee, A.D.; Adam, M.; Antoni, G.; Cutler, C.S.; Fujibayashi, Y.; Jeong, J.M.; Mach, R.H.; Mindt, T.L.; Pike, V.W.; et al. Open letter to journal editors on: International Consensus Radiochemistry Nomenclature Guidelines. *EJNMMI Radiopharm. Chem.* **2019**, *4*, 7. [CrossRef]
7. Sanli, Y.; Sanli, O.; Has Simsek, D.; Subramaniam, R.M. ^{68}Ga-PSMA PET/CT and PET/MRI in high-risk prostate cancer patients. *Nucl. Med. Commun.* **2018**, *39*, 871–880. [CrossRef]
8. Grubnic, S.; Vinnicombe, S.J.; Norman, A.R.; Husband, J.E. MR evaluation of normal retroperitoneal and pelvic lymph nodes. *Clin. Radiol.* **2002**, *57*, 193–200. [CrossRef]
9. Hofman, M.S.; Lawrentschuk, N.; Francis, R.J.; Tang, C.; Vela, I.; Thomas, P.; Rutherford, N.; Martin, J.M.; Frydenberg, M.; Shakher, R.; et al. Prostate-specific membrane antigen PET-CT in patients with high-risk prostate cancer before curative-intent surgery or radiotherapy (proPSMA): A prospective, randomised, multicentre study. *Lancet* **2020**, *395*, 1208–1216. [CrossRef]
10. Hövels, A.M.; Heesakkers, R.A.; Adang, E.M.; Jager, G.J.; Strum, S.; Hoogeveen, Y.L.; Severens, J.L.; Barentsz, J.O. The diagnostic accuracy of CT and MRI in the staging of pelvic lymph nodes in patients with prostate cancer: A meta-analysis. *Clin. Radiol.* **2008**, *63*, 387–395. [CrossRef]
11. Hoffmann, M.A.; Wieler, H.J.; Baues, C.; Kuntz, N.J.; Richardsen, I.; Schreckenberger, M. The Impact of ^{68}Ga-PSMA PET/CT and PET/MRI on the Management of Prostate Cancer. *Urology* **2019**, *130*, 1–12. [CrossRef] [PubMed]

12. Maurer, T.; Gschwend, J.E.; Rauscher, I.; Souvatzoglou, M.; Haller, B.; Weirich, G.; Wester, H.J.; Heck, M.; Kübler, H.; Beer, A.J.; et al. Diagnostic Efficacy of (^{68})Gallium-PSMA Positron Emission Tomography Compared to Conventional Imaging for Lymph Node Staging of 130 Consecutive Patients with Intermediate to High Risk Prostate Cancer. *J. Urol.* **2016**, *195*, 1436–1443. [CrossRef]
13. Hoffmann, M.A.; Buchholz, H.G.; Wieler, H.J.; Miederer, M.; Rosar, F.; Fischer, N.; Müller-Hübenthal, J.; Trampert, L.; Pektor, S.; Schreckenberger, M. PSA and PSA Kinetics Thresholds for the Presence of ^{68}Ga-PSMA-11 PET/CT-Detectable Lesions in Patients with Biochemical Recurrent Prostate Cancer. *Cancers* **2020**, *12*, 398. [CrossRef] [PubMed]
14. Herrmann, K.; Bluemel, C.; Weineisen, M.; Schottelius, M.; Wester, H.J.; Czernin, J.; Eberlein, U.; Beykan, S.; Lapa, C.; Riedmiller, H.; et al. Biodistribution and radiation dosimetry for a probe targeting prostate-specific membrane antigen for imaging and therapy. *J. Nucl. Med.* **2015**, *56*, 855–861. [CrossRef] [PubMed]
15. Cornford, P.; Bellmunt, J.; Bolla, M.; Briers, E.; De Santis, M.; Gross, T.; Henry, A.M.; Joniau, S.; Lam, T.B.; Mason, M.D.; et al. EAU-ESTRO-SIOG Guidelines on Prostate Cancer. Part II: Treatment of Relapsing, Metastatic, and Castration-Resistant Prostate Cancer. *Eur. Urol.* **2017**, *71*, 630–642. [CrossRef]
16. Hoffmann, M.A.; Miederer, M.; Wieler, H.J.; Ruf, C.; Jakobs, F.M.; Schreckenberger, M. Diagnostic performance of ^{68}Gallium-PSMA-11 PET/CT to detect significant prostate cancer and comparison with ^{18}FEC PET/CT. *Oncotarget* **2017**, *14*, 111073–111083. [CrossRef]
17. Epstein, J.I.; Egevad, L.; Amin, M.B.; Delahunt, B.; Srigley, J.R.; Humphrey, P.A.; Grading Committee. The 2014 International Society of Urological Pathology (ISUP) Consensus Conference on Gleason Grading of Prostatic Carcinoma: Definition of Grading Patterns and Proposal for a New Grading System. *Am. J. Surg. Pathol.* **2016**, *40*, 244–252. [CrossRef]
18. Alberts, I.; Sachpekidis, C.; Dijkstra, L.; Prenosil, G.; Gourni, E.; Boxler, S.; Gross, T.; Thalmann, G.; Rahbar, K.; Rominger, A.; et al. The role of additional late PSMA-ligand PET/CT in the differentiation between lymph node metastases and ganglia. *Eur. J. Nucl. Med. Mol. Imaging* **2020**, *47*, 642–651. [CrossRef]
19. Fendler, W.P.; Eiber, M.; Beheshti, M.; Bomanji, J.; Ceci, F.; Cho, S.; Giesel, F.; Haberkorn, U.; Hope, T.A.; Kopka, K.; et al. ^{68}Ga-PSMA PET/CT: Joint EANM and SNMMI procedure guideline for prostate cancer imaging: Version 1.0. *Eur. J. Nucl. Med. Mol. Imaging* **2017**, *44*, 1014–1024. [CrossRef]
20. Afshar-Oromieh, A.; Sattler, L.P.; Mier, W.; Hadaschik, B.A.; Debus, J.; Holland-Letz, T.; Kopka, K.; Haberkorn, U. The Clinical Impact of Additional Late PET/CT Imaging with ^{68}Ga-PSMA-11 (HBED-CC) in the Diagnosis of Prostate Cancer. *J. Nucl. Med.* **2017**, *58*, 750–755. [CrossRef]
21. Schmuck, S.; Nordlohne, S.; von Klot, C.A.; Henkenberens, C.; Sohns, J.M.; Christiansen, H.; Wester, H.J.; Ross, T.L.; Bengel, F.M.; Derlin, T. Comparison of standard and delayed imaging to improve the detection rate of [^{68}Ga]PSMA I&T PET/CT in patients with biochemical recurrence or prostate-specific antigen persistence after primary therapy for prostate cancer. *Eur. J. Nucl. Med. Mol. Imaging* **2017**, *44*, 960–968. [CrossRef] [PubMed]
22. Schmuck, S.; Mamach, M.; Wilke, F.; von Klot, C.A.; Henkenberens, C.; Thackeray, J.T.; Sohns, J.M.; Geworski, L.; Ross, T.L.; Wester, H.J.; et al. Multiple Time-Point ^{68}Ga-PSMA I&T PET/CT for Characterization of Primary Prostate Cancer: Value of Early Dynamic and Delayed Imaging. *Clin. Nucl. Med.* **2017**, *42*, 286–293. [CrossRef]
23. Beheshti, M.; Paymani, Z.; Brilhante, J.; Geinitz, H.; Gehring, D.; Leopoldseder, T.; Wouters, L.; Pirich, C.; Loidl, W.; Langsteger, W. Optimal time-point for ^{68}Ga-PSMA-11 PET/CT imaging in assessment of prostate cancer: Feasibility of sterile cold-kit tracer preparation? *Eur. J. Nucl. Med. Mol. Imaging* **2018**, *45*, 1188–1196. [CrossRef] [PubMed]
24. Sahlmann, C.O.; Meller, B.; Bouter, C.; Ritter, C.O.; Ströbel, P.; Lotz, J.; Trojan, L.; Meller, J.; Hijazi, S. Biphasic ^{68}Ga-PSMA-HBED-CC-PET/CT in patients with recurrent and high-risk prostate carcinoma. *Eur. J. Nucl. Med. Mol. Imaging* **2016**, *43*, 898–905. [CrossRef]
25. Freitag, M.T.; Radtke, J.P.; Hadaschik, B.A.; Kopp-Schneider, A.; Eder, M.; Kopka, K.; Haberkorn, U.; Roethke, M.; Schlemmer, H.P.; Afshar-Oromieh, A. Comparison of hybrid (^{68})Ga-PSMA PET/MRI and (^{68})Ga-PSMA PET/CT in the evaluation of lymph node and bone metastases of prostate cancer. *Eur. J. Nucl. Med. Mol. Imaging* **2016**, *43*, 70–83. [CrossRef]

26. Kunikowska, J.; Kujda, S.; Królicki, L. ^{68}Ga-PSMA PET/CT in Recurrence Prostate Cancer. Should We Perform Delayed Image in Cases of Negative 60 Minutes Postinjection Examination? *Clin. Nucl. Med.* **2020**, *45*, e213–e214. [CrossRef]
27. Rosar, F.; Buchholz, H.G.; Michels, S.; Hoffmann, M.A.; Piel, M.; Waldmann, C.M.; Rösch, F.; Reuss, S.; Schreckenberger, M. Image quality analysis of 44Sc on two preclinical PET scanners: A comparison to ^{68}Ga. *EJNMMI Phys.* **2020**, *7*, 16. [CrossRef]
28. Luiting, H.B.; van Leeuwen, P.J.; Busstra, M.B.; Brabander, T.; van der Poel, H.G.; Donswijk, M.L.; Vis, A.N.; Emmett, L.; Stricker, P.D.; Roobol, M.J. Use of gallium-68 prostate-specific membrane antigen positron-emission tomography for detecting lymph node metastases in primary and recurrent prostate cancer and location of recurrence after radical prostatectomy: An overview of the current literature. *BJU Int.* **2020**, *125*, 206–214. [CrossRef]
29. Han, S.; Woo, S.; Kim, Y.J.; Suh, C.H. Impact of ^{68}Ga-PSMA PET on the Management of Patients with Prostate Cancer: A Systematic Review and Meta-analysis. *Eur. Urol.* **2018**, *74*, 179–190. [CrossRef]
30. Krohn, T.; Verburg, F.A.; Pufe, T.; Neuhuber, W.; Vogg, A.; Heinzel, A.; Mottaghy, F.M.; Behrendt, F.F. [(^{68})Ga]PSMA-HBED uptake mimicking lymph node metastasis in coeliac ganglia: An important pitfall in clinical practice. *Eur. J. Nucl. Med. Mol. Imaging* **2015**, *42*, 210–214. [CrossRef]
31. Derlin, T.; Schmuck, S.; Juhl, C.; Zörgiebel, J.; Schneefeld, S.M.; Walte, A.C.A.; Hueper, K.; von Klot, C.A.; Henkenberens, C.; Christiansen, H.; et al. PSA-stratified detection rates for [^{68}Ga]THP-PSMA, a novel probe for rapid kit-based ^{68}Ga-labeling and PET imaging, in patients with biochemical recurrence after primary therapy for prostate cancer. *Eur. J. Nucl. Med. Mol. Imaging* **2018**, *45*, 913–922. [CrossRef] [PubMed]
32. Afshar-Oromieh, A.; Hetzheim, H.; Kübler, W.; Kratochwil, C.; Giesel, F.L.; Hope, T.A.; Eder, M.; Eisenhut, M.; Kopka, K.; Haberkorn, U. Radiation dosimetry of (^{68})Ga-PSMA-11 (HBED-CC) and preliminary evaluation of optimal imaging timing. *Eur. J. Nucl. Med. Mol. Imaging* **2016**, *43*, 1611–1620. [CrossRef] [PubMed]
33. Haupt, F.; Dijkstra, L.; Alberts, I.; Sachpekidis, C.; Fech, V.; Boxler, S.; Gross, T.; Holland-Letz, T.; Zacho, H.D.; Haberkorn, U.; et al. ^{68}Ga-PSMA-11 PET/CT in patients with recurrent prostate cancer-a modified protocol compared with the common protocol. *Eur. J. Nucl. Med. Mol. Imaging* **2020**, *47*, 624–631. [CrossRef]
34. Annunziata, S.; Pizzuto, D.A.; Treglia, G. Diagnostic Performance of PET Imaging Using Different Radiopharmaceuticals in Prostate Cancer According to Published Meta-Analyses. *Cancers* **2020**, *12*, 2153. [CrossRef]
35. Werner, R.A.; Derlin, T.; Lapa, C.; Sheikbahaei, S.; Higuchi, T.; Giesel, F.L.; Behr, S.; Drzezga, A.; Kimura, H.; Buck, A.K.; et al. 18F-Labeled, PSMA-Targeted Radiotracers: Leveraging the Advantages of Radiofluorination for Prostate Cancer Molecular Imaging. *Theranostics* **2020**, *10*, 1–16. [CrossRef]
36. Eder, M.; Neels, O.; Müller, M.; Bauder-Wüst, U.; Remde, Y.; Schäfer, M.; Hennrich, U.; Eisenhut, M.; Afshar-Oromieh, A.; Haberkorn, U.; et al. Novel Preclinical and Radiopharmaceutical Aspects of [^{68}Ga]Ga-PSMA-HBED-CC: A New PET Tracer for Imaging of Prostate Cancer. *Pharmaceuticals* **2014**, *7*, 779–796. [CrossRef]
37. Strauss, L.G.; Conti, P.S. The applications of PET in clinical oncology. *J. Nucl. Med.* **1991**, *32*, 623–648.

3

Open Versus Robotic Cystectomy: A Propensity Score Matched Analysis Comparing Survival Outcomes

Marco Moschini [1,2,3], Stefania Zamboni [3], Francesco Soria [1,4], Romain Mathieu [1,5], Evanguelos Xylinas [6], Wei Shen Tan [7,8], John D. Kelly[7,8], Giuseppe Simone [9], Anoop Meraney [10], Suprita Krishna [11], Badrinath Konety [11], Agostino Mattei [3], Philipp Baumeister [3], Livio Mordasini [3], Francesco Montorsi [2], Alberto Briganti [2], Andrea Gallina [2], Armando Stabile [2], Rafael Sanchez-Salas [12], Xavier Cathelineau [12], Michael Rink [13], Andrea Necchi [14], Pierre I. Karakiewicz [15], Morgan Rouprêt [16], Anthony Koupparis [17], Wassim Kassouf [18], Douglas S. Scherr[19], Guillaume Ploussard [20], Stephen A. Boorjian [21], Yair Lotan [22], Prasanna Sooriakumaran [8,23] and Shahrokh F. Shariat [1,24,25,*]

1 Department of Urology, Comprehensive Cancer Center, Medical University of Vienna, Vienna General Hospital, A-1090 Vienna, Austria
2 Department of Urology, Urological Research Institute, San Raffaele Scientific Institute, 20132 Milan, Italy
3 Department of Urology, Luzerner Kantonsspital, Spitalstrasse, 6000 Luzern, Switzerland
4 Division of Urology, Department of Surgical Sciences, University of Studies of Torino, 10124 Turin, Italy
5 Department of Urology, Rennes University Hospital, 35000 Rennes, France
6 Department of Urology Bichat Hospital, Paris Descartes University, 75877 Paris, France
7 Division of Surgery and Intervention Science, University College London, London WC1E 6BT, UK
8 Department of Uro-Oncology, University College London Hospital NHS Foundation Trust, London W1T 4EU, UK
9 Department of Urology, "Regina Elena" National Cancer Institute, 00128 Rome, Italy
10 Urology Division, Hartford Healthcare Medical Group, Hartford, CT 06106, USA
11 Department of Urology, University of Minnesota, Minneapolis, MN 55455, USA
12 Department of Urology, L'Institut Mutualiste Montsouris, Université Paris Descartes, 75014 Paris, France
13 Department of Urology, University Medical Center Hamburg-Eppendorf, 20251 Hamburg, Germany
14 Fondazione IRCCS Istituto Nazionale dei Tumori, 20133 Milan, Italy
15 Cancer Prognostics and Health Outcomes Unit, University of Montreal Health Centre, Montreal, QC H4A 3J1, Canada
16 Sorbonne Université, GRC no. 5, ONCOTYPE-URO, AP-HP, Hôpital Pitié-Salpêtrière, F-75013 Paris, France
17 Bristol Urological Institute, North Bristol NHS Trust, Southmead Hospital, Bristol BS10 5NB, UK
18 Department of Urology, McGill University Health Center, Montreal, QC H4A3J1, Canada
19 Department of Urology, Weill Cornell Medical College, New York-Presbyterian Hospital, New York, NY 10038, USA
20 Department of Urology, La Croix du sud Hospital, 314000 Toulouse, France
21 Department of Urology, Mayo Clinic, 200 First Street Southwest, Rochester, MN 55905, USA
22 Department of Urology, University of Texas Southwestern Medical Center, Dallas, TX 75390, USA
23 Department of Molecular Medicine and Surgery, Karolinska Institutet, 17177 Stockholm, Sweden
24 Department of Urology, Weill Cornell Medical College, New York Presbyterian Hospital, New York, NY 10021, USA
25 Department of Urology, The University of Texas M.D. Anderson Cancer Center, Houston, TX 77030, USA
* Correspondence: shahrokh.shariat@meduniwien.ac.at

Abstract: Background: To assess the differential effect of robotic assisted radical cystectomy (RARC) versus open radical cystectomy (ORC) on survival outcomes in matched analyses performed on a large multicentric cohort. Methods: The study included 9757 patients with urothelial bladder cancer (BCa) treated in a consecutive manner at each of 25 institutions. All patients underwent radical cystectomy with bilateral pelvic lymphadenectomy. To adjust for potential selection bias, propensity score matching 2:1 was performed with two ORC patients matched to one RARC patient.

The propensity-matched cohort included 1374 patients. Multivariable competing risk analyses accounting for death of other causes, tested association of surgical technique with recurrence and cancer specific mortality (CSM), before and after propensity score matching. Results: Overall, 767 (7.8%) patients underwent RARC and 8990 (92.2%) ORC. The median follow-up before and after propensity matching was 81 and 102 months, respectively. In the overall population, the 3-year recurrence rates and CSM were 37% vs. 26% and 34% vs. 24% for ORC vs. RARC (all p values > 0.1), respectively. On multivariable Cox regression analyses, RARC and ORC had similar recurrence and CSM rates before and after matching (all p values > 0.1). Conclusions: Patients treated with RARC and ORC have similar survival outcomes. This data is helpful in consulting patients until long term survival outcomes of level one evidence is available.

Keywords: bladder cancer; robotic-assisted; open; radical cystectomy; survival; propensity score

---

1. Introduction

Bladder cancer (BCa) is the second most common genitourinary malignancy with 81,190 estimated new diagnoses for 2018 in the United States alone [1]. Radical cystectomy (RC) with bilateral pelvic lymph node dissection (PLND) is the standard treatment for muscle invasive and very high risk non-muscle invasive BCa [2]. However, this procedure is associated with significant perioperative mortality and morbidity as a direct consequence of the complexity of the procedure and the characteristics of the population which is generally older and suffering from multiple comorbidities when compared to other surgical patients [3]. Minimally invasive surgeries, such as robotic assisted radical cystectomy (RARC), have been designed to improve surgical morbidity. Indeed, robotic-assisted radical surgery in urology has been shown to be associated with decreased blood loss, need for transfusion, and length of stay compared to open RC (ORC) in most studies [4–10].

While these perioperative benefits are generally accepted, the differential impact of RARC compared to ORC on survival outcomes remains debated with widely diverging opinions [4,11,12]. The RAZOR trial [13], a randomized, open-label, non-inferiority, phase 3 trial comparing ORC and RARC, found that RARC was non-inferior to open cystectomy for 2-year progression-free survival but did not report overall survival.

Given the shortage of prospective randomized trials comparing RARC to ORC, controlled data regarding the oncological risks and benefits are needed from well-designed retrospective multicenter studies.

Therefore, to address this unmet need, we collected complete data from BCa patients treated at academic centers to determine the impact of on survival outcomes of RARC compared to the standard ORC. We performed a propensity-matched analysis to limit the impact of selection bias on survival outcomes.

2. Experimental Section

2.1. Patients and Methods

We collected the data from 9757 patients treated with RC for non-metastatic UCB at 25 institutions. Patients were staged preoperatively with cross sectional imaging (mostly computerized tomography), bone scan when indicated and chest X-ray. Surgical specimens were processed according to standard pathologic procedures at each institution. Tumors were staged according to the 2009 American Joint Committee on Cancer-Union Internationale Centre le Cancer (AJCC/UICC) TNM classification. Tumor grade was assigned according to the 2003 WHO/International Society of Urologic Pathology (ISUP) consensus classification. STSM was defined as the presence of tumor at inked areas of soft tissue on the RC specimen [14,15]. Urethral and ureteral margins were not considered as STSM.

Lymphovascular invasion (LVI) was defined as the presence of tumor cells within an endothelium-lined space without underlying muscular walls [16,17].

2.2. *Primary and Secondary End Points*

The primary end-point was to compare survival outcomes of RARC with ORC. The secondary end-point was to evaluate survival outcomes of BCa patients treated with RARC. Overall recurrence and cancer-specific mortality (CSM) were defined as disease recurrence and death from disease, respectively.

2.3. *Statistical Analyses*

Descriptive statistics of categorical variables focused on frequencies and proportions. Means, medians, and interquartile ranges (IQR) were reported for continuously coded variables. The Mann–Whitney and chi-square tests were used to compare the statistical significance of differences in medians and proportions, respectively. Fine and Gray multivariable competing risk analyses tested the impact surgical technique and survival outcomes. Owing to inherent differences between patients undergoing ORC and RARC in terms of baseline patient and disease characteristics, we used a 2:1 propensity score matched analysis to adjust for the effects of these differences. The use of the propensity score method reduces the customary bias associated with the conventional multivariable modeling approach. The variables adjusted for were administration of neoadjuvant chemotherapy (NAC), grade, pathological T stage, lymph node status and age at surgery Subgroup analyses were performed. Statistical significance was considered at $p < 0.05$. Statistical analyses were performed using SPSS v.22.0 (IBM Corp., Armonk, NY, USA) and STATA 14 (Stata Corp., College Station, TX, USA).

3. Results

3.1. *Clinicopathologic Characteristics (Entire Cohort)*

Demographics and pathologic characteristics of the cohort stratified by surgical approach are shown in Table 1. Overall, 767 (7.8%) patients were treated with RARC and 8990 (92.2%) with ORC and most of the patients were men (n = 7775, 80%); median age was: 68 years (IQR: 60–74). About half of the patients (n = 4248, 45%) harbored pathological stage T3-T4, 6.7% had positive STSM (n = 639) and 24% (n = 2276) had lymph node metastases. There were no differences in age at surgery and gender between RARC and ORC patients (all p values > 0.1). Conversely, patients treated with RARC were more likely treated with NAC (26% vs. 3.6%) compared to patients treated with ORC and had less advanced diseases (pT3-pT4 stage: 40% vs. 46% and lymph node metastasis 22% vs. 24%). RARC patients were less likely to receive adjuvant chemotherapy compared to ORC patients (13% vs. 21%).

Table 1. Clinicopathologic demographics of 9757 patients with bladder cancer treated with radical cystectomy according type of surgery.

Variables	Overall (n = 9757, 100%)	RARC (n = 767, 7.8%)	ORC (n = 8990, 92%)	p Value
Age, years				
Mean	67	67	67	0.2
Median (IQR)	68 (60–74)	68 (62–74)	68 (60–74)	
Gender				
Male	7775 (79%)	612 (80%)	7163 (80%)	0.9
Female	1981 (20%)	115 (20%)	1827 (20%)	
Neoadjuvant chemotherapy	520 (5.3%)	198 (26%)	322 (3.6%)	<0.001

Table 1. *Cont.*

Variables	Overall (n = 9757, 100%)	RARC (n = 767, 7.8%)	ORC (n = 8990, 92%)	p Value
Pathological T stage				
pT0-pT1	2908 (31%)	368 (48%)	2540 (29%)	<0.001
pT2	2239 (24%)	93 (12%)	2146 (25%)	
pT3-pT4	4248 (45%)	305 (40%)	3943 (46%)	
High grade	8734 (94%)	361 (76%)	8373 (94%)	<0.001
LNI	2276 (24%)	158 (22%)	2118 (24%)	0.001
Nodes removed, number				
Mean	20	21	20	0.001
Median (IQR)	16 (10–26)	20 (13–28)	16 (9–25)	
Positive surgical margins	639 (6.7%)	107 (10.0%)	532 (6.3%)	<0.001
LVI	3007 (33%)	25 (27%)	2982 (34%)	0.2
Adjuvant chemotherapy	1828 (19%)	85 (13%)	1743 (20.9%)	<0.001

RARC: robotic assisted radical cystectomy, ORC: open radical cystectomy, IQR: interquartile range, LNI: lymph node invasion, LVI: lymphovascular invasion.

3.2. Clinicopathologic Characteristics (Adjusted Cohort)

Demographics and pathologic characteristics of the cohort after propensity matching, stratified by surgical approach are reported in Table 2. After the propensity matching, 420 (33%) patients were treated with RARC and 840 (67%) with ORC; no differences were recorded between ORC and RARC patients considering age, gender, NAC usage, pathological T stage, pathologic grade, and lymph node invasion (all $p > 0.1$). On the other hand, patients treated with RARC recorded higher rate of positive STSM compared to ORC group (11% vs. 6.3%).

Table 2. Clinicopathologic characteristics of 1374 patients with bladder cancer treated with radical cystectomy, comparing robot assisted radical cystectomy (RARC) and open radical cystectomy (ORC) cohorts after propensity matching.

Variables	Overall (n = 1374, 100%)	RARC (n = 420, 33%)	ORC (n = 840, 67%)	p Value
Age, years				
Mean	66	66	66	0.9
Median (IQR)	67 (59–73)	67 (61–72)	67 (51–72)	
Gender				
Male	1003 (80%)	365 (80%)	728 (79%)	0.9
Female	257 (20%)	93 (20%)	188 (21%)	
Neoadjuvant chemotherapy	456 (33%)	1162 (35%)	294 (32%)	0.2
Pathological T stage				
pT0-pT1	535 (39%)	189 (41%)	346 (38%)	0.4
pT2	208 (15%)	52 (11%)	156 (17%)	
pT3-pT4	631 (46%)	217 (47%)	414 (52%)	
High grade	1075 (78%)	348 (76%)	727 (79%)	0.1
Nodes removed, number				
Mean	19	22	17	0.001
Median (IQR)	16 (10–25)	19 (14–28)	14 (8–24)	

Table 2. *Cont.*

Variables	Overall (n = 1374, 100%)	RARC (n = 420, 33%)	ORC (n = 840, 67%)	p Value
LNI	318 (23%)	109 (24%)	209 (23%)	0.6
Positive surgical margins	115 (8.4%)	52 (11%)	63 (7.0%)	0.006
LVI	302 (32%)	23 (45%)	282 (32%)	0.04
Adjuvant chemotherapy	211 (16%)	45 (12%)	166 (18%)	0.004

RARC: robotic assisted radical cystectomy, ORC: open radical cystectomy, IQR: interquartile range, LNI: lymph node invasion, LVI: lymphovascular invasion.

3.3. *Survival Analyses in the Entire Cohort (Unadjusted Cohort)*

The median follow-ups before and after propensity matching were 81 and 102 months, respectively. The 3-year recurrence rates, CSM and OM were 37% vs. 26%, 34% vs. 24% and 47% vs. 34% for ORC vs. RARC (Figure 1, all p values > 0.1), respectively. On multivariable Cox regression analyses adjusting for standard clinico-pathologic characteristics, no significant differences were found between RARC and ORC in overall recurrence and CSM (Table 3, p > 0.1).

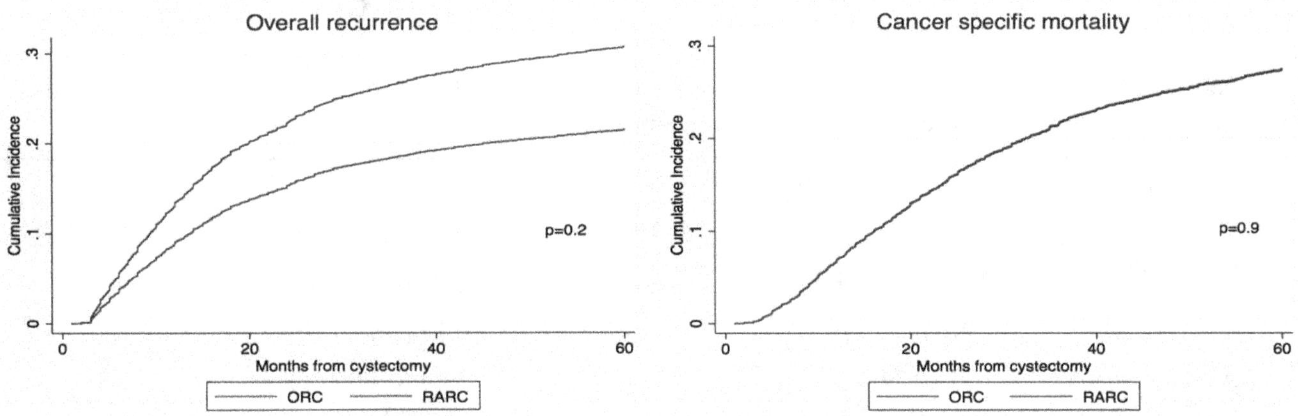

Figure 1. Cumulative incidence of recurrence and cancer specific mortality on overall population of patients with non-metastatic bladder cancer (BCa) treated with radical cystectomy according the type of surgery (ORC vs. RARC).

Table 3. Multivariable competing risk analyses predicting the risk of overall recurrence and cancer specific mortality (CSM) in patients treated with radical cystectomy in overall patients.

Variables	Overall Recurrence		CSM	
	HR (CI 95%)	p Value	HR (CI 95%)	p Value
Gender (male vs. female)	1.07 (0.97–1.17)	0.1	1.15 (1.04–1.27)	0.005
Age, years	1.00 (0.99–1.00)	0.5	1.00 (0.99–1.00)	0.052
RARC approach	0.65 (0.34–1.26)	0.2	1.00 (0.45–2.24)	0.9
pT stage				
pT0-pT1	Ref	Ref	Ref	Ref
pT2	1.35 (1.18–1.55)	<0.001	1.49 (1.27–1.73)	<0.001
pT3-4	2.10 (1.84–2.40)	<0.001	2.62 (2.27–3.03)	<0.001
pN+	1.68 (1.51–1.86)	<0.001	2.09 (1.88–2.33)	<0.001
Nodes removed	0.99 (0.99–1.00)	0.3	0.99 (0.99–1.00)	0.04
High grade vs. low	2.53 (1.73–3.71)	<0.001	2.37 (1.56–3.60)	<0.001

Table 3. *Cont.*

Variables	Overall Recurrence		CSM	
	HR (CI 95%)	p Value	HR (CI 95%)	p Value
LVI	1.44 (1.31–1.57)	<0.001	1.33 (1.21–1.46)	<0.001
Positive surgical margins	1.43 (1.25–1.65)	<0.001	1.64 (1.42–1.90)	<0.001
Neoadjuvant chemotherapy	1.69 (1.36–2.10)	<0.001	1.45 (1.15–1.85)	0.002
Adjuvant chemotherapy	1.18 (1.06–1.31)	0.001	0.89 (0.80–0.99)	0.03

CSM: cancer specific mortality, HR: Hazard ratio, CI: confidence interval, RARC: robotic assisted radical cystectomy, LVI: lymphovascular invasion.

3.4. *Survival Analyses after Propensity Matching (Adjusted Cohort)*

The 3-year recurrence and CSM were 31% vs. 29% and 27% vs. 26% for ORC vs. RARC, respectively (Figure 2, all p values > 0.3), respectively. On multivariable Cox regression analyses adjusting for standard clinicopathologic characteristics, RARC was again associated with similar overall recurrence and CSM compared to ORC (Table 4, $p > 0.3$).

Table 4. Multivariable competing risk analyses predicting the risk of overall recurrence and CSM in patients treated with radical cystectomy after propensity matching.

Variables	Overall Recurrence		CSM	
	HR (CI 95%)	p Value	HR (CI 95%)	p Value
Gender (male vs. female)	1.09 (0.80–1.48)	0.6	1.23 (0.91–1.67)	0.1
Age, years	1.00 (0.99–1.01)	0.5	1.01 (0.99–1.02)	0.09
RARC approach	0.76 (0.39–1.47)	0.4	1.34 (0.49–2.36)	0.8
pT stage				
pT0-1	Ref	Ref	Ref	Ref
pT2	1.21 (0.77–1.90)	0.3	1.34 (0.84–2.15)	0.2
pT3-4	1.57 (1.04–2.37)	0.03	2.17 (1.40–3.35)	<0.001
pN+	1.43 (1.05–1.94)	0.02	2.33 (1.71–3.16)	<0.001
Nodes removed	0.99 (0.98–1.00)	0.3	0.98 (0.97–0.99)	0.01
High grade vs. low	3.20 (1.55–6.59)	0.002	3.60 (1.62–7.98)	0.002
LVI	1.85 (1.37–2.49)	<0.001	1.27 (0.96–1.70)	0.09
Positive surgical margins	1.12 (0.74–1.69)	0.5	1.30 (0.84–2.01)	0.2
Neoadjuvant chemotherapy	1.96 (1.51–2.54)	<0.001	1.34 (1.02–1.76)	0.03
Adjuvant chemotherapy	1.29 (0.94–1.77)	0.1	0.77 (0.56–1.06)	0.1

CSM: cancer specific mortality, HR: Hazard ratio, CI: confidence interval, RARC: robotic assisted radical cystectomy, LVI: lymphovascular invasion.

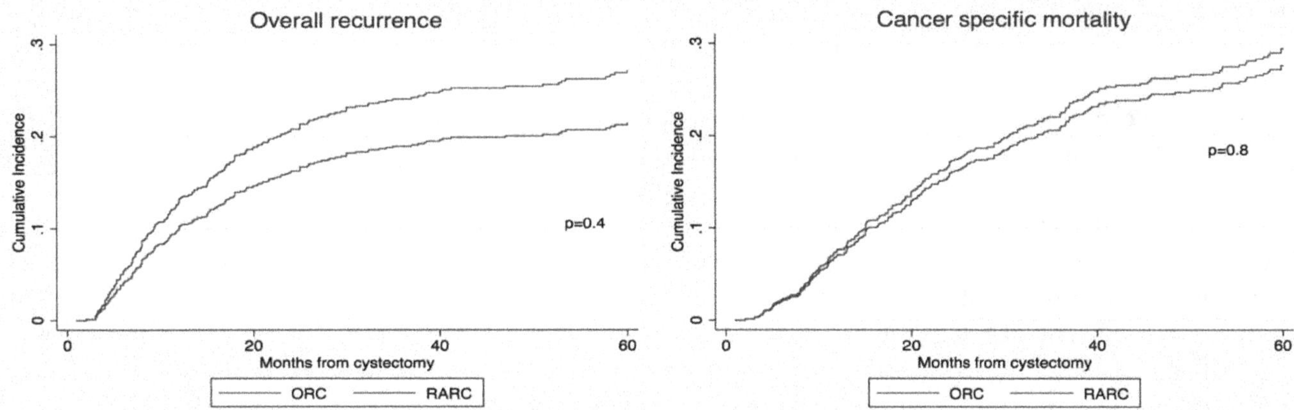

Figure 2. Cumulative incidence of recurrence and cancer specific mortality of patients with non-metastatic BCa treated with radical cystectomy according the type of surgery (ORC vs. RARC) after 2:1 propensity matching for age, pathological T stage, pathological N stage, neoadjuvant chemotherapy (NAC) and grade.

4. Discussion

The adoption of RARC is growing rapidly, but the majority of radical cystectomies continues to be performed by a conventional open approach. The majority of the current data from RARC series which tested perioperative and short term oncological outcomes did not test equivalence regarding long term survival outcomes [18–21]. Several retrospective series raised, indeed, some concerns regarding the oncological safety of the robotic approach [22]. On the other hand, two different prospective trials found no differences in survival outcomes between the two surgical approaches [13,23].

In this multicenter study, we evaluated the survival outcomes of the largest international cohort of bladder cancer patients treated with either ORC or RARC. Patients were treated in both European and American referral centers, collecting data from almost 1000 RARC and matching them with almost 9000 ORC patients. This manuscript follows two previous publications [10,21] from the same collaboration, evaluating for the first time the impact of survival and on peri-operative outcomes demonstrating an advantage of RARC in blood loss and length of stay. New centers were added to this manuscript in respect of the previous publications and the match of the final database was performed separately for each study on the bases of the main aim of each project.

We found that RARC and ORC share similar survival outcomes, both on univariable and multivariable analyses controlled for established prognostic factors. We performed propensity matching to minimize the risk of selection bias adjusting for pathological stage, lymph node status, and age at surgery. Even in this setting we confirmed that the RARC approach is associated with similar recurrence and CSM rates compared to ORC. These results were obtained with a median follow-up before and after propensity matching of 81 and 102 months, respectively. Similarly to our previous manuscript [21], we found a positive surgical margin status higher than 10% in patients treated with RARC. However, this was consistently higher than in patients treated with RARC compared to patients treated with ORC. Despite these differences, this had no impact on survival outcomes when adjusted for all the available confounders in the multivariable model.

Our results confirm the findings of the RAZOR trial [13], an open label, randomized, phase 3, non-inferiority trial comparing RARC versus ORC. A total of 152 patients were included in the ORC group and compared to 150 patients treated with RARC, reporting similar 2-year progression free survival rates. Bochner et al. [23], in a prospective, randomized trial compared 60 and 58 patients treated with RARC and ORC, respectively. No differences were found considering recurrence, cancer survival, or overall survival. Previously, Bochner et al. [18] reported in a single center prospective randomized trial, an advantage in terms of mean intraoperative blood loss for the RARC group but longer operative times compared to ORC. However, no survival outcomes were reported. Similarly, in the prospective trial of Khan et al. [24] and Nix et al. [20] survival outcomes were not analyzed. Given the paucity of prospective data analyzing survival outcomes of RARC patients, new long term level one evidence are required.

Several retrospective series focused on mid-long-term survival outcomes [22,25]. Nguyen at al. [22] analyzed 383 consecutive patients treated with ORC (120) or RARC (263) between 2001 and 2014 at a single institution. With a median follow up of 30 months (for ORC) and 23 months (for RARC), they reported similar recurrence rates with an increasing risk of experiencing extrapelvic lymph node recurrence and peritoneal carcinomatoses for RARC patients. Our analyses did not include the type of recurrence limiting our ability to test this aspect; but we found a similar overall recurrence risk for patients treated with RARC when compared to ORC.

Hu et al. [25], using the SEER database compared 439 patients treated with RARC and 7308 treated with ORC. These authors observed an increasing trend in RARC utilization over the study period and with a median follow up of 44 months, they found no survival differences between the two techniques. However, as recognized by the authors themselves, they analyzed only a small RARC cohort treated by many different centers in their learning in some cases. In a recent systematic review and meta-analyses [26], five studies with a total of 540 participants were included. Authors found no differences in disease progression and local recurrences between patients treated with RARC and ORC. Finally, a recent large retrospective study analyzed the outcomes of RARC versus ORC in the selected population of patients who had received perioperative chemotherapy (in the neoadjuvant or adjuvant setting). No difference was found in multivariable analyses in the rate of positive surgical margins, rate of neobladder diversion, recurrence, and overall survival [27].

Our study represents the largest multicenter collaboration analyzing survival outcomes of patients affected by bladder cancer analyzing the effect of the RARC approach. Our analyses differentiate itself from previous reports including referral centers but excluding low case volume and learning curves which may lead to suboptimal outcomes. Our study comprises the largest available cohort to date analyzing survival outcomes in RARC patients. Despite several strengths, our study is not devoid of limitations. First and foremost, we recognize that our study is limited by its observational nature, and thus our results should be interpreted within the limits of its retrospective design. Second, we did not perform a central review of all specimens and therefore relied on the dedication and attention of the local uro-pathologists. Third, we did not include data regarding urinary diversion that might have an influence on survival outcomes. On the other hand, previous literature failed to prove any differences regarding different urinary diversion in RARC patients supporting the hypothesis of similar survival outcomes between these two groups [28]. Patients treated in academic centers are more prone to be treated with RARC as compared to ORC [8], moreover, differences exist regarding tumor characteristics, patient characteristics, and year of surgery (with an increasing tendency to perform a RARC) [29,30]. These elements can only partially be adjusted for with a propensity match analysis; we are aware that our results need to be confirmed in a controlled randomized trial. In this regard, a high proportion of RARC patients were found with pT0 disease at RC specimen, that might indicate a selection bias that can be only partially mitigated by the propensity matching analyses.

5. Conclusions

Patients treated with RARC were found with an increased rate of positive surgical margin compared to those treated with ORC. However, no differences regarding overall recurrence rate and survival were found between the two study groups. These results were confirmed in propensity score matched analyses adjusted for all the major confounders. High quality prospective trials are warranted to support the long-term oncological safety of RARC.

Author Contributions: M.M.: conceptualization, methodology, validation, formal analysis, investigation, data curation, writing original draft preparation, writing—review and editing; S.Z.: conceptualization, methodology, validation, formal analysis, investigation, data curation, writing—review and editing; F.S., R.M., E.X., W.S.T.,

J.D.K., G.S., A.M. (Anoop Meraney), S.K., B.K., A.M. (Agostino Mattei), P.B., L.M., F.M., A.B., A.G., A.S., R.S.-S., X.C., M.R., A.N., P.I.K., M.R. A.K., W.K., D.S.S., G.P., S.A.B., Y.L., P.S.: methodology, validation, data curation, writing—review and editing; S.F.S.: conceptualization, methodology, validation, investigation, data curation, writing—review and editing, project administration.

Acknowledgments: On behalf of the European Association of Urology-Young Academic Urologists (EAU-YAU), Urothelial carcinoma working group.

References

1. Siegel, R.L.; Miller, K.D.; Jemal, A. Cancer statistics, 2018. *CA Cancer J. Clin.* **2018**, *68*, 7–30. [CrossRef] [PubMed]
2. Babjuk, M.; Böhle, A.; Burger, M.; Capoun, O.; Cohen, D.; Compérat, E.M.; Hernández, V.; Kaasinen, E.; Palou, J.; Rouprêt, M.; et al. EAU Guidelines on Non-Muscle-invasive Urothelial Carcinoma of the Bladder: Update 2016. *Eur. Urol.* **2016**, *71*, 447–461. [CrossRef] [PubMed]
3. Moschini, M.; Simone, G.; Stenzl, A.; Gill, I.S.; Catto, J. Critical Review of Outcomes from Radical Cystectomy: Can Complications from Radical Cystectomy Be Reduced by Surgical Volume and Robotic Surgery? *Eur. Urol. Focus* **2016**, *2*, 19–29. [CrossRef] [PubMed]
4. Challacombe, B.J.; Bochner, B.H.; Dasgupta, P.; Gill, I.; Guru, K.; Herr, H.; Mottrie, A.; Pruthi, R.; Redorta, J.P.; Wiklund, P. The Role of Laparoscopic and Robotic Cystectomy in the Management of Muscle-Invasive Bladder Cancer with Special Emphasis on Cancer Control and Complications. *Eur. Urol.* **2011**, *60*, 767–775. [CrossRef] [PubMed]
5. Yu, H.-Y.; Hevelone, N.D.; Lipsitz, S.R.; Kowalczyk, K.J.; Nguyen, P.L.; Choueiri, T.K.; Kibel, A.S.; Hu, J.C. Comparative Analysis of Outcomes and Costs Following Open Radical Cystectomy Versus Robot-Assisted Laparoscopic Radical Cystectomy: Results From the US Nationwide Inpatient Sample. *Eur. Urol.* **2012**, *61*, 1239–1244. [CrossRef] [PubMed]
6. Styn, N.R.; Montgomery, J.S.; Wood, D.P.; Hafez, K.S.; Lee, C.T.; Tallman, C.; He, C.; Crossley, H.; Hollenbeck, B.K.; Weizer, A.Z. Matched comparison of robotic-assisted and open radical cystectomy. *Urology* **2012**, *79*, 1303–1309. [CrossRef]
7. Ng, C.K.; Kauffman, E.C.; Lee, M.-M.; Otto, B.J.; Portnoff, A.; Ehrlich, J.R.; Schwartz, M.J.; Wang, G.J.; Scherr, D.S. A Comparison of Postoperative Complications in Open versus Robotic Cystectomy. *Eur. Urol.* **2010**, *57*, 274–282. [CrossRef]
8. Hanna, N.; Leow, J.J.; Sun, M.; Friedlander, D.F.; Seisen, T.; Abdollah, F.; Lipsitz, S.R.; Menon, M.; Kibel, A.S.; Bellmunt, J.; et al. Comparative effectiveness of robot-assisted vs. open radical cystectomy. *Urol. Oncol. Semin. Orig. Investig.* **2018**, *36*, 88.e1–88.e9. [CrossRef]
9. Hussein, A.A.; May, P.R.; Jing, Z.; Ahmed, Y.E.; Wijburg, C.J.; Canda, A.E.; Dasgupta, P.; Khan, M.S.; Menon, M.; Peabody, J.O.; et al. Outcomes of Intracorporeal Urinary Diversion after Robot-Assisted Radical Cystectomy: Results from the International Robotic Cystectomy Consortium. *J. Urol.* **2018**, *199*, 1302–1311. [CrossRef]
10. Soria, F.; Moschini, M.; D'Andrea, D.; Abufaraj, M.; Foerster, B.; Mathiéu, R.; Gust, K.M.; Gontero, P.; Simone, G.; Meraney, A.; et al. Comparative Effectiveness in Perioperative Outcomes of Robotic versus Open Radical Cystectomy: Results from a Multicenter Contemporary Retrospective Cohort Study. *Eur. Urol. Focus* **2018**. [CrossRef]
11. Martin, A.D.; Nunez, R.N.; Pacelli, A.; Woods, M.E.; Davis, R.; Thomas, R.; Andrews, P.E.; Castle, E.P. Robot-assisted radical cystectomy: Intermediate survival results at a mean follow-up of 25 months. *BJU Int.* **2010**, *105*, 1706–1709. [CrossRef]
12. Jonsson, M.N.; Adding, L.C.; Hosseini, A.; Schumacher, M.C.; Volz, D.; Nilsson, A.; Carlsson, S.; Wiklund, N.P. Robot-Assisted Radical Cystectomy with Intracorporeal Urinary Diversion in Patients with Transitional Cell Carcinoma of the Bladder. *Eur. Urol.* **2011**, *60*, 1066–1073. [CrossRef] [PubMed]
13. Parekh, D.J.; Reis, I.M.; Castle, E.P.; Gonzalgo, M.L.; Woods, M.E.; Svatek, R.S.; Weizer, A.Z.; Konety, B.R.; Tollefson, M.; Krupski, T.L.; et al. Robot-assisted radical cystectomy versus open radical cystectomy in patients with bladder cancer (RAZOR): An open-label, randomised, phase 3, non-inferiority trial. *Lancet* **2018**, *391*, 2525–2536. [CrossRef]

14. Novara, G.; Svatek, R.S.; Karakiewicz, P.I.; Skinner, E.; Ficarra, V.; Fradet, Y.; Lotan, Y.; Isbarn, H.; Capitanio, U.; Bastian, P.J.; et al. Soft Tissue Surgical Margin Status is a Powerful Predictor of Outcomes After Radical Cystectomy: A Multicenter Study of More Than 4400 Patients. *J. Urol.* **2010**, *183*, 2165–2170. [CrossRef] [PubMed]
15. Xylinas, E.; Rink, M.; Novara, G.; Green, D.A.; Clozel, T.; Fritsche, H.M.; Guillonneau, B.; Lotan, Y.; Kassouf, W.; Tilki, D.; et al. Predictors of survival in patients with soft tissue surgical margin involvement at radical cystectomy. *Ann. Surg. Oncol.* **2013**, *20*, 1027–1034. [CrossRef] [PubMed]
16. Mathieu, R.; Lucca, I.; Rouprêt, M.; Briganti, A.; Shariat, S.F. The prognostic role of lymphovascular invasion in urothelial carcinoma of the bladder. *Nat. Rev. Urol.* **2016**, *13*, 471–479. [CrossRef]
17. Shariat, S.F.; Khoddami, S.M.; Saboorian, H.; Koeneman, K.S.; Sagalowsky, A.I.; Cadeddu, J.A.; McConnell, J.D.; Holmes, M.N.; Roehrborn, C.G. Lymphovascular Invasion is a Pathological Feature of Biologically Aggressive Disease in Patients Treated with Radical Prostatectomy. *J. Urol.* **2004**, *171*, 1122–1127. [CrossRef]
18. Bochner, B.H.; Sjoberg, D.D.; Laudone, V.P. A Randomized Trial of Robot-Assisted Laparoscopic Radical Cystectomy. *N. Engl. J. Med.* **2014**, *371*, 389–390. [CrossRef]
19. Parekh, D.J.; Messer, J.; Fitzgerald, J.; Ercole, B.; Svatek, R. Perioperative outcomes and oncologic efficacy from a pilot prospective randomized clinical trial of open versus robotic assisted radical cystectomy. *J. Urol.* **2013**, *189*, 474–479. [CrossRef]
20. Nix, J.; Smith, A.; Kurpad, R.; Nielsen, M.E.; Wallen, E.M.; Pruthi, R.S. Prospective randomized controlled trial of robotic versus open radical cystectomy for bladder cancer: Perioperative and pathologic results. *Eur. Urol.* **2010**, *57*, 196–201. [CrossRef]
21. Moschini, M.; Soria, F.; Mathieu, R.; Xylinas, E.; D'Andrea, D.; Tan, W.S.; Kelly, J.D.; Simone, G.; Tuderti, G.; Meraney, A.; et al. Propensity-score-matched comparison of soft tissue surgical margins status between open and robotic-assisted radical cystectomy. *Urol. Oncol. Semin. Orig. Investig.* **2019**, *37*, 179.e1–179.e7. [CrossRef] [PubMed]
22. Nguyen, D.P.; Awamlh, B.A.H.A.; Wu, X.; O'Malley, P.; Inoyatov, I.M.; Ayangbesan, A.; Faltas, B.M.; Christos, P.J.; Scherr, D.S. Recurrence Patterns After Open and Robot-assisted Radical Cystectomy for Bladder Cancer. *Eur. Urol.* **2015**, *68*, 399–405. [CrossRef] [PubMed]
23. Bochner, B.H.; Dalbagni, G.; Marzouk, K.H.; Sjoberg, D.D.; Lee, J.; Donat, S.M.; Coleman, J.A.; Vickers, A.; Herr, H.W.; Laudone, V.P. Randomized Trial Comparing Open Radical Cystectomy and Robot-assisted Laparoscopic Radical Cystectomy: Oncologic Outcomes. *Eur. Urol.* **2018**, *74*, 465–471. [CrossRef] [PubMed]
24. Khan, M.S.; Gan, C.; Ahmed, K.; Ismail, A.F.; Watkins, J.; Summers, J.A.; Peacock, J.L.; Rimington, P.; Dasgupta, P. A Single-centre Early Phase Randomised Controlled Three-arm Trial of Open, Robotic, and Laparoscopic Radical Cystectomy (CORAL). *Eur. Urol.* **2016**, *69*, 613–621. [CrossRef] [PubMed]
25. Hu, J.C.; Chughtai, B.; O'Malley, P.; Halpern, J.A.; Mao, J.; Scherr, D.S.; Hershman, D.L.; Wright, J.D.; Sedrakyan, A. Perioperative Outcomes, Health Care Costs, and Survival After Robotic-assisted Versus Open Radical Cystectomy: A National Comparative Effectiveness Study. *Eur. Urol.* **2016**, *70*, 195–202. [CrossRef] [PubMed]
26. Sathianathen, N.J.; Kalapara, A.; Frydenberg, M.; Lawrentschuk, N.; Weight, C.J.; Parekh, D.; Konety, B.R. Robotic Assisted Radical Cystectomy vs Open Radical Cystectomy: Systematic Review and Meta-Analysis. *J. Urol.* **2018**. [CrossRef] [PubMed]
27. Necchi, A.; Pond, G.R.; Smaldone, M.C.; Pal, S.K.; Chan, K.; Wong, Y.-N.; Viterbo, R.; Sonpavde, G.; Harshman, L.C.; Crabb, S.; et al. Robot-assisted Versus Open Radical Cystectomy in Patients Receiving Perioperative Chemotherapy for Muscle-invasive Bladder Cancer: The Oncologist's Perspective from a Multicentre Study. *Eur. Urol. Focus* **2018**, *4*, 937–945. [CrossRef]
28. Pyun, J.H.; Kim, H.K.; Cho, S.; Kang, S.G.; Cheon, J.; Lee, J.G.; Kim, J.J.; Kang, S.H. Robot-Assisted Radical Cystectomy with Total Intracorporeal Urinary Diversion: Comparative Analysis with Extracorporeal Urinary Diversion. *J. Laparoendosc. Adv. Surg. Tech.* **2016**, *26*, 349–355. [CrossRef]
29. Leow, J.J.; Reese, S.W.; Jiang, W.; Lipsitz, S.R.; Bellmunt, J.; Trinh, Q.-D.; Chung, B.I.; Kibel, A.S.; Chang, S.L. Propensity-Matched Comparison of Morbidity and Costs of Open and Robot-Assisted Radical Cystectomies: A Contemporary Population-Based Analysis in the United States. *Eur. Urol.* **2014**, *66*, 569–576. [CrossRef]
30. Monn, M.F.; Cary, K.C.; Kaimakliotis, H.Z.; Flack, C.K.; Koch, M.O. National trends in the utilization of robotic-assisted radical cystectomy: An analysis using the Nationwide Inpatient Sample. *Urol. Oncol. Semin. Orig. Investig.* **2014**, *32*, 785–790. [CrossRef]

4

Consensus Definition and Prediction of Complexity in Transurethral Resection or Bladder Endoscopic Dissection of Bladder Tumours

Mathieu Roumiguié [1], Evanguelos Xylinas [2], Antonin Brisuda [3], Maximillian Burger [4], Hugh Mostafid [5], Marc Colombel [6], Marek Babjuk [3], Joan Palou Redorta [7], Fred Witjes [8] and Bernard Malavaud [1,*]

1 Department of Urology, Institut Universitaire du Cancer, 31059 Toulouse CEDEX 9, France; Roumiguie.Mathieu@iuct-oncopole.fr
2 Department of Urology, Hôpital Cochin, APHP, 75014 Paris, France; evanguelos.xylinas@aphp.fr
3 Department of Urology, 2nd Faculty of Medicine, Charles University, Teaching Hospital Motol, 15006 Prague, Czech Republic; antonin.brisuda@fnmotol.cz (A.B.); Marek.Babjuk@fnmotol.cz (M.B.)
4 St. Josef, Klinik für Urologie, Caritas-Krankenhaus, 93053 Regensburg, Germany; mburger@caritasstjosef.de
5 Department of Urology, Royal Surrey County Hospital, Surrey, Guildford GU2 7RF, UK; hugh.mostafid@nhs.net
6 Department of Urology, Hôpital Edouard Herriot, 69437 Lyon, France; marc.colombel@chu-lyon.fr
7 Department of Urology, Fundacio Puigvert, 08025 Barcelona, Spain; jpalou@fundacio-puigvert.es
8 Department of Urology, Radboud UMC, 6525 GA Nijmegen, The Netherlands; Fred.Witjes@radboudumc.nl
* Correspondence: malavaud.bernard@iuct-oncopole.fr

Simple Summary: Transurethral resection of bladder tumours may be technically challenging. Complexity was defined by consensus from the literature by a panel of ten senior urologists as "any TURBT/En-bloc dissection that results in incomplete resection and/or prolonged surgery (>1 h) and/or significant (Clavien-Dindo ≥ 3) perioperative complications". Patient and tumour's characteristics that suggested to by the panel to relate to complex surgery were collected and then ranked by Delphi consensus. They were tested in the prediction of complexity in 150 clinical scenarios. After univariate and logistic regression analyses, significant characteristics were organized into a checklist that predicts complexity. Receiver operating characteristics (ROC) curves of the regression model and the corresponding calibration curve showed adequate discrimination (AUC = 0.916) and good calibration. The resulting Bladder Complexity Checklist can be used to deliver optimal preoperative information and personalise the organisation of surgery.

Abstract: Ten senior urologists were interrogated to develop a predictive model based on factors from which they could anticipate complex transurethral resection of bladder tumours (TURBT). Complexity was defined by consensus. Panel members then used a five-point Likert scale to grade those factors that, in their opinion, drove complexity. Consensual factors were highlighted through two Delphi rounds. Respective contributions to complexity were quantitated by the median values of their scores. Multivariate analysis with complexity as a dependent variable tested their independence in clinical scenarios obtained by random allocation of the factors. The consensus definition of complexity was "any TURBT/En-bloc dissection that results in incomplete resection and/or prolonged surgery (>1 h) and/or significant (Clavien-Dindo ≥ 3) perioperative complications". Logistic regression highlighted five domains as independent predictors: patient's history, tumour number, location, and size and access to the bladder. Receiver operating characteristic (ROC) analysis confirmed good discrimination (AUC = 0.92). The sum of the scores of the five domains adjusted to their regression coefficients or Bladder Complexity Score yielded comparable performance (AUC = 0.91, C-statistics, $p = 0.94$) and good calibration. As a whole, preoperative factors identified by expert judgement were organized to quantitate the risk of a complex TURBT, a crucial requisite to personalise patient information, adapt human and technical resources to individual situations and address TURBT variability in clinical trials.

Keywords: bladder cancer; transurethral resection; en-bloc resection

---

1. Introduction

Bladder cancer is the seventh most prevalent cancer worldwide [1] and the sixth leading cause of cancer in the EU, where it entails a significant burden in healthcare organization and cost [2]. Most patients present with non-muscle invasive bladder cancer (NMIBC), for which endoscopic resection or en-bloc dissection of bladder tumours, collectively referred to as transurethral resection of bladder tumour (TURBT), initiate the treatment and inform the risks of recurrence and progression. Pathology also provides information on the adequacy of surgery that is visually complete resection and presence of muscle at the resection base [3]. Although this is the most common procedure in oncologic urology, with over 120,000 new cases across Europe annually [2], few reports have addressed how individual characteristics may challenge the successful completion of surgery [4,5]. In addition, the reported variability of residual disease [6] and higher performances of experienced surgeons [7] emphasize the demands of "good-quality" TURBT [7]. Moreover, quality represents latent information for the non-expert, contrary to clinical complications that are self-evident, closely monitored by the public and insurers and used as proxy for quality metrics [8].

Any system capable to document how individual presentations influence surgical outcomes would be of high clinical relevance. Therefore, the objective of the present consensus was to detail and organize the factors based on which experienced urologists anticipate a complex TURBT.

2. Results

2.1. Step 1: Definition of Complexity

A PubMed search of "transurethral resection" (of) "bladder" and "morbidity" or "complication", or "mortality" or "death" yielded 585, 664, 9 and 95 articles, respectively. Of these, 89 articles relevant to the process of defining complexity were analysed, obtaining 36 articles (Table S(1) which were instrumental in highlighting adequacy, operative time and morbidity as the three drivers that characterize a complex surgery, as opposed to an uneventful procedure [4,8–42].

After a single round of circulation, all panellists validated the following definition of a complex TURBT: "any TURBT/En-bloc dissection that results in incomplete resection and/or prolonged surgery (>1 h) and/or significant (Clavien-Dindo ≥ 3) perioperative complications".

2.2. Step 2: Items That Drive Complexity

Eighty-five characteristics that were suggested by the panellists to influence surgery were organized into six chapters consistent with standard medical practice: patient's characteristics and history, tumour characteristics, access to the bladder, bladder anatomy and surgical environment.

Their relevance was researched in two Delphi rounds, which showed consensus for 42 characteristics in the first round (Figures S1–S4) and 83 in the second (Figures 1–4). For any characteristic or item, the median opinion of the panel (Figures 1–4) was then used as the metrics to weight its individual contribution to complexity.

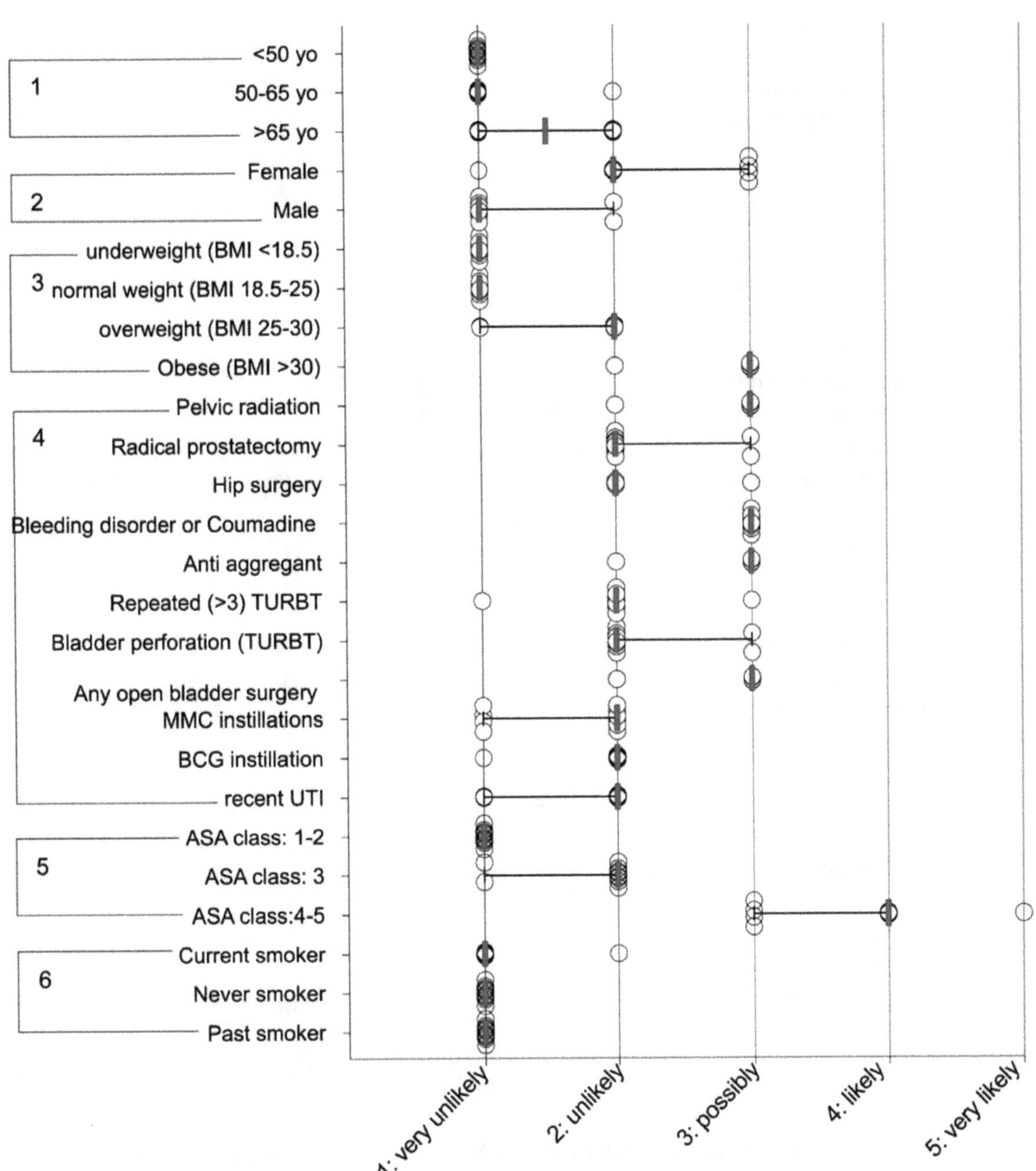

Figure 1. Distribution of the scores regarding the likelihood of incomplete resection and/or prolonged surgery (>1 h) and/or significant (Clavien-Dindo ≥ 3) perioperative complications according to patient's characteristics. ((1) age, (2) sex, (3) weight and body mass index (BMI), (4) patient's history, (5) American Society of Anaesthesiologists' (ASA) physical status classification, (6) tobacco smoking. MMC: Mitomycin C, Bacille Calmette Guérin (BCG), TURBT: transurethral resection of bladder tumour.

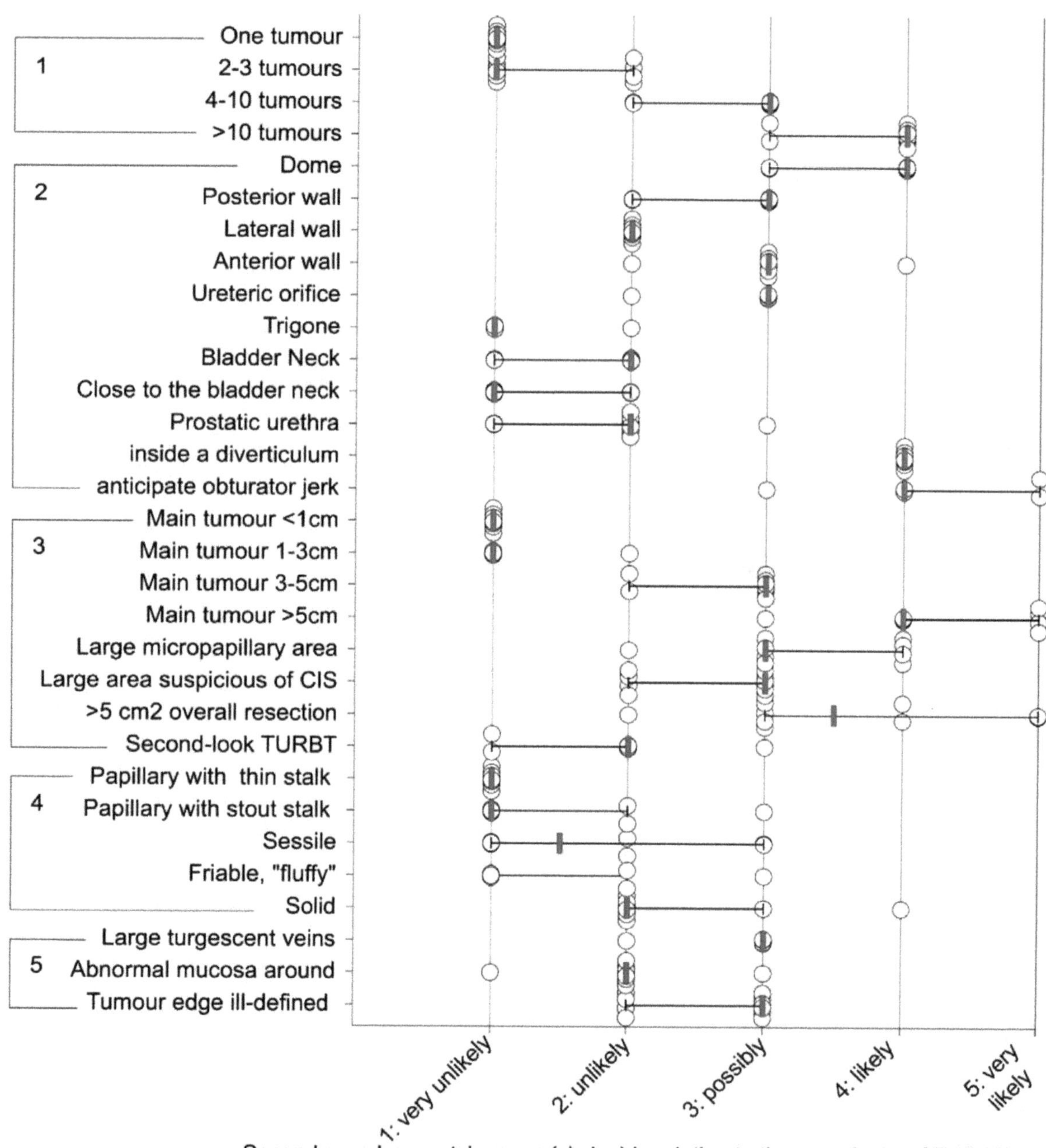

Figure 2. Distribution of the scores regarding the likelihood of incomplete resection and/or prolonged surgery (>1 h) and/or significant (Clavien-Dindo ≥ 3) perioperative complications according to tumour's characteristics: ((1) number, (2) location, (3) size, (4) structure, (5) surroundings. CIS: carcinoma in situ.

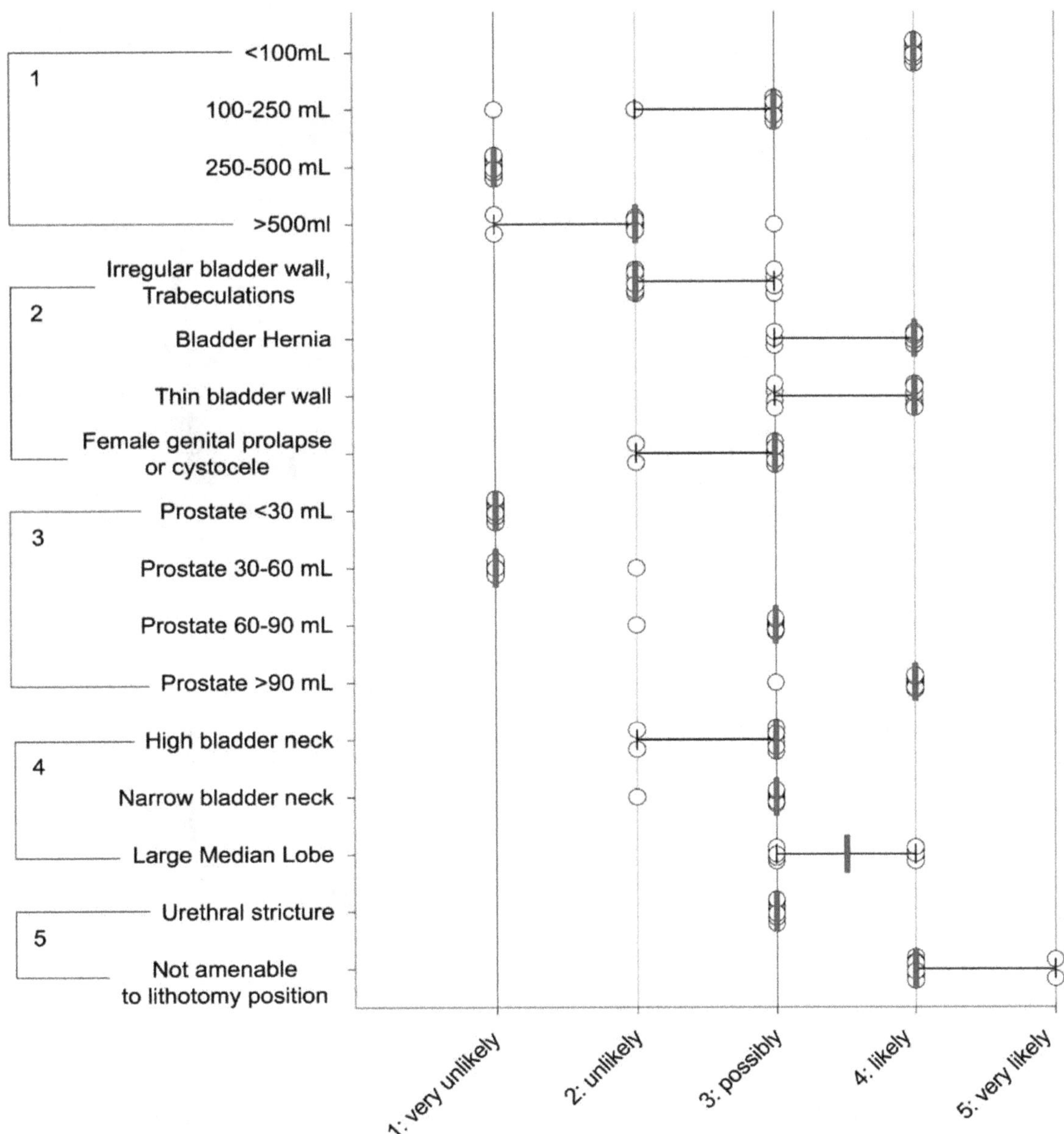

Figure 3. Distribution of the scores regarding the likelihood of incomplete resection and/or prolonged surgery (>1 h) and/or significant (Clavien-Dindo ≥ 3) perioperative complications according to bladder characteristics and access to the bladder cavity: ((1) bladder capacity, (2) bladder structure, (3) prostate volume, (4) bladder neck, (5) others.

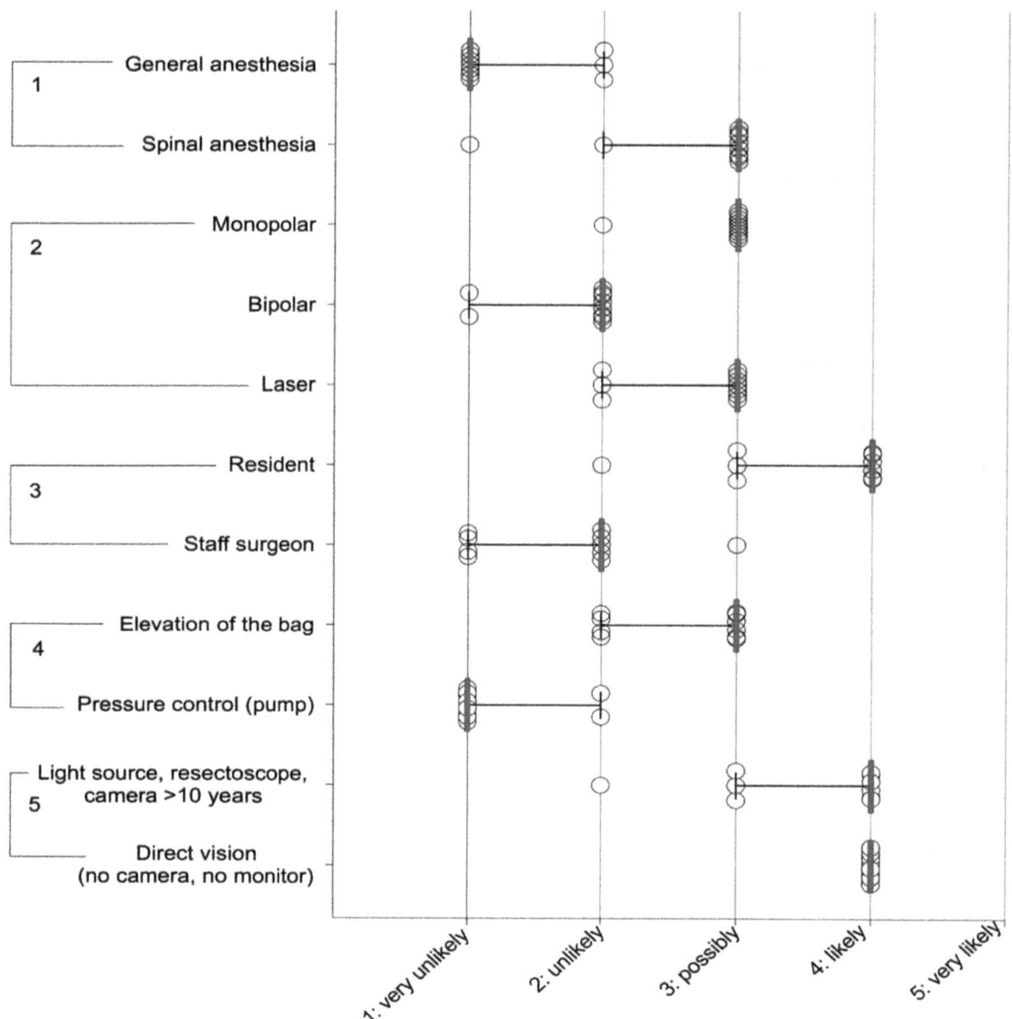

Figure 4. Distribution of the scores regarding the likelihood of incomplete resection and/or prolonged surgery (>1 h) and/or significant (Clavien-Dindo ≥ 3) perioperative complications according to the surgical environment: ((1) anaesthesia, (2) energy, (3) operator, (4) bladder irrigation, (5) instruments.

2.3. *Step 3: Construction, Discrimination and Accuracy of the Bladder Complexity Checklist Sum*

2.3.1. Clinical Scenarios

Smoking, underweight, normal weight and American Society of Anaesthesiologists (ASA) class 1–2 or 3 that in the panel's opinions did not relate to the complexity of TURBT were not included in the scenarios, although age and sex that were also considered of little influence were retained, as they are standards in medical reporting. Although the surgical environment was consistently considered to have bearing on the odds of a complex surgery, the corresponding items were not included in the scenarios, as they were considered circumstantial rather than constitutive of the case. As a whole, 150 scenarios that included 9 items organized 5 five domains (Table 1) were presented to the panel. The members were strongly consistent in their anticipation of complexity, as consensus was observed for 131/150 (87.3%) scenarios that were by design confirmed for univariate and multivariate analysis.

Table 1. Univariate analysis of the scores of preoperative characteristics in a cohort of 131 random scenarios for which the panel was consistent in its anticipation of complexity.

Domain of Interest	Feature	Number of Items	Median Score, (95%CI)		Mann–Whitney *U*-Test
			TURBT Unlikely to Be Complex (n = 73)	TURBT Likely to Be Complex (n = 58)	
Patient's characteristics	Age	3	1 (1–(1)	1 (1–(1)	n.s. ($p = 0.85$)
	Sex	2	1 (1–(1)	1 (1–2)	n.s. ($p = 0.72$)
Patient's history		12	1 (1–2)	2 (1–2)	n.s. ($p = 0.07$)
Tumour's characteristics	Number	3	1 (1–(1)	3 (3–4)	$p = 0.002$
	Location	10	3 (2–3)	4 (3–4)	$p < 0.0001$
	Size	5	2 (1–3)	3 (3–3)	$p < 0.0001$
	Structure	5	2 (2–3)	2 (2–3)	n.s. ($p = 0.97$)
Bladder Anatomy		8	3 (2–3)	3 (2–3)	n.s. ($p = 0.82$)
Access to the Bladder cavity		13	1 (1–3)	3 (3–4)	$p < 0.0001$

n.s. not significant.

2.3.2. Discrimination and Accuracy

In univariate analysis, the items that informed the tumour characteristics (number, location, size) and access to the bladder were significantly associated with complexity (Table 1). Patient's history that did not reach statistical relevance still qualified for multivariate analysis ($p = 0.07$).

Five domains (Table 2) that in logistic regression were independent predictors of complexity, i.e., history, tumour number, location, and size and access to the bladder cavity, were used to develop the probability function that modelled the probability of a complex surgery.

Table 2. Logistic regression analysis showing independent relationships between the complexity of TURBT and patient history, tumour number, main tumour location and size and factors restraining the access to the bladder cavity.

Independent Variables	Regression Coefficient	Std. Error	z	$p > \|z\|$	95% CI of the Regression Coefficient	
Patient History	0.99	0.32	3.11	0.002	0.37	1.61
Tumour Number	0.96	0.23	4.18	0.000	0.51	1.41
Main Tumour Location	1.44	0.33	4.42	0.000	0.80	2.09
Main Tumour Size	1.04	0.26	3.98	0.000	0. 53	1.55
Access	1.10	0.26	4.31	0.000	0. 60	1.60
Intercept value	−13.34	2.31	−5.77	0.000	−17.87	−8.81

$$p(complex) = \frac{1}{1+\exp(13.34-0.99xHistory-0.96xTuNumber-1.44xMainTuLocation-1.04xMainTuSize-1.1xAccess)} \quad (1)$$

This function showed good discrimination (AUC: 0.92 (95%CI: 0.87–0.96) in receiver operating characteristic (ROC) analysis (Figure 5).

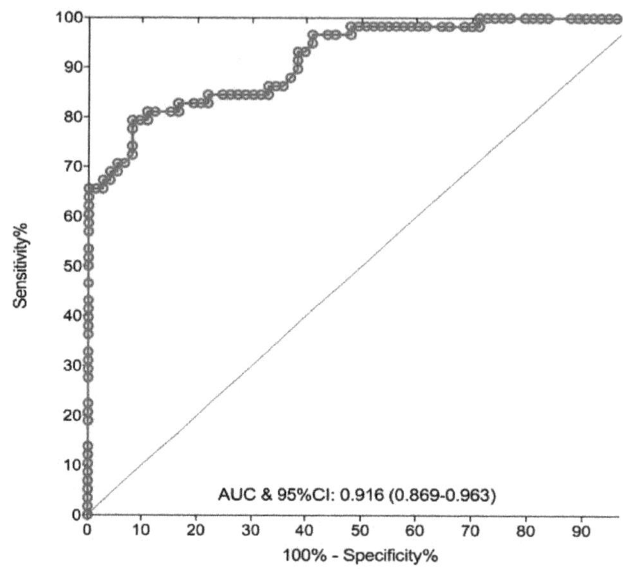

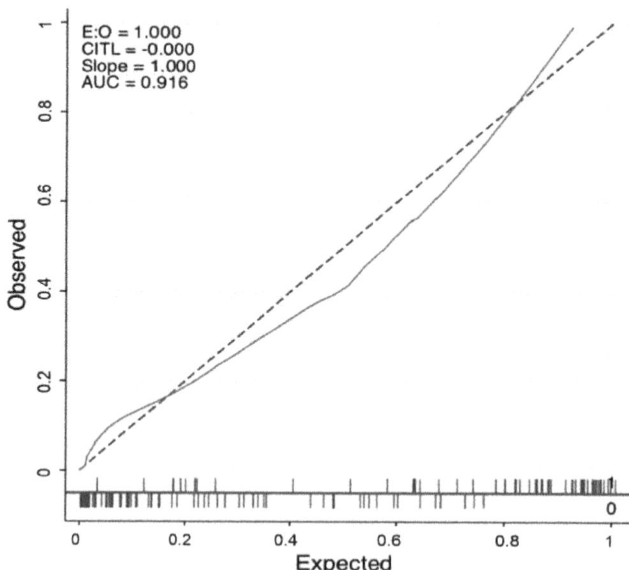

Figure 5. Receiver operating characteristics (ROC) curves of the regression model with the corresponding calibration curve showing adequate discrimination (AUC = 0.916) and good calibration, with calibration slope of 1 and calibration in the large (CITL) of 0, indicating that the predicted prevalence of complexity was in keeping with the observed prevalence (CITL) and that the model was not over fitted (slope).

The simplification offered by the Bladder Complexity Checklist Sum (BCCS, Table 3) yielded comparable performance (C-Statistics $p = 0.94$, Figure 6).

Table 3. Checklist detailing the five domains related to the prediction of a complex transurethral resection of bladder tumours by the panel. The Bladder Complexity Score (BCS) was calculated as the sum of the weight-adjusted scores. Increments in BCS relate to the positive and negative predictive values of experiencing a complex surgery, that is, "any TURBT/En-bloc dissection that results in incomplete resection and/or prolonged surgery (>1 h) and/or significant (Clavien-Dindo ≥ 3) perioperative complications".

	Patient's Characteristics		Tumour's Characteristics		
Weight-Adjusted Scores	**Medical History**	**Bladder Access**	**Number**	**Size**	**Location**
1	No Relevant History	No relevant features	1–3	<3 cm	
1.5					Trigon
2	Hip Surgery Radical Prostatectomy Repeated TURBT (>3) Prior Bladder perforation MMC or BCG instillations UTI	Large bladder (>500 mL) Irregular bladder wall, Trabeculations		Recent TURBT (second-look)	
3	Obese BMI > 30 Pelvic Radiation Any open bladder surgery Bleeding disorder or Coumadin or Anti-aggregant	Urethral stricture High or narrow bladder neck Large Median lobe Large prostate (60–90 mL) Small bladder (100–250 mL) Female prolapse or cystocele	4–10	3–5 cm Large micropapillary area or suspicious for CIS (>5 cm^2)	Prostatic urethra Bladder neck Lateral wall
4	ASA class 4–5	Not amenable to lithotomy position Very small bladder (<100 mL) Very large prostate (>90 mL) Bladder hernia Thin bladder wall	>10	>5 cm	
4.5					Posterior or Anterior wall Ureteric orifice
6					Dome Anticipate obturator jerk Diverticulum

Abbreviations: UTI: urinary tract infection.

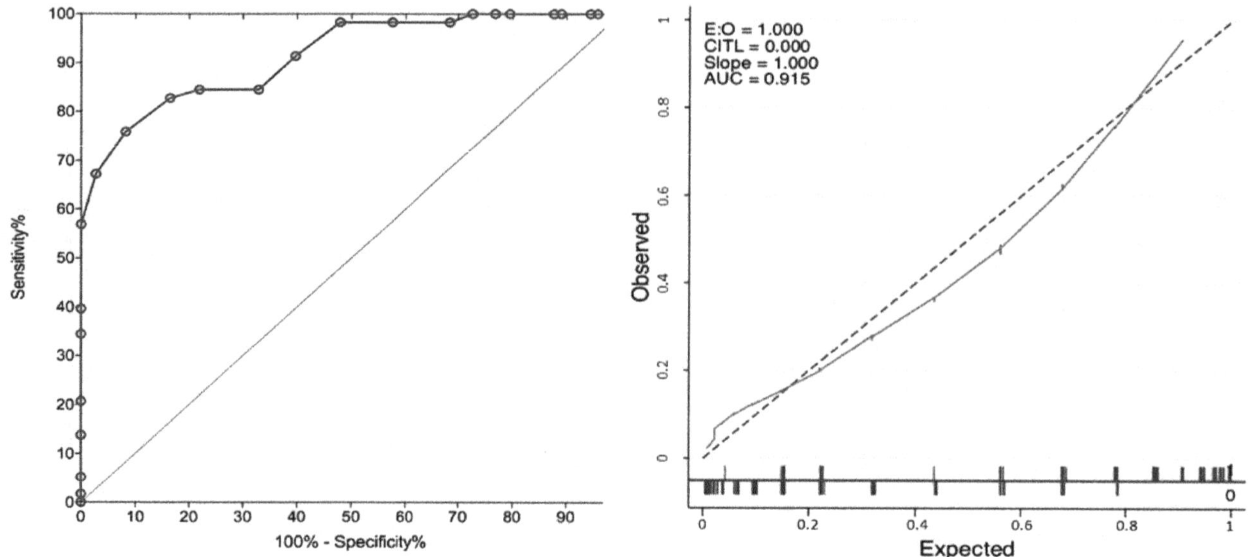

Figure 6. ROC curves of the Bladder Complexity Checklist Sum (BCCS) and the corresponding calibration curve showing similar discrimination and calibration performances compared to the regression model.

Both instruments showed good calibration (Figure 3, Figure 4).

Figure 7 illustrates the balance between positive and negative predictive values according to increments in BCCS.

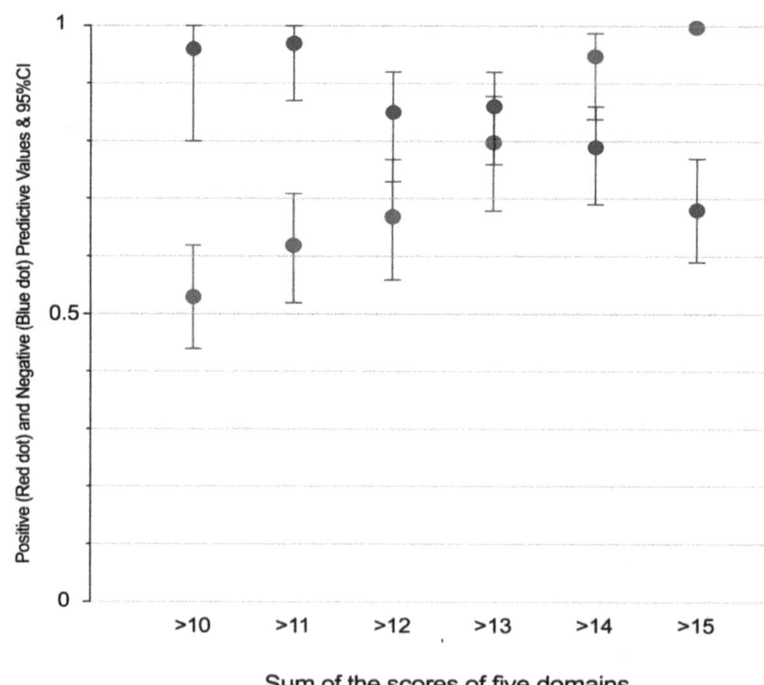

Figure 7. Negative (**blue**) and positive (**red**) predictive values (NPV and PPV) of increments in the BCCS.

3. Discussion

Anticipation is essential to adapt staff and technical resources to individual challenges of clinical situations. The adoption of standardized instruments of evaluation for major urological procedures [43] spurred us to develop similar instruments for TURBT, the most common procedure in oncologic urology [2].

The first step contextualized complexity, a concept adapted to the rationalization of healthcare [44]. A PubMed search highlighted three dimensions that characterize a complex surgery, as opposed to a satisfactory and uneventful procedure. Adequacy was recently introduced in the European Association of Urology (EAU) guidelines to insist on the importance of complete resection of all visible tumours with the detrusor muscle in the specimen, a surrogate marker of resection quality that controls the risk of early recurrence [9] and may impact adjuvant treatment [11]. Surgery longer than one hour was included following a large population-based report from the American College of Surgeons National Surgical Quality Improvement Program (NSQIP), where it related to postoperative complications independently from age, comorbidities, tumour size and ASA classification [31]. Lastly, postoperative complications requiring surgical, endoscopic or radiological intervention—that is, Grade III and higher in the recently TURBT-adapted Clavien–Dindo classification [29]—were also considered, as they were recently shown [33] to affect a significant minority of patients (8.1%, of which 15% were Grade III and higher). Reminiscent of other major oncologic procedures (e.g., trifecta in kidney and prostate surgery), the consensus therefore encompassed the three reported qualifiers of complexity, oncological, procedural and postoperative into a multidimensional definition.

The second step researched robust clinical predictors. To that end, we relayed on expert judgement, a valuable instrument when other methods are intractable for scientific or practicable reasons [45]. TURBT appears to fall in that category, as although many factors are known to impact surgery and its outcomes [4,5,46], some important ones were not detailed in population-based series (e.g., position of the tumour) or were so infrequent as to elude detection (e.g., diverticulum). Conversely, experienced urologists are bound to encounter them along their career and to drive some operational conclusions as to the influence they may have on their management. This was confirmed by the extensive list of items drawn from experience and by the broad consensus of the panel on their relative contributions to complexity.

Most of the items that carried a "possibly", "likely" or "very likely" risk of complication were consistent with the current literature. Conversely, some that had eluded cohorts [33] and population-based registries [4,31] made sense to the practising physician, notably, the access to the bladder cavity or the position of the tumours, with TURBT at the dome considered as "likely" to result in visually incomplete, lengthy or morbid surgery, compared to "very unlikely" for the trigon. The increments in scores with tumour sizes presented according to the current US procedural terminology (Figure 2) were in keeping with the increasing risks of complication and 30-day reoperation rates reported in two large NSQIP population-based studies [4,31]. A similar correlation was observed for the number of tumours, that is also a central parameter in the EAU/European Organisation for Research and Treatment of Cancer (EORTC) risk stratification of progression and recurrence [3].

Overall, high consistency between the literature or the practical constraints of surgery and the Delphi scores vindicated the present approach to anticipate complex TURBT.

However relevant, no single factor could possibly drive the entirety of the surgical challenge, which spurred us to the third step to analyse their respective contributions in random scenarios. Although the panel acknowledged the influence of technology in TURBT (Figure 4), elements pertaining to the surgical environment that were considered as adaptive rather than constitutive were not considered in the scenarios. Consistent with the format of clinical presentations, scenarios included age and sex, although they are considered of little bearing in TURBT (Figure 1). To account for the risk of cognitive overload [47], only four aspects were considered: patient's history, tumour and bladder anatomy and access. Although this resulted in a high prevalence of complex cases (58/131 (44.2%) scenarios were classified as "possibly", "likely" or "very likely" to result in incomplete resection or prolonged surgery (>1 h) or significant complications), random scenarios were preferred to collecting real-life clinical cases in the construction of the score, as this ensured that even rare situations were not overlooked.

On univariate analysis, tumour number, size, and location and access to the bladder cavity significantly related to complexity (Table 1). Although not significant in univariate analysis ($p = 0.07$), patient's history still qualified for multivariate analysis, where all five aspects independently related to complexity.

As measured by their regression coefficients (Table 2), although patients' history and bladder contributed to a lesser extent, tumour characteristics carried most of the information, thereby emphasizing the classical emphasis on thorough preoperative evaluation. The regression model showed excellent discrimination on ROC analysis (AUC: 0.92), while the calibration curve confirmed its accuracy (Figure 5).

The Bladder Complexity Checklist was then developed to facilitate the recording of significant characteristics in the clinic (Table 3). For illustration purposes, the case of a 75-year-old female patient with a thin bladder wall, showing a single 3 cm tumour of the dome would yield a sum of 15, consistent with a predictive value for complexity (PPV) of 100% (Figure 7). Summing the weight-adjusted scores of the Bladder Complexity Checklist carried similar discrimination and accuracy as the logistic model (Figure 4). This is to our knowledge the first effort to quantitatively inform with a simple clinical instrument the multidimensional complexity of TURBT. It could readily complement the other checklists proposed to control the quality of the procedure [37] or the step-by-step management of NMIBC [14].

Overall, the present methodology highlighted the factors that drove the anticipation by experienced surgeons of a complex TURBT. It would be amenable to other procedures where the surgical outcome relates to a large number of factors accessible to preoperative evaluation (e.g., radical prostatectomy, kidney transplantation). It also emphasized the variability in complexity of a procedure that is still widely regarded as menial.

The ability to anticipate and document complexity has important practical consequences. First, the Bladder Complexity Checklist could be instrumental in personalising the human and technical resources required for the most common procedure in oncologic urology [2]. This has become an absolute requisite in the current era of value-based care [48], where most procedural terminologies and reimbursement policies for TURBT consider the size and number of tumours compounded by comorbidity indexes, but overlook essential predictors such as the position of the tumour, a key descriptor of complexity in the present consensus. The Bladder Complexity Checklist Sum that organises and quantitates all relevant clinical information could also be used to drive the adaptation of health resources according to increments of complexity and support complexity-adapted coverage from health insurances.

Second, quantitating the difficulties entailed by a "good-quality" TURBT [7] would offer a solid ground to confront the morbidity and oncological outcome of a potentially complex procedure. Documenting variability is also important when analysing the benefits of different systems of resection or evaluating adjuvant treatments in research protocols [11]. Although all controlled trials to date overlooked the bias of complexity, we believe that crucial information such as the complexity score or, at the very least, a minimal dataset including size, number and position of the tumours should be documented and balanced in clinical research.

Third, measuring complexity that amounts to weighting the risks of the procedure would constitute an important instrument to inform the patient and therefore control part of his anxiety [49]. The constraints of information also include the training and experience of the surgical staff [50]. A large study from the NSQIP concluded that residents' involvement in urology procedures was not associated with increased complications, although it significantly increased the operative time [27].

Regarding TURBT, the relation between time and complications [31] and surgeon experience and the presence of the detrusor muscle in the specimen [9] vindicated the panel's prudent assessment of residents' participation (Figure 4). This observation also has direct bearing on the organisation of care in academic hospitals, in terms not only of informed consent [50] but also of organizing the list so that cases showing high complexity receive proper attention in terms of consultant supervision and position on the surgical list [50].

Several limitations should be considered. First, it is recommended for health indicators to include panellists of different origins, from public health experts to patients' representatives [51]. Here, the sole urologists' perspective was adopted, which certainly contributed to the high degree of consensus and the strong consistency with clinicians' experience. With 10 experts, the panel positioned at the first quartile of the distribution of panellists in a systematic review [51] of the Delphi methodology and was in line with the number of experts invited to develop other multidimensional instruments in urology [43].

Second, the model was not validated in the clinics, where a lower prevalence of complex cases may be anticipated. However, the review of 416 diagnostic studies showed that a lower prevalence improved specificity and had no systemic effect on sensitivity [52], suggesting that the current model would retain its relevance in the real-life setting. Third, important predictors such as the position or the multiplicity of tumours are best defined by preoperative flexible cystoscopy [53], which is optional when the diagnosis can be ascertained by medical imaging [3]. Last, the process yielded a large number of items (Table 3) that may require streamlining after the first returns of clinical experience.

4. Materials and Methods

The present Delphi method followed the recommendations of a systematic review for the development of healthcare quality indicators [51]. Six urologists designed the study into three separate work packages: definition of complexity, outline of the factors that drive complexity and evaluation of their respective contributions in clinical scenarios. Four panellists were then invited to broaden the scope of ages and experiences (Table 4). As a whole, the panel comprised 10 board-certified urologists with over 202 years of combined experience.

Table 4. Panel participants' characteristics and experience in urology.

Expert	Country	Age	Urology * (Years)	Oncology * (Years)	FEBU	PhD	Head of Urology **	National Association of Urology	European Association of Urology
1	F	36	4	2	-	-	0	Member NMIBC guidelines panel	Member
2	F	38	5	3	Yes	Yes	-	Board member NMIBC guidelines panel	Chairman YAU Board member YOU & ESOU
3	CZ	39	14	-	Yes	Yes	-	Member	Member
4	D	45	19	14	Yes	Yes	6	Board Member in charge of Research	Vice-Chairman NMIBC guidelines panel
5	UK	53	20	20	Yes	-	0	Member	Member NMIBC guidelines panel
6	F	58	26	26	-	Yes	-	Member	Board Member ESOU
7	CZ	58	27	22	-	Yes	10	President of National Urological Society	Chairman NMIBC guidelines panel Member Education office of the ESU

Table 4. *Cont.*

Expert	Country	Age	Urology * (Years)	Oncology * (Years)	FEBU	PhD	Head of Urology **	National Association of Urology	European Association of Urology
8	F	59	26	25	Yes	Yes	5	Member	EAU Board Member ESU Member
9	E	61	33	20	Yes	Yes	2	Member	EAU Board member Director of ESU NMIBC Guidelines panel
10	NL	62	28	28	-	Yes	22	Chairman bladder cancer guidelines office	Chairman MIBC guidelines panel, ESU Member

* Years since board certification, that is, 202 years of combined experience in urology and 160 years in oncology. ** Years since head of department or unit. FEBU: Fellow of the European Board of Urology, ESU European School of Urology, YAU: Young Academic Urologists, ESOU: European Society of Oncologic Urology, NMIBC: non-muscle invasive bladder cancer, MIBC: muscle-invasive bladder cancer.

4.1. Step 1: Consensus Definition of Complexity

Reports on morbidity or mortality of TURBT were researched in the PubMed database (English language, 4/2009–4/2019, key words: "transurethral resection (of) bladder", "morbidity", "complication" "mortality" or "death"). A senior author (BM) reviewed all abstracts and analysed the articles of potential relevance before proposing to the panel a working definition of complexity in TURBT (Table S1).

4.2. Step 2: Listing the Items That Drive Complexity

4.2.1. Collection of the Factors Related to Complexity

Experts collected the factors that in their opinion could impact TURBT. All suggested items were considered and organized into domains, consistent with the medical usage and segmented according to the literature into a comprehensive list of items.

4.2.2. Delphi Validation

The panellists scored the items using a five-point Likert scale, classifying from "very unlikely" to "very likely" the risk of complexity entailed by the individual items (Table 5). After the first Delphi round, they were informed of the panel's distribution of the scores and requested in the second round to confirm or adjust their personal evaluation.

Consensus on an item was reached when the opinions across the panel were so consistent that the 95% confidence interval of their distribution was bounded within two consecutive scores. In subsequent analyses, the median value of the opinions or Median Opinion (MO) was used to weight the contribution of an item to complexity.

Table 5. Questions and Likert scores for complexity and patient and tumour's characteristics and surgical environment.

Domains	Question	Likert Scores
Patient and tumour and bladder characteristics	How likely is this characteristic to negatively impact TURBT, that is, to result in incomplete resection or prolonged surgery (>1 h) or significant intra- or postoperative complications (Clavien-Dindo Grade III and higher)?	(1) It is VERY UNLIKELY to impact TURBT
		(2) It is UNLIKELY to impact TURBT
		(3) It may OCCASIONALLY impact TURBT
		(4) It is LIKELY to impact TURBT
		(5) It is VERY LIKELY to impact TURBT
Surgical Environment	How likely is the following element of the surgical environment to influence the risk of TURBT resulting in either three situations, i.e., incomplete resection according to the operator, or prolonged surgery (>1 h) or significant intra- (bleeding that requires transfusion, laparotomy) or postoperative complications (Clavien-Dindo Grade III and higher)?	(1) It is VERY LIKELY TO REDUCE the risk
		(2) It is LIKELY TO REDUCE the risk
		(3) It is NOT EXPECTED TO INFLUENCE the risk in either way
		(4) It is LIKELY TO INCREASE the risk
		(5) It is VERY LIKELY TO INCREASE the risk
Clinical scenarios	In the following scenario, will TURBT result in incomplete resection or prolonged surgery (>1 h) or significant intra- or postoperative complications (Clavien-Dindo Grade III and higher)?	(1) This is VERY UNLIKELY to happen
		(2) This is UNLIKELY to happen
		(3) This may OCCASIONALLY happen
		(4) This is LIKELY to happen
		(5) This IS VERY LIKELY to happen

4.3. *Step 3: Construction of the Bladder Complexity Checklist*

4.3.1. Construction of Clinical Scenarios

To acknowledge the multifactorial nature of complexity in medicine, items that reached consensus were then organized along clinical scenarios constructed by their random allocation within their respective domains of interest: patient's history, tumour number, main tumour size, location, and structure, access to the bladder cavity. One hundred and fifty scenarios were constructed (Table S2) and validated for clinical consistency (e.g., refuting the association of 30 mL prostate and female genital prolapse) by a senior author (B.M.). In keeping with the epidemiology of bladder cancer, twice as many scenarios were developed for male than female patients [54].

The panellists were requested to follow an adapted five-point Likert scale (Table 5) to answer the question: in the following scenario will TURBT result in incomplete resection or prolonged surgery (>1 h) or significant intra or postoperative complications (Clavien-Dindo Grade III and higher)?

Consensus was reached when the 95% confidence interval of the answers strictly showed "unlikely" as the upper bound (concluded as a scenario unlikely to be complex) or "possibly" as the lower bound (concluded as a possibly complex scenario). Otherwise, the answers were considered inconclusive, and the scenario was not considered for further analyses.

4.3.2. Discrimination of Individual Items in the Prediction of Complexity

On univariate analysis, the two-tailed Mann–Whitney U-test tested in the 150 scenarios the relationship between the domains of interest and complexity, dichotomized as "very unlikely or unlikely" or "possibly, likely or very likely".

Logistic regression was conducted, with the domains showing $p < 0.1$ on univariate analyses as predictors and complexity as a dependent variable. The probability of a complex surgery was estimated from the probability function. In keeping with the logistic regression model [55], it acknowledges the contributions of all independent domains (Table 2) by their respective regression coefficients adjusted to the specifics of the case by the median opinions of the panel (e.g., the respective contributions to complexity of a single tumour compared to 4 to10 tumours were 0.96 and 0.96×3, respectively, as shown in Figure 2).

Following the structure of the probability function:

$$probability = \frac{1}{1 + \exp(-x)} \tag{2}$$

where x is the sum of the intercept value of the logistic regression and of the scores of the independent domains multiplied by their regression coefficients, for any domain, the product of its regression coefficient by the score of its descriptor correlates with the probability of a complex surgery. This was used to simplify the function into a checklist (Table 3) where the respective inputs of the items were similarly quantitated by the product of the regression coefficient of their domains by the scores summarizing the median opinions of the panel (e.g., location on the anterior wall of the bladder; median opinion: 3 (Figure 2), regression coefficient of tumour location: 1.44 (Table 2), product: 3×1.44, approximated for ease of use to 4.5).

In any clinical situation, recording the most significant item in patient's history and access to the bladder, in complement to the tumour number, main tumour location and size, calculated the Bladder Complexity Checklist Sum.

ROC curves of the model and of the Bladder Complexity Checklist Sum were compared by the C-statistics. Ultimately, calibration curves illustrated their accuracies in the estimation of the probability of complexity in individual scenarios [56].

STATA/MP was used for statistics (StataCorp, College Station, TX-USA), significance was set at $p < 0.05$.

5. Conclusions

Preoperative factors that relate to complex TURBT were identified by expert judgement and organized into the Bladder Complexity Checklist to facilitate the evaluation of the risk of a complex TURBT, a crucial requisite to personalise patient's information, adapt human and technical resources to individual situations and address TURBT variability in clinical trials.

Supplementary Materials
Figure S1: First-round distribution of the experts' scores regarding the influence of the characteristics of the patient on the likelihood of complex TURBT; Figure S2: First-round distribution of the experts' scores regarding the influence of the characteristics of the tumour on the likelihood of complex TURBT; Figure S3: First-round distribution of the experts' scores regarding the influence on the likelihood of complex TURBT of bladder characteristics and access; Figure S4: First-round distribution of the experts' scores regarding the influence of the surgical environment on the risk of TURBT or En-Bloc resection resulting in either three situations: incomplete resection according to the operator, prolonged surgery (>1 h) or significant intra- (bleeding that requires transfusion, laparotomy) or postoperative complications (Clavien-Dindo Grade III and higher); Table S1: Articles (English language, 4/2009-4/2019) found relevant to the definition of complexity in transurethral resection of bladder tumours; Table S2: 150 scenarios constructed for univariate and multivariate analyses of clinical features in relation to complexity.

Author Contributions: Conceptualization: E.X., M.C., M.B. (Marek Babjuk), J.P.R., F.W., B.M.; methodology M.R., B.M.; investigations: M.R., E.X., A.B., M.B. (Maximillian Burger), H.M., M.C., M.B. (Marek Babjuk), J.P.R., F.W., B.M.; writing—original draft preparation: M.R., B.M.; writing—review and editing: B.M.; supervision: B.M. All authors have read and agreed to the published version of the manuscript.

Acknowledgments: The authors express their gratitude to Doctor Thomas Filleron for critical discussion on the methodology and to Professor Laurent Boccon-Gibod for his comments and review of the manuscript.

References

1. Bray, F.; Ferlay, J.; Soerjomataram, I.; Siegel, R.L.; Torre, L.A.; Jemal, A. Global cancer statistics 2018: GLOBOCAN estimates of incidence and mortality worldwide for 36 cancers in 185 countries. *CA Cancer J. Clin.* **2018**, *68*, 394–424. [CrossRef] [PubMed]
2. Leal, J.; Luengo-Fernandez, R.; Sullivan, R.; Witjes, J.A. Economic Burden of Bladder Cancer Across the European Union. *Eur. Urol.* **2016**, *69*, 438–447. [CrossRef] [PubMed]
3. Babjuk, M.; Burger, M.; Comperat, E.M.; Gontero, P.; Mostafid, A.H.; Palou, J.; van Rhijn, B.W.G.; Roupret, M.; Shariat, S.F.; Sylvester, R.; et al. European Association of Urology Guidelines on Non-muscle-invasive Bladder Cancer (TaT1 and Carcinoma In Situ) - 2019 Update. *Eur. Urol.* **2019**, *76*, 639–657. [CrossRef] [PubMed]
4. Pereira, J.F.; Pareek, G.; Mueller-Leonhard, C.; Zhang, Z.; Amin, A.; Mega, A.; Tucci, C.; Golijanin, D.; Gershman, B. The Perioperative Morbidity of Transurethral Resection of Bladder Tumor: Implications for Quality Improvement. *Urology* **2019**, *125*, 131–137. [CrossRef] [PubMed]
5. Hollenbeck, B.K.; Miller, D.C.; Taub, D.; Dunn, R.L.; Khuri, S.F.; Henderson, W.G.; Montie, J.E.; Underwood, W.; Wei, J.T., 3rd; Wei, J.T. Risk factors for adverse outcomes after transurethral resection of bladder tumors. *Cancer* **2006**, *106*, 1527–1535. [CrossRef]
6. Cumberbatch, M.G.K.; Foerster, B.; Catto, J.W.F.; Kamat, A.M.; Kassouf, W.; Jubber, I.; Shariat, S.F.; Sylvester, R.J.; Gontero, P. Repeat Transurethral Resection in Non-muscle-invasive Bladder Cancer: A Systematic Review. *Eur. Urol.* **2018**, *73*, 925–933. [CrossRef]
7. Mariappan, P.; Finney, S.M.; Head, E.; Somani, B.K.; Zachou, A.; Smith, G.; Mishriki, S.F.; N'Dow, J.; Grigor, K.M.; Edinburgh Urological Cancer G. Good quality white-light transurethral resection of bladder tumours (GQ-WLTURBT) with experienced surgeons performing complete resections and obtaining detrusor muscle reduces early recurrence in new non-muscle-invasive bladder cancer: Validation across time and place and recommendation for benchmarking. *BJU Int.* **2012**, *109*, 1666–1673.
8. Ghali, F.; Moses, R.A.; Raffin, E.; Hyams, E.S. What factors are associated with unplanned return following transurethral resection of bladder tumor? An analysis of a large single institution's experience. *Scand. J. Urol.* **2016**, *50*, 370–373. [CrossRef]

9. Mariappan, P.; Zachou, A.; Grigor, K.M.; Edinburgh Uro-Oncology Group. Detrusor muscle in the first, apparently complete transurethral resection of bladder tumour specimen is a surrogate marker of resection quality, predicts risk of early recurrence, and is dependent on operator experience. *Eur. Urol.* **2010**, *57*, 843–849. [CrossRef]
10. Gan, C.; Patel, A.; Fowler, S.; Catto, J.; Rosario, D.; O'Brien, T. Snapshot of transurethral resection of bladder tumours in the United Kingdom Audit (STUKA). *BJU Int.* **2013**, *112*, 930–935. [CrossRef]
11. Prasad, N.N.; Muddukrishna, S.N. Quality of transurethral resection of bladder tumor procedure influenced a phase III trial comparing the effect of KLH and mitomycin C. *Trials* **2017**, *18*, 123. [CrossRef] [PubMed]
12. Skrzypczyk, M.A.; Nyk, L.; Szostek, P.; Szemplinski, S.; Borowka, A.; Dobruch, J. The role of endoscopic bladder tumour assessment in the management of patients subjected to transurethral bladder tumour resection. *Eur. J. Cancer Care (Engl.)* **2017**, *26*. [CrossRef] [PubMed]
13. Del Rosso, A.; Pace, G.; Masciovecchio, S.; Saldutto, P.; Galatioto, G.P.; Vicentini, C. Plasmakinetic bipolar versus monopolar transurethral resection of non-muscle invasive bladder cancer: A single center randomized controlled trial. *Int. J. Urol.* **2013**, *20*, 399–403. [CrossRef] [PubMed]
14. Pan, D.; Soloway, M.S. The importance of transurethral resection in managing patients with urothelial cancer in the bladder: Proposal for a transurethral resection of bladder tumor checklist. *Eur. Urol.* **2012**, *61*, 1199–1203. [CrossRef]
15. Venkatramani, V.; Panda, A.; Manojkumar, R.; Kekre, N.S. Monopolar versus bipolar transurethral resection of bladder tumors: A single center, parallel arm, randomized, controlled trial. *J. Urol.* **2014**, *191*, 1703–1707. [CrossRef]
16. Wu, Y.P.; Lin, T.T.; Chen, S.H.; Xu, N.; Wei, Y.; Huang, J.B.; Sun, X.L.; Zheng, Q.S.; Xue, X.Y.; Li, X.D. Comparison of the efficacy and feasibility of en bloc transurethral resection of bladder tumor versus conventional transurethral resection of bladder tumor: A meta-analysis. *Medicine (Baltimore)* **2016**, *95*, e5372. [CrossRef]
17. Zhang, K.Y.; Xing, J.C.; Li, W.; Wu, Z.; Chen, B.; Bai, D.Y. A novel transurethral resection technique for superficial bladder tumor: Retrograde en bloc resection. *World J. Surg. Oncol.* **2017**, *15*, 125. [CrossRef]
18. Herkommer, K.; Hofer, C.; Gschwend, J.E.; Kron, M.; Treiber, U. Gender and body mass index as risk factors for bladder perforation during primary transurethral resection of bladder tumors. *J. Urol.* **2012**, *187*, 1566–1570. [CrossRef]
19. Golan, S.; Baniel, J.; Lask, D.; Livne, P.M.; Yossepowitch, O. Transurethral resection of bladder tumour complicated by perforation requiring open surgical repair—Clinical characteristics and oncological outcomes. *BJU Int.* **2011**, *107*, 1065–1068. [CrossRef]
20. Carmignani, L.; Picozzi, S.; Stubinski, R.; Casellato, S.; Bozzini, G.; Lunelli, L.; Arena, D. Endoscopic resection of bladder cancer in patients receiving double platelet antiaggregant therapy. *Surg. Endosc.* **2011**, *25*, 2281–2287. [CrossRef]
21. Zhao, C.; Tang, K.; Yang, H.; Xia, D.; Chen, Z. Bipolar Versus Monopolar Transurethral Resection of Nonmuscle-Invasive Bladder Cancer: A Meta-Analysis. *J. Endourol.* **2016**, *30*, 5–12. [CrossRef] [PubMed]
22. Sugihara, T.; Yasunaga, H.; Horiguchi, H.; Matsui, H.; Nishimatsu, H.; Nakagawa, T.; Fushimi, K.; Kattan, M.W.; Homma, Y. Comparison of perioperative outcomes including severe bladder injury between monopolar and bipolar transurethral resection of bladder tumors: A population based comparison. *J. Urol.* **2014**, *192*, 1355–1359. [CrossRef] [PubMed]
23. Allard, C.B.; Meyer, C.P.; Gandaglia, G.; Chang, S.L.; Chun, F.K.; Gelpi-Hammerschmidt, F.; Hanske, J.; Kibel, A.S.; Preston, M.A.; Trinh, Q.D. The Effect of Resident Involvement on Perioperative Outcomes in Transurethral Urologic Surgeries. *J. Surg. Educ.* **2015**, *72*, 1018–1025. [CrossRef] [PubMed]
24. Patel, H.D.; Ball, M.W.; Cohen, J.E.; Kates, M.; Pierorazio, P.M.; Allaf, M.E. Morbidity of urologic surgical procedures: An analysis of rates, risk factors, and outcomes. *Urology* **2015**, *85*, 552–559. [CrossRef]
25. Avallone, M.A.; Sack, B.S.; El-Arabi, A.; Charles, D.K.; Herre, W.R.; Radtke, A.C.; Davis, C.M.; See, W.A. Ten-Year Review of Perioperative Complications After Transurethral Resection of Bladder Tumors: Analysis of Monopolar and Plasmakinetic Bipolar Cases. *J. Endourol.* **2017**, *31*, 767–773. [CrossRef]
26. Rambachan, A.; Matulewicz, R.S.; Pilecki, M.; Kim, J.Y.; Kundu, S.D. Predictors of readmission following outpatient urological surgery. *J. Urol.* **2014**, *192*, 183–188. [CrossRef]

27. Matulewicz, R.S.; Pilecki, M.; Rambachan, A.; Kim, J.Y.; Kundu, S.D. Impact of resident involvement on urological surgery outcomes: An analysis of 40,000 patients from the ACS NSQIP database. *J. Urol.* **2014**, *192*, 885–890. [CrossRef]
28. Picozzi, S.; Marenghi, C.; Ricci, C.; Bozzini, G.; Casellato, S.; Carmignani, L. Risks and complications of transurethral resection of bladder tumor among patients taking antiplatelet agents for cardiovascular disease. *Surg. Endosc.* **2014**, *28*, 116–121. [CrossRef]
29. De Nunzio, C.; Franco, G.; Cindolo, L.; Autorino, R.; Cicione, A.; Perdona, S.; Falsaperla, M.; Gacci, M.; Leonardo, C.; Damiano, R.; et al. Transuretral resection of the bladder (TURB): Analysis of complications using a modified Clavien system in an Italian real life cohort. *Eur. J. Surg. Oncol.* **2014**, *40*, 90–95. [CrossRef]
30. Valerio, M.; Cerantola, Y.; Fritschi, U.; Hubner, M.; Iglesias, K.; Legris, A.S.; Lucca, I.; Vlamopoulos, Y.; Vaucher, L.; Jichlinski, P. Comorbidity and nutritional indices as predictors of morbidity after transurethral procedures: A prospective cohort study. *Can. Urol. Assoc. J.* **2014**, *8*, E600–E604. [CrossRef]
31. Matulewicz, R.S.; Sharma, V.; McGuire, B.B.; Oberlin, D.T.; Perry, K.T.; Nadler, R.B. The effect of surgical duration of transurethral resection of bladder tumors on postoperative complications: An analysis of ACS NSQIP data. *Urol. Oncol.* **2015**, *33*, e19–e24. [CrossRef] [PubMed]
32. Di Paolo, P.L.; Vargas, H.A.; Karlo, C.A.; Lakhman, Y.; Zheng, J.; Moskowitz, C.S.; Al-Ahmadie, H.A.; Sala, E.; Bochner, B.H.; Hricak, H. Intradiverticular bladder cancer: CT imaging features and their association with clinical outcomes. *Clin. Imaging* **2015**, *39*, 94–98. [CrossRef] [PubMed]
33. Gregg, J.R.; McCormick, B.; Wang, L.; Cohen, P.; Sun, D.; Penson, D.F.; Smith, J.A.; Clark, P.E.; Cookson, M.S.; Barocas, D.A.; et al. Short term complications from transurethral resection of bladder tumor. *Can. J. Urol.* **2016**, *23*, 8198–8203.
34. Cornu, J.N.; Herrmann, T.; Traxer, O.; Matlaga, B. Prevention and Management Following Complications from Endourology Procedures. *Eur. Urol. Focus* **2016**, *2*, 49–59. [CrossRef]
35. Bolat, D.; Gunlusoy, B.; Degirmenci, T.; Ceylan, Y.; Polat, S.; Aydin, E.; Aydogdu, O.; Kozacioglu, Z. Comparing the short-term outcomes and complications of monopolar and bipolar transurethral resection of non-muscle invasive bladder cancers: A prospective, randomized, controlled study. *Arch. Esp. Urol.* **2016**, *69*, 225–233. [CrossRef]
36. Bansal, A.; Sankhwar, S.; Goel, A.; Kumar, M.; Purkait, B.; Aeron, R. Grading of complications of transurethral resection of bladder tumor using Clavien-Dindo classification system. *Indian. J. Urol.* **2016**, *32*, 232–237. [CrossRef] [PubMed]
37. Anderson, C.; Weber, R.; Patel, D.; Lowrance, W.; Mellis, A.; Cookson, M.; Lang, M.; Barocas, D.; Chang, S.; Newberger, E.; et al. A 10-Item Checklist Improves Reporting of Critical Procedural Elements during Transurethral Resection of Bladder Tumor. *J. Urol.* **2016**, *196*, 1014–1020. [CrossRef]
38. Konishi, T.; Washino, S.; Nakamura, Y.; Ohshima, M.; Saito, K.; Arai, Y.; Miyagawa, T. Risks and complications of transurethral resection of bladder tumors in patients receiving antiplatelet and/or anticoagulant therapy: A retrospective cohort study. *BMC Urol.* **2017**, *17*, 118. [CrossRef]
39. Prader, R.; De Broca, B.; Chevallier, D.; Amiel, J.; Durand, M. Outcome of Transurethral Resection of Bladder Tumor: Does Antiplatelet Therapy Really Matter? Analysis of a Retrospective Series. *J. Endourol.* **2017**, *31*, 1284–1288. [CrossRef]
40. Caras, R.J.; Lustik, M.B.; Kern, S.Q.; McMann, L.P.; Sterbis, J.R. Preoperative Albumin Is Predictive of Early Postoperative Morbidity and Mortality in Common Urologic Oncologic Surgeries. *Clin. Genitourin. Cancer* **2017**, *15*, e255–e262. [CrossRef]
41. Naspro, R.; Lerner, L.B.; Rossini, R.; Manica, M.; Woo, H.H.; Calopedos, R.J.; Cracco, C.M.; Scoffone, C.M.; Herrmann, T.R.; de la Rosette, J.J.; et al. Perioperative antithrombotic therapy in patients undergoing endoscopic urologic surgery: Where do we stand with current literature? *Minerva. Urol. Nefrol.* **2018**, *70*, 126–136.
42. Suskind, A.M.; Zhao, S.; Walter, L.C.; Boscardin, W.J.; Finlayson, E. Mortality and Functional Outcomes After Minor Urological Surgery in Nursing Home Residents: A National Study. *J. Am. Geriatr. Soc.* **2018**, *66*, 909–915. [CrossRef]
43. Ficarra, V.; Novara, G.; Secco, S.; Macchi, V.; Porzionato, A.; De Caro, R.; Artibani, W. Preoperative aspects and dimensions used for an anatomical (PADUA) classification of renal tumours in patients who are candidates for nephron-sparing surgery. *Eur. Urol.* **2009**, *56*, 786–793. [CrossRef] [PubMed]

44. Broer, T.; Bal, R.; Pickersgill, M. Problematisations of Complexity: On the Notion and Production of Diverse Complexities in Healthcare Interventions and Evaluations. *Sci. Cult. (Lond.)* **2017**, *26*, 135–160. [CrossRef] [PubMed]
45. Werner, C.; Bedford, T.; Cooke, R.M.; Hanea, A.M.; Morales-Napoles, O. Expert judgement for dependence in probabilistic modelling: A systematic literature review and future research directions. *Eur. J. Operat. Res.* **2017**, *258*, 801–819. [CrossRef]
46. Fernandez, M.I.; Brausi, M.; Clark, P.E.; Cookson, M.S.; Grossman, H.B.; Khochikar, M.; Kiemeney, L.A.; Malavaud, B.; Sanchez-Salas, R.; Soloway, M.S.; et al. Epidemiology, prevention, screening, diagnosis, and evaluation: Update of the ICUD-SIU joint consultation on bladder cancer. *World J. Urol.* **2019**, *37*, 3–13. [CrossRef] [PubMed]
47. Croskerry, P. From mindless to mindful practice—Cognitive bias and clinical decision making. *N. Engl. J. Med.* **2013**, *368*, 2445–2448. [CrossRef]
48. Peard, L.; Goodwin, J.; Hensley, P.; Dugan, A.; Bylund, J.; Harris, A.M. Examining and Understanding Value: The Impact of Preoperative Characteristics, Intraoperative Variables, and Postoperative Complications on Cost of Robot-Assisted Laparoscopic Radical Prostatectomy. *J. Endourol.* **2019**, *33*, 541–548. [CrossRef]
49. Bromwich, D. Plenty to worry about: Consent, control, and anxiety. *Am. J. Bioeth.* **2012**, *12*, 35–36. [CrossRef]
50. Wiseman, O.J.; Wijewardena, M.; Calleary, J.; Masood, J.; Hill, J.T. 'Will you be doing my operation doctor?' Patient attitudes to informed consent. *Ann. R. Coll. Surg. Engl.* **2004**, *86*, 462–464. [CrossRef]
51. Boulkedid, R.; Abdoul, H.; Loustau, M.; Sibony, O.; Alberti, C. Using and reporting the Delphi method for selecting healthcare quality indicators: A systematic review. *PLoS ONE* **2011**, *6*, e20476. [CrossRef] [PubMed]
52. Leeflang, M.M.; Rutjes, A.W.; Reitsma, J.B.; Hooft, L.; Bossuyt, P.M. Variation of a test's sensitivity and specificity with disease prevalence. *CMAJ* **2013**, *185*, E537–E544. [CrossRef] [PubMed]
53. Dalgaard, L.P.; Zare, R.; Gaya, J.M.; Redorta, J.P.; Roumiguie, M.; Filleron, T.; Malavaud, B. Prospective evaluation of the performances of narrow-band imaging flexible videoscopy relative to white-light imaging flexible videoscopy, in patients scheduled for transurethral resection of a primary NMIBC. *World J. Urol.* **2019**, *37*, 1615–1621. [CrossRef] [PubMed]
54. Cumberbatch, M.G.K.; Jubber, I.; Black, P.C.; Esperto, F.; Figueroa, J.D.; Kamat, A.M.; Kiemeney, L.; Lotan, Y.; Pang, K.; Silverman, D.T.; et al. Epidemiology of Bladder Cancer: A Systematic Review and Contemporary Update of Risk Factors in 2018. *Eur. Urol.* **2018**, *74*, 784–795. [CrossRef] [PubMed]
55. Vollmer, R.T. Multivariate statistical analysis for pathologist. Part I, The logistic model. *Am. J. Clin. Pathol.* **1996**, *105*, 115–126. [CrossRef]
56. Steyerberg, E.W.; Vickers, A.J.; Cook, N.R.; Gerds, T.; Gonen, M.; Obuchowski, N.; Pencina, M.J.; Kattan, M.W. Assessing the performance of prediction models: A framework for traditional and novel measures. *Epidemiology* **2010**, *21*, 128–138. [CrossRef]

5

Do Younger Patients with Muscle-Invasive Bladder Cancer have Better Outcomes?

Florian Janisch [1,2], Hang Yu [1], Malte W. Vetterlein [1], Roland Dahlem [1], Oliver Engel [1], Margit Fisch [1], Shahrokh F. Shariat [2,3,4,5,6,7], Armin Soave [1] and Michael Rink [1,*]

1 Department of Urology, Medical University of Hamburg, Martinistraße 52, 20246 Hamburg, Germany; drfjanisch@gmail.com (F.J.); yuhang.seu@outlook.com (H.Y.); malte.vetterlein@googlemail.com (M.W.V.); r.dahlem@uke.de (R.D.); o.engel@uke.de (O.E.); m.fisch@uke.de (M.F.); armin.soave@googlemail.com (A.S.)
2 Department of Urology, Medical University of Vienna, Währinger Gürtel 18-20, 1090 Vienna, Austria; sfshariat@gmail.com
3 Institute for Urology and Reproductive Health, Sechenov University, Bolshaya Pirogovskaya str. 2-4, 119991 Moscow, Russia
4 Department of Urology, Weill Cornell Medical School, 1300 York Avenue, New York, NY 10065, USA
5 Department of Urology, University of Texas Southwestern Medical Center, 5323 Harry Hines Blvd, Dallas, TX 75390, USA
6 Karl Landsteiner Institute of Urology and Andrology, Franziskanergasse 4, a 3100 St. Poelten, Austria
7 Department of Urology, Second Faculty of Medicine, Charles University, Ovocný trh 5, Prague 1-116 36, Czech Republic
* Correspondence: m.rink@uke.de

Abstract: Urothelial cancer of the bladder (UCB) is usually a disease of the elderly. The influence of age on oncological outcomes remains controversial. This study aims to investigate the impact of age on UCB outcomes in Europe focusing particularly on young and very young patients. We collected data of 669 UCB patients treated with RC at our tertiary care center. We used various categorical stratifications as well as continuous age to investigate the association of age and tumor biology as well as endpoints with descriptive statistics and Cox regression. The median age was 67 years and the mean follow-up was 52 months. Eight patients (1.2%) were ≤40 years old and 39 patients (5.8%) were aged 41–50 years, respectively. In multivariable analysis, higher continuous age and age above the median were independent predictors for disease recurrence, and cancer-specific and overall mortality (all p-values ≤ 0.018). In addition, patients with age in the oldest tertile group had inferior cancer-specific and overall survival rates compared to their younger counterparts. Young (40–50 years) and very young (≤40 years) patients had reduced hazards for all endpoints, which, however, were not statistically significant. Age remains an independent determinant for survival after RC. Young adults did, however, not have superior outcomes in our analyses. Quality of life and complications are endpoints that need further evaluation in patients undergoing RC.

Keywords: bladder cancer; age; urothelial carcinoma; radical cystectomy; outcome; survival

---

1. Introduction

With an incidence of over 80,000 new cases and over 17,000 deaths estimated to occur in 2019 in the United States alone, urothelial cancer of the bladder (UCB) is the second leading genitourinary malignancy and a potentially lethal disease [1]. Compared with other malignancies, UCB is usually a disease of the elderly with a peak incidence among those in their 70s [2,3]. In fact, in general there is an increasing life expectancy in the US and Europe and in consequence, a potential further rise in UCB diagnoses is expected in the next few decades [4,5]. Ageing trends are of major scientific and clinical importance in any cancer including UCB, as the optimal management has great impact for each individuum and the public health system in general, especially in an expensive disease as UCB [6].

Despite the overwhelming incidence in elderly patients, UCB does also occur in a non-negligible number of young patients [3]. While the development of UCB in the elderly has been suggested to be driven by a cumulative lifetime exposure to environmentally, occupationally, or individually acquired carcinogens (e.g., smoking) [7–9], the factors for UCB in young patients remain rather inconclusive. Not only the diagnosis of UCB, particularly the need of RC with all its negative effects on quality of life has a significant impact on the psyche and more, especially in the younger. RC is more frequently offered in younger patients, due to their longer life expectancy, lower frailty resulting in lower adverse events and the superiority in survival outcomes of early compared to delayed RC [10]. Recent reports suggest superior UCB-specific outcomes in young and adolescent patients (15–39 years) [11].

The impact of patient age on oncological outcomes remains controversial and regional variabilities may be present that need to be considered in patient counselling and treatment planning. The aim of this study was to evaluate the impact of age on UCB outcomes after RC in a consecutive cohort of European patients, particularly focusing on the young and very young. We hypothesized that younger patients may have better oncologic outcomes as their disease may be earlier in their natural history and different as it may not have a large mutational burden.

2. Material and Methods

2.1. Patient Population

We retrospectively reviewed the medical records of 789 consecutive patients treated with RC and bilateral pelvic lymphadenectomy for UCB between 1996 and 2011 at our institution. Guideline adherent indications for RC were muscle invasive UCB or recurrent Ta, T1, or carcinoma in situ (CIS) refractory to transurethral resection of the bladder (TURB) with or without intravesical chemo- or immunotherapy. As neoadjuvant chemotherapy may be more frequently administered in younger patients, implementing an inherent bias of natural UCB history in age analyses, these patients were excluded upfront ($n = 8$). Moreover, 75 patients were excluded because of missing variables or follow-up, 30 patients with RC for non-malignant indication for RC, and seven patients with advanced, bladder infiltrating prostate cancer. In total, 669 patients remained for analyses. Overall, 147 patients (20.0%) received adjuvant chemotherapy (95% platinum-based) at the clinicians' discretion in accordance with the guidelines at the time. The study was approved by the local ethics committee.

2.2. Follow-Up Regimen

Follow-up strategy has been previously reported in detail [12,13]. In brief, patients were generally seen every three to four months for the first year after surgery, every six months from the second to fifth year, and annually thereafter. Follow-up included a history, physical examination and serum chemistry evaluation. Diagnostic imaging of the abdomen including the urinary tract and chest radiography were performed at least annually or when clinically indicated. Additional radiographic evaluations were performed when clinically indicated.

2.3. Statistical Analysis

Statistical analyses included demographic data on patients' age, ethnicity, gender, ASA status, pathologic tumor stage and grade, concomitant CIS, lymph node status, margin status, lymphovascular invasion, and adjuvant chemotherapy, respectively.

The co-primary endpoints were recurrence-free survival (RFS), cancer-specific survival (CSS), and overall survival (OS), respectively. Disease recurrence was defined as local failure in the operative site, regional lymph nodes, or distant metastasis. Upper tract urothelial carcinoma was considered a metachronous tumor and not disease recurrence. Patients who did not experience disease recurrence were censored at time of last follow-up for recurrence-free survival analysis. Cancer-specific mortality was defined as death from UCB. The cause of death was determined by the treating physician, by chart review corroborated by death certificates, or by death certificates alone [14]. Perioperative mortality (i.e., death within 30 days of surgery) was censored at time of death for UCB-specific survival analyses.

Age was analyzed as a continuous variable, with a cut-off at median and tertiles, and using the cut-offs of 50 years. (dichotomized) and ≤40, 41–50, and >50 years (three categories), respectively. The different analytic approaches were used to optimally approach the definition of young age. There is no clear determination for UCB patients treated with RC in the urologic literature defining a patient as 'young' or 'very young'. However, there is a consensus among oncological experts that patients <50 years. are usually defined as 'young' and patients <40 years. defined as 'very young' [15]. Using median and tertiles as cut-off, we investigated the effects of age in our study population with homogenous sample distributions. Utilization of the dichotomized cut-off of 50 years. was based on previous reports that indicated superior survival outcomes in patients <50 years. The tri-categorical analyses uses cut-offs of <40 years and <50 years following predefined ranges indicated by the NCI in 2006 [15]. In addition, study results indicate significant outcome differences, suggesting these strata represent an ideal standard [11].

The Kolmogorov–Smirnov test was used to assess the normal distribution of variables. The Fisher's exact test and the chi-square test were used to evaluate the association between categorical variables. Differences in variables with a continuous distribution across categories were assessed using the Mann–Whitney U test (two categories) and Kruskal–Wallis test (three and more categories). Actuarial method was used to estimate RFS, CSS, and OS probabilities and the differences were assessed with the log rank test. Kaplan–Meier estimates were used to graphically display survival functions. Univariable and multivariable Cox regression models addressed time-to-event endpoint analyses. In all models, proportional hazards assumptions were systematically verified using the Grambsch–Therneau residual-based test. Multicollinearity was assessed with the variance inflation factor to test for possible confounding between relevant covariates. All reported *p*-values were two-sided, and statistical significance was set at $p < 0.05$. All statistical tests were performed with IBM SPSS Statistics 25 (IBM Corp., Armonk, NY, USA).

3. Results

3.1. *Association of Age with Clinical–Pathological Characteristics*

The median age of the study cohort was 67 years (interquartile range [IQR]: 59; 73), and 520 (78%) of the patients were male. In total, 622 patients (93.0%) were older than 50 years. Of those being <50 years, 39 patients (5.8%) were aged 41–50 years and 8 patients (1.2%) were younger than 40 years. Tertiles for age were ≤59 years (first tertile), 60–72 years (second tertile), and ≥73 years (third tertile), respectively. The descriptive clinicopathologic characteristics of the study cohort are presented in Table 1.

Table 1. Descriptive characteristics stratified by dichotomy age groups of 669 UCB patients treated with radical cystectomy

	All	Young (≤50)		Elderly (≥51)	*p*-Value	*p*-Value
		≤40	41–50	≥51	≤50 vs. ≥51	≤40 vs. 41–50 vs. ≥51
Patients, *n*	669	8	39	622	-	-
Gender (%)					0.85	0.98
Male	520 (77.7)	6 (75.0)	30 (76.9)	484 (77.8)		
Female	149 (22.3)	2 (25.0)	9 (23.1)	138 (22.2)		
ASA (%)					<0.001	<0.001
1	52 (7.8)	4 (50.0)	7 (18.0)	41 (6.6)		
2	386 (57.7)	3 (37.5)	27 (69.2)	356 (57.2)		
3	225 (33.6)	1 (12.5)	3 (7.7)	221 (35.5)		
4	6 (0.9)	0 (0)	2 (5.1)	4 (0.7)		
Pathological Tumor Stage (%)					0.92	0.34
pT0	73 (10.9)	3 (37.5)	4 (10.3)	66 (10.6)		

Table 1. *Cont.*

	All	Young (≤50)		Elderly (≥51)	*p*-Value	*p*-Value
		≤40	41–50	≥51	≤50 vs. ≥51	≤40 vs. 41–50 vs. ≥51
pTa	26 (3.9)	0 (0)	1 (2.6)	25 (4.0)		
pTis	66 (9.9)	0 (0)	3 (7.7)	63 (10.1)		
pT1	74 (11.1)	1 (12.5)	4 (10.3)	69 (11.1)		
pT2	132 (19.7)	0 (0)	10 (25.6)	122 (19.6)		
pT3	182 (27.2)	4 (50.0)	8 (20.5)	170 (27.3)		
pT4	116 (17.3)	0 (0)	9 (23.1)	107 (17.2)		
Pathological Tumor Grade (%)					0.58	0.42
No grading (pT0)	73 (10.9)	3 (37.5)	4 (10.3)	66 (10.6)		
G2	65 (9.7)	1 (12.5)	6 (15.4)	58 (9.3)		
G3	531 (79.4)	4 (50.0)	29 (74.3)	498 (80.1)		
Concomitant carcinoma in situ (%)					0.051	0.12
Absent	424 (63.4)	7 (87.5)	29 (74.4)	388 (62.4)		
Present	245 (36.6)	1 (12.5)	10 (25.6)	234 (37.6)		
Lymph node status (%)					0.91	0.58
pN0	479 (71.6)	7 (87.5)	27 (69.2)	445 (71.5)		
pN+	190 (28.4)	1 (12.5)	12 (30.8)	177 (28.5)		
Margin status (%)					0.94	0.99
R0	586 (87.6)	7 (87.5)	34 (87.2)	545 (87.6)		
R+	83 (12.4)	1 (12.5)	5 (12.8)	77 (12.4)		
Lymphovascular invasion (%)					0.52	0.62
L0	455 (68.0)	6 (75)	24 (61.5)	425 (68.3)		
L1	214 (32.0)	2 (25)	15 (38.5)	197 (31.7)		
Adjuvant Chemotherapy (%)					0.089	0.21
No	522 (78.0)	6 (75.0)	26 (66.7)	490 (78.8)		
Yes	147 (22.0)	2 (25.0)	13 (33.3)	132 (21.2)		

Comparing patients under and over 50, older patients presented with a significantly higher ASA score ($p < 0.001$). ASA scores increased significantly from patients ≤40 years to patients aged 41–50 and to ≥50 years ($p < 0.001$). There were no statistically significant differences in any other clinical–pathological variables irrespective of the stratification used.

3.2. Association of Age with Disease Recurrence and Survival Outcomes

The median follow-up was 52 months (IQR: 17; 78). During the follow-up period, 192 patients (32.4%) experienced disease recurrence, 175 patients (28.0%) died of UCB, and 257 patients (42.1%) died of any cause. The actuarial recurrence-free survival estimates at 2- and 5-years after RC were 64 ± 2% and 59 ± 2%, respectively. The actuarial cancer-specific survival estimates at 2- and 5-years after RC were 71 ± 2% and 61 ± 3%, respectively. The actuarial overall-specific survival estimates at 2- and 5-years after RC were 62 ± 2% and 50 ± 2%, respectively.

In the Kaplan–Meier analyses, no statistically significant difference was observed in recurrence-free survival ($p = 0.49$; Figure 1A), cancer-specific survival ($p = 0.78$; Figure 1C), and overall survival ($p = 0.67$; Figure 1E) between patients younger than 50 years, and those 50 and above. In categorical age group analyses, there was also no statistically significant difference in recurrence-free survival, cancer-specific survival and overall survival ($p > 0.05$ for all; Figure 1B,D,F) between patients 50 years and above, those between 41–50 years and those 40 and younger.

3.3. Risk Factor Analyses for Disease Recurrence and Survival Outcomes

All variables tested on multicollinearity had an VIF in the range of 1.1–2.9, indicating that no multicollinearity is present between factors included in the cox regression model. The results of univariable Cox regression analyses for different age stratifications are presented in Table 2. Higher continuous age was significantly associated with inferior recurrence-free (Hazard ratio (HR): 1.017; 95%CI: 1.002–1.032; $p = 0.029$), cancer-specific (HR: 1.023; 95%CI: 1.007–1.039; $p = 0.005$), and overall survival (HR: 1.030; 95%CI: 1.016–1.044; $p < 0.001$). In addition, patients older than the median (all $p \leq 0.01$) and patients in the highest age tertile compared to patients in the second tertile (all $p \leq 0.008$) were significantly associated with inferior outcomes for all three endpoints. Analyses according to all age categories (i.e., ≤50 vs >50; ≤40 vs. 41–50 vs. >50, tertiles) revealed that patients in higher age categories were not associated with a higher risk for all endpoints (all $p > 0.05$).

The results of multivariable Cox regression analyses that adjusted for standard UCB clinic-pathological parameters (Table 3) showed that higher continuous age (RFS HR: 1.019; $p = 0.018$; CSS HR: 1.025; $p = 0.004$, and OS HR: 1.030; $p < 0.001$), age above the median of our cohort (RFS HR: 1.472; $p = 0.014$; CSS HR: 1.553; $p = 0.008$; and OS HR: 1.596; $p = 0.001$) and age in the third tertile (≥73 years) compared to the second age tertile (60–72 years) (RFS HR: 1.862; $p = 0.005$; CSS HR: 2.085; $p = 0.001$; OS HR: 2.256; $p < 0.001$) were all independently associated with worse outcomes for all three endpoints. In addition, CSS and OS of patients in the third tertile were also inferior compared to the outcomes of patients in the first age tertile (≤59 years) (CSS HR: 1.545; $p \leq 0.034$; OS HR 1.728; $p = 0.002$).

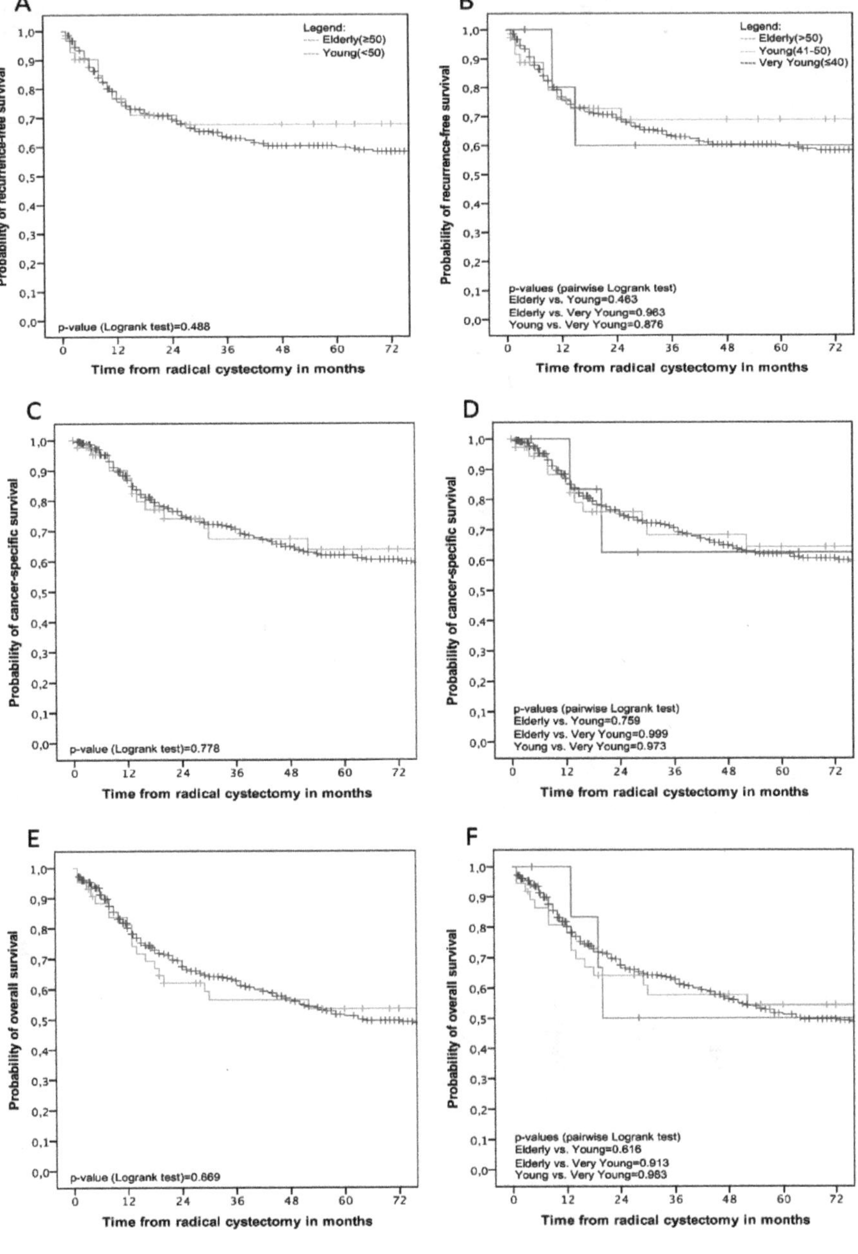

Figure 1. Kaplan–Meier estimates of stratified age groups of elderly (≥50 years.) and young patients (<50 years.) (**A,C,E**), and stratified in three age groups of elderly (>50 years.) young (41–50 years.) and very young (≤40 years.) patients (**B,D,F**) for recurrence-free, cancer-specific, and overall survival, respectively.

Table 2. Univariable cox regression analysis of variable age stratifications predicting recurrence-free survival, cancer-specific survival and overall survival of 669 patients with UCB treated with radical cystectomy

Age Stratifications	RFS			CSS			OS		
	HR	95%CI	*p*-Value	HR	95%CI	*p*-Value	HR	95%CI	*p*-Value
Continuous age	1.017	1.002–1.032	0.029	1.023	1.007–1.039	0.005	1.030	1.016–1.044	<0.001
Median Age	1.454	1.095–1.932	0.010	1.550	1.150–2.088	0.004	1.663	1.299–2.129	<0.001
Age ≤50 vs. >50	1.227	0.684–2.202	0.49	1.084	0.616–1.909	0.78	1.107	0.693–1.767	0.67
Age (three categories)									
≤40 vs. >50	0.818	0.179–3.733	0.80	0.910	0.202–4.111	0.90	0.832	0.242–2.858	0.77
41–50 vs. >50	1.035	0.257–4.170	0.96	1.001	0.248–4.038	0.99	0.946	0.303–2.955	0.92
Age (Tertiles)									
first vs. third tertile	1.242	0.861–1.793	0.25	1.364	0.926–2.008	0.12	1.576	1.137–2.185	0.006
second vs. third tertile	1.699	1.151–2.507	0.008	1.931	1.278–2.917	0.002	2.194	1.546–3.112	<0.001

Abbreviations: RFS = recurrence free survival; CSS = cancer specific survival; OS = overall survival; HR = hazard ratio; CI = confidence interval; UCB = urothelial carcinoma of the bladder.

Table 3. Multivariable cox regression analysis of the effect of age on predicting recurrence-free survival, cancer-specific survival and overall survival of 669 patients with UCB and treated with radical cystectomy

Age Stratifications	RFS			CSS			OS		
	HR	95%CI	*p*-Value	HR	95%CI	*p*-Value	HR	95%CI	*p*-Value
Continuous Age	1.019	1.003–1.035	0.018	1.025	1.008–1.042	0.004	1.030	1.016–1.045	0.000
Median age	1.472	1.081–2.005	0.014	1.553	1.124–2.146	0.008	1.596	1.225–2.080	0.001
Age (Tertiles)									
first vs. third tertile	1.339	0.914–1.962	0.13	1.545	1.033–2.312	0.034	1.728	1.230–2.428	0.002
second vs. third tertile	1.862	1.211–2.864	0.005	2.085	1.328–3.276	0.001	2.256	1.541–3.304	<0.001

All multivariable analyses were adjusted for the following co-variables: gender, ASA score, pathological tumor stage, pathological tumor grade, concomitant carcinoma in situ, lymph node status, margin status, lymphovascular invasion, and adjuvant chemotherapy. Abbreviations: RFS = recurrence free survival; CSS = cancer specific survival; OS = overall survival; HR = hazard ratio; CI = confidence interval; UCB = urothelial carcinoma of the bladder.

4. Discussion

We found that young patients did not present with more favorable tumor biological features compared to their older counterparts. In addition, we did not find significantly superior survival outcomes for all three endpoints in favor of young patients. Therefore, we reject our hypothesis that young UCB patients with MIBC have better outcomes post-RC than the normal MIBC patient. This is in contrast to previous studies that reported better oncological outcomes in younger UCB populations [11,16,17]. Differences in results between our study and previous reports may be explained by different definition of young age, diverse race/ethnicity or distinct socioeconomic status, etc. [18]. Indeed, we found that higher continuous age and other strata defining patients as elderly were independently associated with inferior survival outcomes. Thus, while one end of the age spectrum does not better, the other end of the spectrum seems to have worse oncologic outcomes. Undeniably, this underscores the validity of our UCB cohort as these findings are in line with those of large, multicentric UCB series [19,20].

The relationship between age and prognosis of UCB remains controversial. In fact, there is no clear definition when a UCB patient is defined to be very young, young, old, or very old. A recent large US study reported that adolescents and young UCB patients (ages 15–39) [11] had superior cancer-specific and overall survival compared to their older counterparts. In another study, patients were stratified using a cut-off of 50 years with superior cancer-specific and overall survival in the younger group [16]. In our study we, therefore, used variable age stratifications and cut-offs to reflect the most comprehensive picture on the impact of age across a wide spectrum of definitions and results. Indeed, using this comprehensive approach, we only found differences in categorized outcome analyses when using the median age or age tertiles of our cohort. Of importance, the median age in our cohort was 67 years and the upper age tertile included patients above 73 years. Thus, despite depicting a statistical significance compared to 'younger patients' in our cohort, our data did not demonstrate superior outcomes in those patients usually defined to be young or very young.

From the biological rationale it intuitively seems reasonable that older patients may experience inferior outcomes. With increasing age, exposure to several environmental, occupational, and individually amenable (e.g., smoking) stressors accumulate over time [7,21,22]. In addition, especially elderly men often experience obstructive lower urinary tract symptoms with incomplete bladder drainage. In consequence, the potentially prolonged contact time to carcinogens excreted in the urine may induce accumulation of cellular events that can lead to neoplastic transformation and subsequently UCB development [20]. Moreover, younger patients tend to be healthier in general, with mostly good immunity and nutrition status, as well as fewer co-morbidities to tolerate the complications of cancers or treatment.

From a clinical perspective, our results are important, as recent studies found very young UCB patients to have a lower hazard of cancer-specific mortality compared to their older counterparts [11], suggesting that organ-sparing approaches may be a viable option in young patients [23–25]. Especially the prospect of incontinence, impotence and/or infertility due to radical cystectomy may lead to delay of therapy or a switch of strategy to a bladder sparing, multimodal approach. However, younger patients are more reluctant to undergo necessary diagnostics and treatments or comply with strict follow-up schedules, possibly affecting outcomes [26]. In agreement with our results, other investigators also found either no difference [27] or even worse outcomes, due to a higher rate of metastases [28], in patients ≤40 years. A potential reason for the disparity in findings of various studies including ours may be due to difference in ethnicities, regional varieties in treatment, different socioeconomic backgrounds, and other factors that we could not all adjust for in our analyses. However, despite our findings not providing a final answer on the influence of a very young age on UCB outcomes treated with RC, our results do generate hypotheses that warrant further investigation of this association in larger, multi-institutional, ideally prospective studies. Indeed, our findings support the surgical approach of radical cystectomy also in young and very-young patients, as our findings underscore the aggressive nature of UCB and no age-group had superior survival outcomes.

Certainly, the reconstruction which affects quality of life and perceived self-image should be adopted to patients' preferences, and general and specific health factors [29].

Our study is not devoid of limitations. First and foremost, the retrospective and single-center nature may inevitably introduce some selection bias. Despite this being a large monocentric cohort of consecutive patients, the overall sample size is still limited, especially in the subgroup of very young patients. Nevertheless, we feel that our study still provides a representative insight on age-dependent prognostic outcomes for Europe. All patients in our study were Caucasians, which should be considered since ethnicity may influence survival in UCB [30,31]. We were unable to collect and adjust analyses for several predisposing risk factors of UCB, including smoking, occupational exposure, family history, insurance status, immunity or nutrition status, adjuvant therapies, or socio-economic factors that also may influence tumor biology or outcomes [22,32,33]. In addition, laboratory and molecular data was not available. However, from the clinical perspective, the latter information is usually not available in daily routine for patient counselling. Age in general does represent a competing risk for death particularly since older patients have a greater frailty and UCB patients often harbor important comorbidities [34–36]. However, due to sample size limitations, we were unable to perform competing-risk analyses. Consequently, a contemporary, European multicenter approach would be warranted to shed further insight on this relevant topic.

5. Conclusions

In conclusion, we found that young age at time of MIBC diagnosis does not result in better outcomes compared to typical age after RC. Higher age, however, remains an important prognostic factor for cancer-related endpoints in UCB and thus needs to be incorporated in therapeutic considerations. Radical cystectomy remains standard treatment for patients with muscle-invasive bladder cancer independent of age. Further studies to assess the differential effect of RC and the different types of urinary diversion on the health-related quality of life and metabolic consequences across age are necessary.

Author Contributions: Conceptualization, F.J. and M.R.; Data curation, M.R. and M.W.V.; Formal analysis, M.R. and H.Y.; Funding acquisition, M.R.; Investigation, F.J., H.Y. and M.R.; Methodology, M.R.; Project administration, A.S.; Resources, R.D.; Supervision, M.R. and M.F.; Validation, F.J., M.W.V. and O.E.; Visualization, A.S.; Writing—original draft, F.J., H.Y. and M.R.; Writing—review & editing, F.J., M.W.V., A.S., O.E., S.F.S., M.F. and M.R.

Acknowledgments: Hang Yu is supported by the China Scholarship Council.

References

1. Siegel, R.L.; Miller, K.D.; Jemal, A. Cancer statistics, 2019. *CA Cancer J. Clin.* **2019**, *69*, 7–34. [CrossRef] [PubMed]
2. Guancial, E.A.; Roussel, B.; Bergsma, D.P.; Bylund, K.C.; Sahasrabudhe, D.; Messing, E.; Mohile, S.G.; Fung, C. Bladder cancer in the elderly patient: Challenges and solutions. *Clin. Interv. Aging* **2015**, *10*, 939–949. [CrossRef] [PubMed]
3. Shariat, S.F.; Milowsky, M.; Droller, M.J. Bladder cancer in the elderly. *Urol. Oncol.* **2009**, *27*, 653–667. [CrossRef] [PubMed]
4. Organization, W.H. *World Health Statistics 2018: Monitoring Health for the SDGs*; WHO: Geneva, Switzerland, 2018.
5. Abdollah, F.; Gandaglia, G.; Thuret, R.; Schmitges, J.; Tian, Z.; Jeldres, C.; Passoni, N.M.; Briganti, A.; Shariat, S.F.; Perrotte, P.; et al. Incidence, survival and mortality rates of stage-specific bladder cancer in United States: A trend analysis. *Cancer Epidemiol.* **2013**, *37*, 219–225. [CrossRef] [PubMed]
6. Leal, J.; Luengo-Fernandez, R.; Sullivan, R.; Witjes, J.A. Economic Burden of Bladder Cancer Across the European Union. *Eur. Urol.* **2016**, *69*, 438–447. [CrossRef] [PubMed]
7. Rink, M.; Crivelli, J.J.; Shariat, S.F.; Chun, F.K.; Messing, E.M.; Soloway, M.S. Smoking and Bladder Cancer: A Systematic Review of Risk and Outcomes. *Eur. Urol. Focus* **2015**, *1*, 17–27. [CrossRef]

8. Rink, M.; Furberg, H.; Zabor, E.C.; Xylinas, E.; Babjuk, M.; Pycha, A.; Lotan, Y.; Karakiewicz, P.I.; Novara, G.; Robinson, B.D.; et al. Impact of smoking and smoking cessation on oncologic outcomes in primary non-muscle-invasive bladder cancer. *Eur. Urol.* **2013**, *63*, 724–732. [CrossRef]
9. Rink, M.; Zabor, E.C.; Furberg, H.; Xylinas, E.; Ehdaie, B.; Novara, G.; Babjuk, M.; Pycha, A.; Lotan, Y.; Trinh, Q.D.; et al. Impact of smoking and smoking cessation on outcomes in bladder cancer patients treated with radical cystectomy. *Eur. Urol.* **2013**, *64*, 456–464. [CrossRef]
10. Denzinger, S.; Fritsche, H.M.; Otto, W.; Blana, A.; Wieland, W.F.; Burger, M. Early versus deferred cystectomy for initial high-risk pT1G3 urothelial carcinoma of the bladder: Do risk factors define feasibility of bladder-sparing approach? *Eur. Urol.* **2008**, *53*, 146–152. [CrossRef]
11. Lara, J.; Brunson, A.; Keegan, T.H.; Malogolowkin, M.; Pan, C.-X.; Yap, S.; deVere White, R. Determinants of survival for adolescents and young adults with urothelial bladder cancer: Results from the California Cancer Registry. *J. Urol.* **2016**, *196*, 1378–1382. [CrossRef]
12. Soave, A.; Dahlem, R.; Hansen, J.; Weisbach, L.; Minner, S.; Engel, O.; Kluth, L.A.; Chun, F.K.; Shariat, S.F.; Fisch, M.; et al. Gender-specific outcomes of bladder cancer patients: A stage-specific analysis in a contemporary, homogenous radical cystectomy cohort. *Eur. J. Surg. Oncol.* **2015**, *41*, 368–377. [CrossRef] [PubMed]
13. Soave, A.; Schmidt, S.; Dahlem, R.; Minner, S.; Engel, O.; Kluth, L.A.; John, L.M.; Hansen, J.; Schmid, M.; Sauter, G.; et al. Does the extent of variant histology affect oncological outcomes in patients with urothelial carcinoma of the bladder treated with radical cystectomy? *Urol. Oncol.* **2015**, *33*, 21.e21–21.e29. [CrossRef] [PubMed]
14. Rink, M.; Fajkovic, H.; Cha, E.K.; Gupta, A.; Karakiewicz, P.I.; Chun, F.K.; Lotan, Y.; Shariat, S.F. Death certificates are valid for the determination of cause of death in patients with upper and lower tract urothelial carcinoma. *Eur. Urol.* **2012**, *61*, 854–855. [CrossRef] [PubMed]
15. Institute, N.C. *Closing the Gap: Research and Care Imperatives for Adolescents and Young Adults with Cancer*; Institute, N.C.: Bethesda, MD, USA, 2006.
16. Feng, H.; Zhang, W.; Li, J.; Lu, X. Different patterns in the prognostic value of age for bladder cancer-specific survival depending on tumor stages. *Am. J. Cancer Res.* **2015**, *5*, 2090. [PubMed]
17. Nayak, J.G.; Gore, J.L.; Holt, S.K.; Wright, J.L.; Mossanen, M.; Dash, A. Patient-centered risk stratification of disposition outcomes following radical cystectomy. *Urol. Oncol. Semin. Orig. Investig.* **2016**, *34*, 235.e217–235.e223. [CrossRef] [PubMed]
18. Isbarn, H.; Jeldres, C.; Zini, L.; Perrotte, P.; Baillargeon-Gagne, S.; Capitanio, U.; Shariat, S.F.; Arjane, P.; Saad, F.; McCormack, M.; et al. A population based assessment of perioperative mortality after cystectomy for bladder cancer. *J. Urol.* **2009**, *182*, 70–77. [CrossRef] [PubMed]
19. Chromecki, T.F.; Mauermann, J.; Cha, E.K.; Svatek, R.S.; Fajkovic, H.; Karakiewicz, P.I.; Lotan, Y.; Tilki, D.; Bastian, P.J.; Volkmer, B.G.; et al. Multicenter validation of the prognostic value of patient age in patients treated with radical cystectomy. *World J. Urol.* **2012**, *30*, 753–759. [CrossRef] [PubMed]
20. Shariat, S.F.; Sfakianos, J.P.; Droller, M.J.; Karakiewicz, P.I.; Meryn, S.; Bochner, B.H. The effect of age and gender on bladder cancer: A critical review of the literature. *BJU Int.* **2010**, *105*, 300–308. [CrossRef] [PubMed]
21. Noon, A.P.; Martinsen, J.I.; Catto, J.W.F.; Pukkala, E. Occupation and Bladder Cancer Phenotype: Identification of Workplace Patterns That Increase the Risk of Advanced Disease Beyond Overall Incidence. *Eur. Urol. Focus* **2018**, *4*, 725–730. [CrossRef] [PubMed]
22. Crivelli, J.J.; Xylinas, E.; Kluth, L.A.; Rieken, M.; Rink, M.; Shariat, S.F. Effect of smoking on outcomes of urothelial carcinoma: A systematic review of the literature. *Eur. Urol.* **2014**, *65*, 742–754. [CrossRef]
23. Mathieu, R.; Lucca, I.; Klatte, T.; Babjuk, M.; Shariat, S.F. Trimodal therapy for invasive bladder cancer: Is it really equal to radical cystectomy? *Curr. Opin. Urol.* **2015**, *25*, 476–482. [CrossRef] [PubMed]
24. Ploussard, G.; Daneshmand, S.; Efstathiou, J.A.; Herr, H.W.; James, N.D.; Rodel, C.M.; Shariat, S.F.; Shipley, W.U.; Sternberg, C.N.; Thalmann, G.N.; et al. Critical Analysis of Bladder Sparing with Trimodal Therapy in Muscle-invasive Bladder Cancer: A Systematic Review. *Eur. Urol.* **2014**, *66*, 120–137. [CrossRef] [PubMed]
25. Knoedler, J.; Frank, I. Organ-sparing surgery in urology: Partial cystectomy. *Curr. Opin. Urol.* **2015**, *25*, 111–115. [CrossRef] [PubMed]

26. Katafigiotis, I.; Sfoungaristos, S.; Martini, A.; Stravodimos, K.; Anastasiou, I.; Mykoniatis, I.; Duvdevani, M.; Constantinides, C. Bladder Cancer to Patients Younger than 30 Years: A Retrospective Study and Review of the Literature. *Urol. J.* **2017**, *84*, 231–235. [CrossRef] [PubMed]
27. Telli, O.; Sarici, H.; Ozgur, B.C.; Doluoglu, O.G.; Sunay, M.M.; Bozkurt, S.; Eroglu, M. Urothelial cancer of bladder in young versus older adults: Clinical and pathological characteristics and outcomes. *Kaohsiung J. Med. Sci.* **2014**, *30*, 466–470. [CrossRef] [PubMed]
28. Yossepowitch, O.; Dalbagni, G. Transitional cell carcinoma of the bladder in young adults: Presentation, natural history and outcome. *J. Urol.* **2002**, *168*, 61–66. [CrossRef]
29. Lee, R.K.; Abol-Enein, H.; Artibani, W.; Bochner, B.; Dalbagni, G.; Daneshmand, S.; Fradet, Y.; Hautmann, R.E.; Lee, C.T.; Lerner, S.P.; et al. Urinary diversion after radical cystectomy for bladder cancer: Options, patient selection, and outcomes. *BJU Int.* **2014**, *113*, 11–23. [CrossRef] [PubMed]
30. Sung, J.M.; Martin, J.W.; Jefferson, F.A.; Sidhom, D.A.; Piranviseh, K.; Huang, M.; Nguyen, N.; Chang, J.; Ziogas, A.; Anton-Culver, H.; et al. Racial and Socioeconomic Disparities in Bladder Cancer Survival: Analysis of the California Cancer Registry. *Clin. Genitourin. Cancer* **2019**. [CrossRef]
31. Gild, P.; Wankowicz, S.A.; Sood, A.; von Landenberg, N.; Friedlander, D.F.; Alanee, S.; Chun, F.K.H.; Fisch, M.; Menon, M.; Trinh, Q.D.; et al. Racial disparity in quality of care and overall survival among black vs. white patients with muscle-invasive bladder cancer treated with radical cystectomy: A national cancer database analysis. *Urol. Oncol.* **2018**, *36*, 469.e1–469.e11. [CrossRef]
32. Dobruch, J.; Daneshmand, S.; Fisch, M.; Lotan, Y.; Noon, A.P.; Resnick, M.J.; Shariat, S.F.; Zlotta, A.R.; Boorjian, S.A. Gender and Bladder Cancer: A Collaborative Review of Etiology, Biology, and Outcomes. *Eur. Urol.* **2016**, *69*, 300–310. [CrossRef]
33. Svatek, R.S.; Shariat, S.F.; Lasky, R.E.; Skinner, E.C.; Novara, G.; Lerner, S.P.; Fradet, Y.; Bastian, P.J.; Kassouf, W.; Karakiewicz, P.I.; et al. The effectiveness of off-protocol adjuvant chemotherapy for patients with urothelial carcinoma of the urinary bladder. *Clin. Cancer Res.* **2010**, *16*, 4461–4467. [CrossRef] [PubMed]
34. Goossens-Laan, C.A.; Leliveld, A.M.; Verhoeven, R.H.; Kil, P.J.; de Bock, G.H.; Hulshof, M.C.; de Jong, I.J.; Coebergh, J.W. Effects of age and comorbidity on treatment and survival of patients with muscle-invasive bladder cancer. *Int. J. Cancer* **2014**, *135*, 905–912. [CrossRef] [PubMed]
35. Megwalu, I.I.; Vlahiotis, A.; Radwan, M.; Piccirillo, J.F.; Kibel, A.S. Prognostic impact of comorbidity in patients with bladder cancer. *Eur. Urol.* **2008**, *53*, 581–589. [CrossRef] [PubMed]
36. Fairey, A.S.; Jacobsen, N.E.; Chetner, M.P.; Mador, D.R.; Metcalfe, J.B.; Moore, R.B.; Rourke, K.F.; Todd, G.T.; Venner, P.M.; Voaklander, D.C.; et al. Associations between comorbidity, and overall survival and bladder cancer specific survival after radical cystectomy: Results from the Alberta Urology Institute Radical Cystectomy database. *J. Urol.* **2009**, *182*, 85–92. [CrossRef] [PubMed]

6

Downstream Neighbor of SON (DONSON) Expression is Enhanced in Phenotypically Aggressive Prostate Cancers

Niklas Klümper [1,2,3], Marthe von Danwitz [1,2], Johannes Stein [1,2], Doris Schmidt [1,2], Anja Schmidt [1,2], Glen Kristiansen [2,4], Michael Muders [2,4], Michael Hölzel [2,3], Manuel Ritter [1,2], Abdullah Alajati [1,2,*,†] and Jörg Ellinger [1,2,*,†]

1 Department of Urology, University Hospital Bonn, 53127 Bonn, Germany; niklas.kluemper@ukbonn.de (N.K.); s4mavond@uni-bonn.de (M.v.D.); johannes.stein@ukbonn.de (J.S.); doris.schmidt@ukbonn.de (D.S.); Anja.Schmidt@ukbonn.de (A.S.); mritter@ukbonn.de (M.R.)

2 Center for Integrated Oncology, University Hospital Bonn, 53127 Bonn, Germany; glen.kristiansen@ukbonn.de (G.K.); michael.muders@ukbonn.de (M.M.); michael.hoelzel@ukbonn.de (M.H.)

3 Institute of Experimental Oncology, University Hospital Bonn, 53127 Bonn, Germany

4 Institute of Pathology, University Hospital Bonn, 53127 Bonn, Germany

* Correspondence: abdullah.alajati@ukbonn.de (A.A.); joerg.ellinger@ukbonn.de (J.E.)

† Joint senior authors.

Simple Summary: Downstream neighbor of SON (DONSON) plays a crucial role in cell cycle progression and in maintaining genomic stability. We identified DONSON to be associated with an aggressive histopathological phenotype and unfavorable survival in prostate cancer (PCa) in different transcriptomic cohorts and on the protein level in our tissue microarray cohort. DONSON expression in the primary tumor was particularly strong in locally advanced, metastasized, and dedifferentiated carcinomas (TNM Stage, Gleason). Highly proliferating tumors exhibited a significant correlation to DONSON expression, and DONSON expression was notably upregulated in distant metastases and androgen-deprivation resistant metastases. In vitro, specific DONSON-knockdown significantly reduced the migration capacity in PC-3 and LNCaP, which further suggests a tumor-promoting role of DONSON in PCa. The results of our comprehensive expression analyses, as well as the functional data obtained after DONSON-depletion, lead us to the conclusion that DONSON is a promising prognostic biomarker with oncogenic properties in PCa.

Abstract: Downstream neighbor of Son (DONSON) plays a crucial role in cell cycle progression and in maintaining genomic stability, but its role in prostate cancer (PCa) development and progression is still underinvestigated. Methods: DONSON mRNA expression was analyzed with regard to clinical-pathological parameters and progression using The Cancer Genome Atlas (TCGA) and two publicly available Gene Expression Omnibus (GEO) datasets of PCa. Afterwards, DONSON protein expression was assessed via immunohistochemistry on a comprehensive tissue microarray (TMA). Subsequently, the influence of a DONSON-knockdown induced by the transfection of antisense-oligonucleotides on proliferative capacity and metastatic potential was investigated. DONSON was associated with an aggressive phenotype in the PCa TCGA cohort, two GEO PCa cohorts, and our PCa TMA cohort as DONSON expression was particularly strong in locally advanced, metastasized, and dedifferentiated carcinomas. Thus, DONSON expression was notably upregulated in distant and androgen-deprivation resistant metastases. In vitro, specific DONSON-knockdown significantly reduced the migration capacity in the PCa cell lines PC-3 and LNCaP, which further suggests a tumor-promoting role of DONSON in PCa. In conclusion, the results of our comprehensive expression analyses, as well as the functional data obtained after DONSON-depletion, lead us to the conclusion that DONSON is a promising prognostic biomarker with oncogenic properties in PCa.

Keywords: prostate carcinoma; DONSON; Downstream Neighbor of SON; biomarker; metastatic spread

1. Introduction

Prostate cancer (PCa) is the most common malignancy in men and contributes significantly to the overall mortality of malignant diseases [1]. Critical steps in PCa progression are the development of castration resistance and metastatic spread. The therapy of these advanced and castration-resistant PCa (CRPC) has improved considerably in recent years, but mortality remains high with limited therapy options in end-stage carcinomas [2,3]. A better understanding of the biology of this multi-facetted carcinoma can help to further improve the therapy of our PCa patients.

The Cancer Genome Atlas (TCGA) platform is a reliable source and an invaluable tool for cancer research [4]. A large cohort of primary PCa (pPCa) has already been comprehensively investigated by the TCGA Research Network, which has certainly contributed to a deeper understanding of this disease [5]. We hypothesized that genes that show a correlation to an unfavorable clinical course, and therefore to particularly aggressive tumors, represent interesting research targets. In an investigative approach, the PCa TCGA dataset was used to determine prognostically relevant genes [4,6], and in the present study, Downstream Neighbor of SON (DONSON) was identified as an interesting target gene for further analyses in PCa. Of note, in a comprehensive pan-cancer analysis of 30 distinct tumor entities using TCGA datasets, we recently found DONSON overexpression to be associated with unfavorable overall survival in diverse entities, suggesting tumor-independent oncogenic properties of this largely unknown gene [7]. Thus, DONSON was found to be a robust biomarker for risk stratification in clear cell renal cell carcinoma (ccRCC), and in vitro, DONSON was linked to a malignant phenotype in ccRCC cell culture models [7,8]. Mechanistically, it is known that DONSON represents a critical replication fork protein required for physiological DNA replication [9]. DONSON is pivotal for genome stability and integrity as severe replication-associated DNA damage was observed after depletion of DONSON [10]. Further, DONSON plays an important role in cell-cycle regulation and the DNA damage response pathway (DDR) signaling cascade [11]. Regulated cell division and the preservation of genomic integrity are essential to maintain cellular homeostasis, and disorders can lead to tumor formation [12].

Considering the apparently decisive role of DONSON on genome integrity and as DONSON seems to be associated with an aggressive PCa phenotype in the transcriptomic TCGA dataset, the question arises whether DONSON also plays an important role in the progression of PCa. However, a differentiated analysis of the role of this gene in PCa is still pending. Therefore, the aim of this study was to thoroughly analyze the expression pattern of DONSON in PCa cohorts and, subsequently, its functional role in vitro in established PCa cell culture models.

2. Results

2.1. *Downstream Neighbor of SON (DONSON) mRNA Expression is Associated with Aggressive PCa*

In order to analyze the relevance of the DONSON in PCa, we comprehensively associated clinical-pathological parameters and the patients' clinical course with the DONSON mRNA expression using the PCa TCGA dataset (n = 532). DONSON expression was significantly enhanced in the carcinoma samples compared to normal adjacent prostatic tissue (NAT) (Figure 1A). DONSON was associated with enhanced local tumor expansion (pT-stage, Figure 1B) and lymphonodal metastatic dissemination (pN-stage, Figure 1C). Furthermore, a strong association of the DONSON expression with the ISUP grading, derived from the PCa-specific grading parameter Gleason score [13], was evident (Figure 1D). After dichotomizing the PCa cohort using the median DONSON expression, there was a strongly reduced progression-free survival (PFS) for the DONSON overexpressing subgroup (Figure 1E). DONSON remained an independent predictor of unfavorable PFS in the PCA TCGA cohort after adjustment for co-variables (TNM; age) using a Cox regression model ($p = 0.001$; HR = 1.87, 95% CI (1.31; 2.68); Table 1). Since PCa with a Gleason score of 7 is particularly difficult to stratify in terms of aggressiveness, we next investigated whether DONSON would have additive prognostic value in this subgroup. In this clinically highly relevant patient cohort, DONSON expression was again significantly associated with shortened PFS and remained an independent predictor of unfavorable clinical course in a multivariate Cox analysis ($p = 0.01$; HR = 3.82, 95% CI [1.44; 10.2]; Table 1) (Figure 1F). Of note, the proliferation marker Ki67 expression had no prognostic value in the Gleason 7 subgroup in univariate and multivariate Cox regression analyses, and DONSON remained an independent predictor of unfavorable PFS after co-adjusting for Ki67 additionally to TNM and age ($p = 0.01$; HR = 4.03, 95% CI [1.49; 10.9]). DONSON overexpression was also associated with worse overall survival (OS). However, the low number of events in the PCa TCGA cohort ($n = 10$) only permits a limited consideration of this important endpoint (Supplementary Figure S1A and Table S1).

Table 1. Multivariate Cox Regression Analyses in the evaluated prostate cancer (PCa) cohorts regarding progression-free survival (PFS).

Multivariate Cox Regression Analyses (TNM, Age)		
Clinical-Pathological Parameters	***p* Value**	**Hazard Ratio (95% CI Low/High)**
PCa TCGA cohort		
DONSON	0.001	1.87 (1.31; 2.68)
T-Stage	0.002	2.11 (1.31; 3.37)
N-Stage	0.60	1.15 (0.69; 1.91)
Age	0.68	1.01 (0.98; 1.04)
PCa TCGA cohort (Gleason = 7)		
DONSON	0.01	3.82 (1.44; 10.2)
T-Stage	0.73	1.16 (0.50; 2.72)
N-Stage	0.52	1.53 (0.42; 5.54)
Age	0.47	1.03 (0.96; 1.10)
PCa TMA cohort		
DONSON	0.13	1.48 (0.89; 2.47)
T-Stage	0.16	1.71 (0.80; 3.65)
N-Stage	0.62	0.76 (0.26; 2.25)
Age	0.98	1.00 (0.94; 1.07)

PC—Prostate cancer, TCGA—The Cancer Genome Atlas, TMA—Tissue microarray, DONSON—Downstream Neighbor of SON.

Since the PCa TCGA dataset set only contains the expression profiles of primary carcinomas, we wanted to investigate further data sets to more precisely examine the role of DONSON during tumor progression. Of note, in a publicly available PCa progression cohort (GSE21032) [14], DONSON expression was strongly upregulated in the metastatic samples compared to pPCA, which might hint towards a role DONSON plays during the metastatic process (Figure 2A). Interestingly, comparing the sites of the metastatic samples, DONSON expression was significantly enhanced in locally extensive and distant metastatic samples (bone, brain, lung) compared to lymphonodal metastases (LNPC) (Figure 2B). In accordance with this, DONSON expression was strongly enhanced in $n = 25$ androgen-deprivation resistant metastatic samples (Met(CRPC)) compared to pPCa in a second PCa progression cohort (GSE6919, Figure 2C) [15–17]. It is known that fast-growing carcinomas indicate a particularly aggressive phenotype. The proliferation marker Ki-67 is therefore evaluated for assessing tumor aggressiveness, e.g., in breast carcinoma [18], and was also described as a risk stratifier in PCa patients [19]. Of note, we observed a significant positive correlation between DONSON and the proliferative activity of the carcinomas measured by Ki-67 in all of the three independent cohorts (Figure 2D–F).

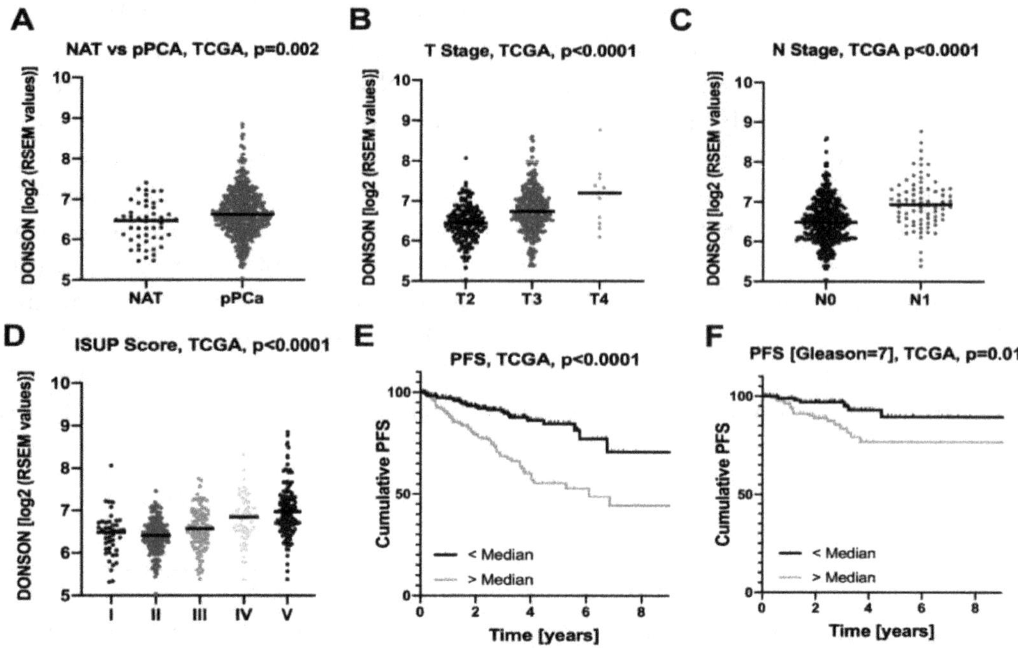

Figure 1. DONSON is associated with clinical-pathological parameters of malignancy and progression-free survival (PFS) using the PCa TCGA dataset (**A**) DONSON expression is enhanced in primary PCa compared to normal adjacent prostatic glands (NAT). DONSON is associated with locally advanced tumor expansion (T Stage), positive lymphonodal metastatic status (N Stage) and the dedifferentiation ISUP score (**B–D**). (**E,F**) DONSON overexpressing PCa exhibit a shortened PFS when analyzing the whole (**E**) or only the clinically relevant (**F**) subgroup of Gleason 7 carcinomas of the PCa TCGA cohort.

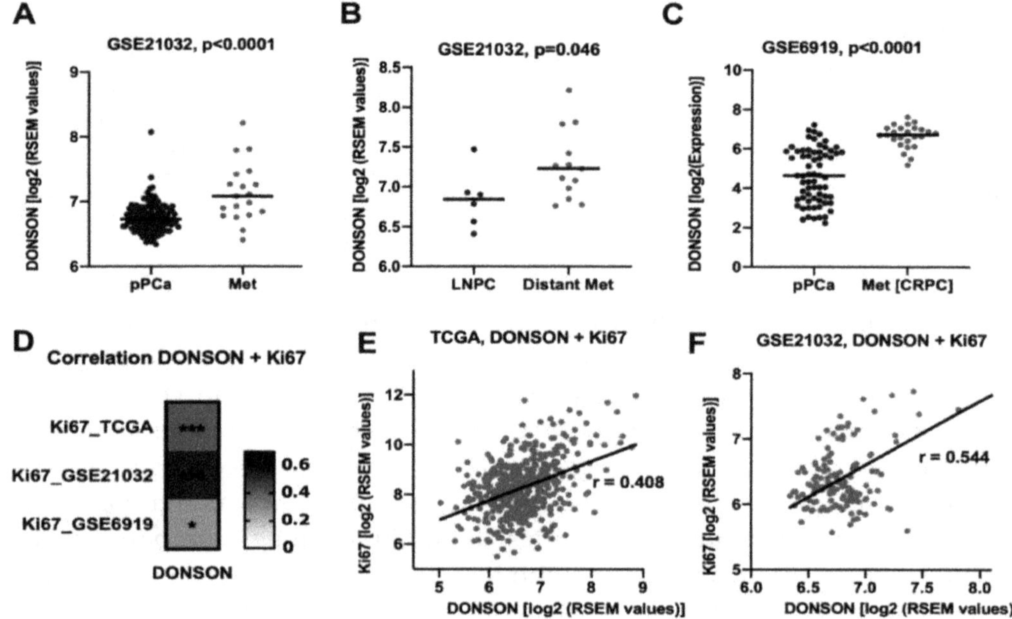

Figure 2. (**A–C**), DONSON expression is significantly increased in metastatic samples compared to primary PCA, which was particularly evident in distant (**B**) and androgen-deprivation resistant metastases (Met [CRPC], (**C**). (**D**), Correlation heatmap depicting DONSON´s significant correlation to the proliferative activity of PCa in three cohorts. (**E,F**), Scatter plots with regression line included visualize the distribution of the TCGA and GSE21032 cohort with regard to the DONSON and Ki67 expression (parametric Pearson´s r is specified). * $p < 0.05$, *** $p < 0.001$.

2.2. *DONSON Protein Expression on a PCa Tissue Microarray (TMA)*

To test the prognostic potential of DONSON at the protein level, we stained and evaluated a large PCa TMA cohort immunohistochemically against DONSON. DONSON was expressed in the cytoplasm, which is in accordance with the staining pattern observed in the PCa and normal prostate gland specimens of The Human Protein Atlas cohort (HPA, www.proteinatlas.org) [20,21] (Figure 3A). Immunocytochemical DONSON staining in PC-3 cells with and without DONSON knockdown, induced via transfection of specific antisense oligonucleotides, was performed to confirm the cytoplasmic staining pattern and antibody specificity (Supplementary Figure S2). Interestingly, DONSON revealed a heterogeneous expression throughout the investigated cohort (DONSON expression negative/weak $n = 48$; DONSON expression moderate/strong $n = 68$). Of note, enhanced DONSON expression was associated with an advanced pT-stage (Figure 3B). In addition, the aggressive Gleason ≥ 8 PCa (ISUP IV+V) exhibited a significantly increased DONSON expression compared to Gleason ≤ 7 (ISUP I-III) (Figure 3C). No further significant associations between DONSON and clinical pathological parameters were evident, which may be due to the low sample size.

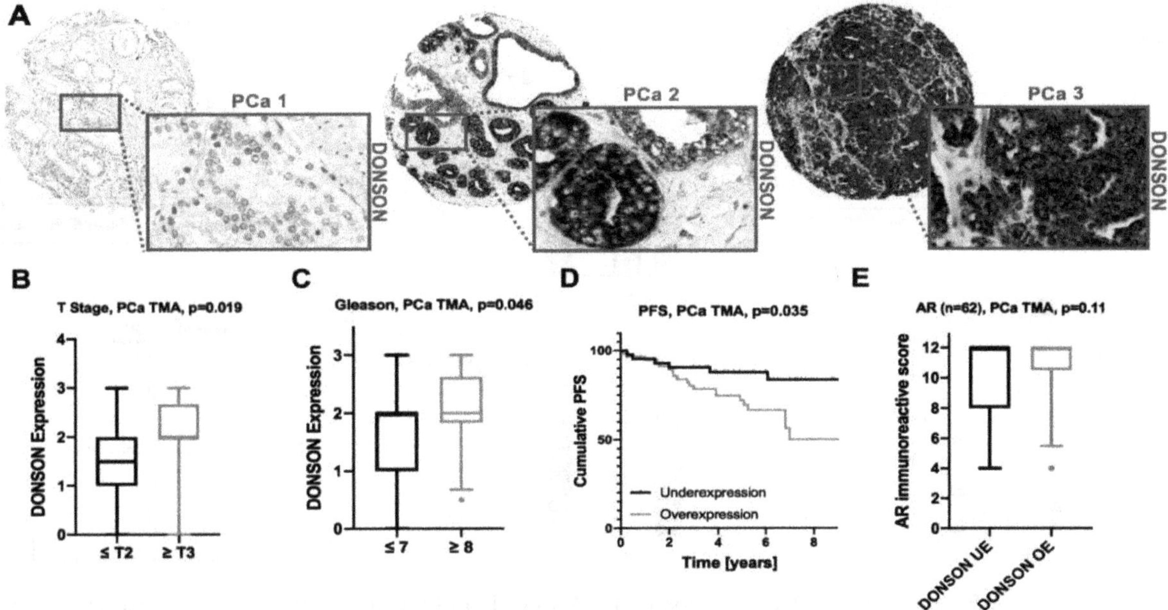

Figure 3. Immunohistochemical staining (IHC) against DONSON on a comprehensive PCa TMA with subsequent expression analysis (**A**), Representative images of the heterogeneous DONSON expression throughout the primary PCa cohort are depicted in three cases; 10× and 40× objective magnification. PCa 1 represents a well-differentiated DONSON-negative carcinoma. PCa 2 + 3 represent cases with particularly strong DONSON protein expression, wherein PCa 3 additionally exhibits an aggressive phenotype with fusing glands and components of a solid carcinoma. (**B**,**C**), DONSON expression is associated with advanced T Stage and Gleason score. (**D**), DONSON overexpression, defined as DONSON moderate/high (Score ≥ 2), predicts shortened PFS compared to the negative/low expression subgroup. (**E**), A strong statistical tendency for an increased nuclear AR expression was evident in the DONSON overexpressing subgroup; overexpression = OE, underexpression = UE.

In line with its potential as a risk stratifier in the PCa TCGA cohort, DONSON overexpression also showed a significant association with progression-free survival (PFS) at the protein level in the investigated cohort (Figure 3D). Further, a strong statistical trend was seen for DONSON to be an independent predictor of unfavorable PFS ($p = 0.13$; HR 1.48, 95% CI (0.89; 2.47); Table 1) measured by multivariate Cox regression co-adjusting the TNM stage and age.

The androgen receptor (AR) signaling pathway plays a crucial role in the progression of PCa, and nuclear expression of AR predicts an unfavorable clinical outcome and shorter time to the development of castration resistance [22]. Interestingly, in the examined PCa cohort, a strong trend for increased AR expression (studied earlier in [23]) in the DONSON overexpressing subgroup was evident (Figure 3E). In accordance with this, in both PCa progression cohorts a significant correlation of AR and DONSON mRNA expression was observed (GSE21032: Pearson's r = 0.204, p-value = 0.012; GSE6919: Pearson's r = 0.549, p-value < 0.0001).

2.3. Functional Characterization of DONSON In Vitro

In order to investigate the functional role of DONSON in vitro, we used the antisense locked nucleic acid (LNA) GapmeR system to induce efficient and specific DONSON-knockdowns in established PCa cell culture models. The prostate cancer cell lines PC-3, LNCaP, C4-2B, and DU-145 were screened for their DONSON baseline expression under standard conditions (Figure 4A). As LNCap and PC-3 expressed the highest DONSON protein levels, they have been chosen for further investigations. Thus, via transfection of the specific antisense oligonucleotides, we were able to induce efficient DONSON-depletion assessed by qRT-PCR, Western blotting, and immunocytochemistry (Figure 4B,C, Figure S2).

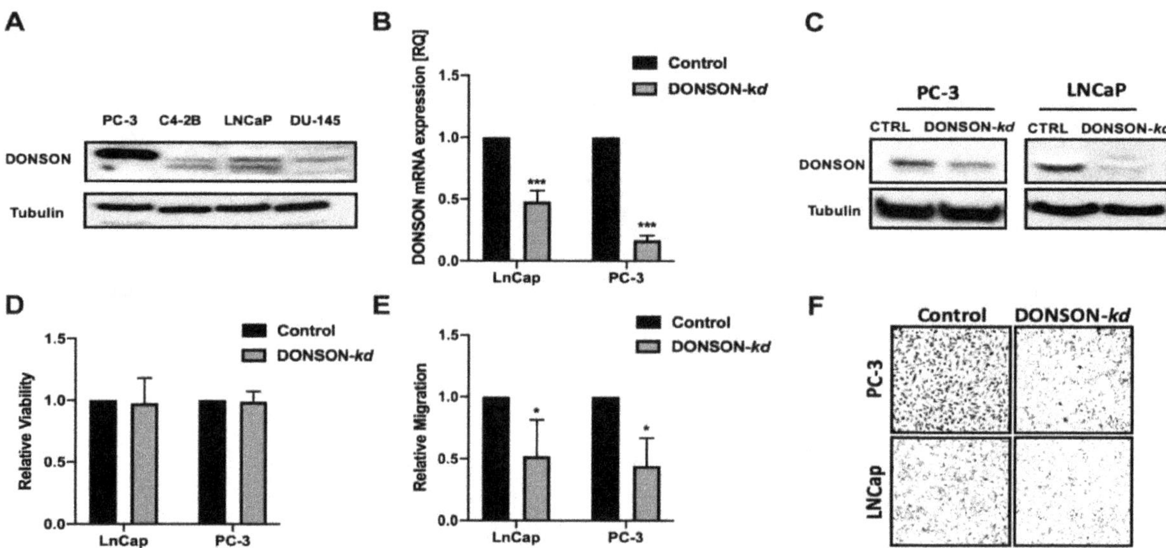

Figure 4. Effect of specific DONSON-depletion in the PCa cell lines LNCaP and PC-3. (**A**), Screening Western Blot for DONSON in four broadly used PCa cell lines. (**B**,**C**), Induction of efficient Antisense LNA GapmeR-mediated DONSON knockdowns in LNCaP and PC-3 with subsequent validation via qPCR (**B**) and Western Blotting (**C**). (**D**,**E**) DONSON-depletion did not affect cell viability but specifically reduced the cellular motility in a Boyden Chamber Migration Assay. (**F**), Membranes depicted in 10× objective magnification. Each experiment was performed in biological triplicates. * $p < 0.05$, *** $p < 0.001$.

After establishing efficient DONSON-depletion in both cell culture models, we aimed to investigate the dependence of important parameters of malignancy towards DONSON. In the conducted cell proliferation and cytotoxicity assay, no growth effects were evident in die DONSON-depleted PCa cells compared to the negative control (Figure 4D). Next, we explored the impact of DONSON-knockdown on the migration capacity of the investigated metastasizing PCa cells via Boyden chamber migration assays. Of note, a strong impairment of their migration capacity was seen after DONSON-knockdown (Figure 4E,F), which is thought to be an essential trait for metastatic spread and an important attribute conferring to an aggressive phenotype.

3. Discussion

To date, the role of DONSON in PCa has not been explored. In this study, we were able to identify the relatively unknown gene DONSON as a promising risk stratifier with oncogenic properties in the PCa cell culture model. DONSON was an independent predictor of a shortened PFS in the comprehensive PCa TCGA cohort and correlated with the clinical-pathological parameters (pT-stage, lymphonodal status, ISUP/Gleason score). In the group of Gleason 7 carcinomas, which plays a crucial role clinically due to the intermediate aggressiveness with regard to the prognosis and need for therapy, DONSON also shows an additive prognostic potential in the multivariate Cox analysis.

The prognostic potential of DONSON has been validated at the protein level in a large PCa TMA cohort, highlighting its potential as a robust biomarker. Of note, the DONSON protein was localized in the cytoplasm of the PCa samples, which was in accordance with the staining pattern observed in The Human Protein Atlas and as described previously for clear cell renal cell carcinoma tissue [7,8]. Staining specificity was confirmed via immunocytochemistry in PC-3 cells with and without DONSON knockdown. Nevertheless, due to its function in DNA replication and repair, an additional nuclear expression would have been expected. During the S phase, nuclear DONSON foci were observed [9]. However, the DNA replication and S phase only describes a small part of the cell cycle, and thus the localization of DONSON could differ during the G1 phase [24]. Furthermore, as the overall knowledge regarding DONSON is sparse, it may have additional functions, also inside the cytoplasm. As this was not the scope of our study, further investigations regarding its subcellular localization, trafficking, and exact biological function are needed to clarify this.

Interestingly, the PCa TMA cohort showed a heterogeneous picture, with some tumors being DONSON-negative while others, especially Gleason 8 and higher carcinomas, strongly overexpressed DONSON. It has to be mentioned that only a strong statistical trend was seen for DONSON to be an independent predictor of unfavorable PFS in this cohort (HR 1.46, 95% CI; 0.86–2.48; $p = 0.17$), which may be due to a relatively low sample size compared to the PCa TCGA cohort (PFS Follow-up PCa TMA cohort $n = 103$ (29 events); PCa TCGA cohort $n = 497$ (93 events)).

In addition, two independent PCa progression cohorts showed a significant increase in DONSON expression in the metastatic samples compared to pPCA, which was particularly evident in distant metastases and androgen-deprivation resistant metastases. The crucial step in PCa progression is displayed by the development of metastases and a castration-resistant status during androgen-deprivation therapy (ADT). Among the different mechanisms of CRPC development, aberrant androgen receptor (AR) signaling is thought to be a major player [22,25]. An association between DONSON and AR expression was observed in the PCa progression and the PCa tissue microarray (TMA) cohorts on both transcriptional and translational levels. However, the exact interaction of DONSON and the AR signaling pathway and a possible link between DONSON and the development of castration-resistance requires further functional investigations. In addition, the proliferative activity measured by Ki67 expression, which is also an established prognostic biomarker in PCa and other cancers [18,19], was significantly correlated with DONSON expression, which seems comprehensible due to the predicted function of DONSON as part of the replisome [10,26]. Thus, renal cell carcinoma cell lines showed decreased proliferative capacity after oligonucleotide-mediated DONSON knockdown [7,8]. However, in our PCa cell culture model, no influence on proliferation could be detected after DONSON-depletion, which suggests an additional unknown function of DONSON, but this requires further investigation. In our cell culture model, DONSON-depletion led to potent inhibition of cell motility, which is recognized as a surrogate for the metastatic capacity in vitro. This provides evidence that DONSON plays a role during the metastatic process, which could ultimately explain its significant upregulation in the metastatic samples in both PCa progression cohorts and the N+ pPCa samples (PCa TCGA).

Taxane-based therapy is a backbone of PCa therapy and preferentially attacks tumor cells with an increased cell division rate as well as limited DNA damage repair capacity. As DONSON plays a pivotal role in both cellular processes, replication, and maintaining genome stability, it could be an interesting therapeutic target for combination therapies [10,11]. Therefore, we think that our study on DONSON in PCa, as well as the fact that DONSON overexpression seems to mediate tumor-independent oncogenic properties, could be a starting point for further basic and oncological research on DONSON.

Thus, the results of our comprehensive expression analyses, as well as the functional data obtained after DONSON-depletion, lead us to the conclusion that DONSON is a promising prognostic biomarker with oncogenic properties in PCa.

4. Materials and Methods

4.1. Transcriptome Data Assembly

Log2 transformed RNA sequencing data generated by IlluminaHiSeq (Illumina, San Diego, CA, USA) and publicly available by the TCGA Research Network were downloaded via the UCSC Xena browser (http://xena.ucsc.edu, PCa $n = 497$, plus normal adjacent kidney tissue (NAT) $n = 52$; Table S1) [4,5].

Microarray data (Affymetrix Human Genome U95C Array; Affymetrix, Santa Clara, CA, USA) from the first prostate cancer progression cohort for DONSON, KI67, and AR were downloaded via Gene Expression Omnibus (GEO, http://www.ncbi.nlm.nih.gov/geo/, GSE6919) [15]. The expression profiles of 25 androgen-deprivation resistant metastatic samples derived from four patients were obtained from different metastatic sites and were thereby used as individual samples (pPCa $n = 66$, Met(CRPC) $n = 25$). Normalized log2 mRNA (DONSON, Ki67, AR) expression data and the clinical features of the second investigated progression cohort were obtained from http://cbio.mskcc.org/cancergenomics/prostate/, which included primary PCa and metastatic samples (GSE21032, pPCa $n = 131$, Met $n = 19$) [14].

4.2. Immunohistochemistry

A tissue microarray (TMA) from paraffin-embedded prostate tissue was assessed as described previously [23,27,28] (Supplementary Table S2). Paraffin sections of 5 μm thickness were cut and stained with the polyclonal DONSON-antibody (HPA039558, Atlas Antibodies, dilution 1:50; Sigma Aldrich, St. Louis, MO, USA) with the Ventana Benchmark automated staining system (Ventana Medical System, Tuscon, AZ, USA) [7,29–31]. The staining quality and specificity were confirmed by experienced uropathologists, and subsequently, the TMA cohort was stained. Two experienced observers independently scored the DONSON staining intensity with a score ranging negative, weak, moderate, or strong DONSON protein expression (score values 0 to 3) as previously described for PCa specimens [27]. Androgen receptor (AR) expression data, already collected using the immunoreactive score, were also available for a subset of the examined cohort ($n = 62$) [23].

4.3. Antisense LNA GapmeR-Mediated Knockdown

Transfections in both cell lines were conducted using a final concentration of 150 nM in a ratio of 3:1 with the FuGENE HD-Transfection reagent (E2311, Promega Corporation, Madison, WI, USA) in accordance with the producers' instructions and as described previously [7,31]. DONSON GapmeR sequence: 5′-A*C*C*A*G*T*C*A*C*T*C*A*T*T*A*A-3′. Non-targeting negative control GapmeR sequence: 5′-*C*G*T*A**G*T*C*G*A*G*G*A*A*G*T*A-3′.

4.4. Immunocytochemistry

Briefly, 72 h post-transfection, PC-3 cells were harvested and transferred into Cellmatrix (Type I-A) (Fujifilm Wako Chemicals, Osaka, Japan). Subsequently, cells were fixed in 4% paraformaldehyde for 24 h and embedded into paraffin. Afterward, DONSON staining was performed as described in Section 4.2.

4.5. Real-Time PCR

Transcriptional knockdown efficiency was assessed 48 h post-transfection using quantitative real-time PCR. The following primer sequences were used: DONSON forward primer: 5′-gtccagcattgtagggcaac-3′ and reverse primer: 5′-ggctctgctggaaggtacaa-3′; β-Actin forward primer: 5′-CCAACCGCGAGAAGATGA-3′ and reverse primer: 5′-CCAGAGGCGTACAGGGATAG-3′.

4.6. Western Blot

DONSON knockdown efficiency was assessed 72h post-transfection. The following antibodies were used: Anti-DONSON (1:1000, LS-C167506, Rabbit, LSBio, Seattle, WA, USA); Anti-alpha-Tubulin (1:4000, A5316, Mouse, Sigma-Aldrich, St. Louis, MO, USA).

4.7. Cell Proliferation Assays

We used the EZ4U cell proliferation and cytotoxicity assay kit according to the manufacturer's protocol (EZ4U, Biomedica Group, Vienna, Austria).

4.8. Migration Assays

Boyden Chamber Migration Assays (8.0 μm pore size, 353097, Falcon, Corning, Amsterdam, The Netherlands) were performed to assess cell motility and migration. The cells were plated 48 h post-transfection in the upper chamber of the migration inserts with starved RPMI medium (0% FCS), whereas the lower chamber was filled with standard medium containing 10% FCS for chemotactic attraction. The experiment was stopped after 48 h of incubation, the cells being fixed with 4% formaldehyde and colored with hematoxylin. Membranes were scanned, and the cells were counted automatically by nucleus detection using the QuPath software (v0.2.0-m6) [7,32].

4.9. Statistical Analysis

Microsoft Excel (v16), SPPS (v25), and GraphPad Prism (v8) were used for statistical analyses and visualization of the data. The nonparametric Mann–Whitney U or Kruskal–Wallis test were used for group comparisons. Pearson´s correlation coefficients were calculated. Survival analyses were performed using Kaplan Meier estimate curves and log-rank tests. Thus, multivariate Cox regression analyses were performed after co-adjustment of the TNM stage (the only $n = 3$ M1 in PCa TCGA were excluded; in PCa TMA no cM1 cases) and age to evaluate an independent and additive prognostic value on patients' progression-free survival.

4.10. Ethical Approval and Consent to Participate

All patients gave written informed consent for the collection of biomaterials. The study was approved by the Ethics Committee at the Medical Faculty of the Rheinische Friedrich-Wilhelms-University Bonn (number: 273/18; 013/20).

5. Conclusions

In total, our study could show for the first time that DONSON expression is strongly enhanced in phenotypically aggressive PCa and advanced metastatic samples and represents an interesting and robust prognostic biomarker. Further, DONSON could play an important role in the PCa progression and metastatic process supported by functional in vitro analyses.

Author Contributions: Conceptualization, N.K., A.A., and J.E.; methodology, N.K., M.v.D., J.S., D.S., A.S., A.A., and J.E.; validation, N.K., M.v.D., J.S., D.S., A.S., G.K., M.M., M.H., M.R., A.A., and J.E.; investigation, N.K., M.v.D., and J.S.; resources, G.K., M.H., M.R., A.A., and J.E.; writing, N.K., M.v.D., A.A., and J.E.; review and editing, J.S., D.S., A.S., G.K., M.M., M.H., and M.R.; supervision, A.A. and J.E. All authors have read and agreed to the published version of the manuscript.

Acknowledgments: The tissue samples were collected within the framework of the Biobank of the Center for Integrated Oncology Cologne Bonn at the University Hospital Bonn.

References

1. Siegel, R.L.; Miller, K.D.; Jemal, A. Cancer statistics, 2019. *CA Cancer J. Clin.* **2019** *69*, 7–34. [CrossRef]

2. Gillessen, S.; Attard, G.; Beer, T.M.; Beltran, H.; Bjartell, A.; Bossi, A.; Briganti, A.; Bristow, R.G.; Chi, K.N.; Clarke, N.; et al. Management of Patients with Advanced Prostate Cancer: Report of the Advanced Prostate Cancer Consensus Conference. 2019. *Eur. Urol.* **2020**, *77*, 508–547. [CrossRef] [PubMed]
3. Dellis, A.; Zagouri, F.; Liontos, M.; Mitropoulos, D.; Bamias, A.; Papatsoris, A.G. Management of advanced prostate cancer: A systematic review of existing guidelines and recommendations. *Cancer Treat. Rev.* **2019**, *73*, 54–61. [CrossRef] [PubMed]
4. The Cancer Genome Atlas Research Network; Weinstein, J.N.; Collisson, E.A.; Mills, G.B.; Shaw, K.R.M.; Ozenberger, B.A.; Ellrott, K.; Shmulevich, I.; Sander, C.; Stuart, J.M. The Cancer Genome Atlas Pan-Cancer analysis project. *Nat. Genet.* **2013**, *45*, 1113–1120. [CrossRef]
5. Cancer Genome Atlas Research Network The Molecular Taxonomy of Primary Prostate Cancer. *Cell* **2015**, *163*, 1011–1025. [CrossRef] [PubMed]
6. Uhlen, M.; Zhang, C.; Lee, S.; Sjöstedt, E.; Fagerberg, L.; Bidkhori, G.; Benfeitas, R.; Arif, M.; Liu, Z.; Edfors, F.; et al. A pathology atlas of the human cancer transcriptome. *Science* **2017**, *357*, eaan2507. [CrossRef]
7. Klümper, N.; Blajan, I.; Schmidt, D.; Kristiansen, G.; Toma, M.; Hölzel, M.; Ritter, M.; Ellinger, J. Downstream neighbor of SON (DONSON) is associated with unfavorable survival across diverse cancers with oncogenic properties in clear cell renal cell carcinoma. *Transl. Oncol.* **2020**, *13*, 100844. [CrossRef]
8. Yamada, Y.; Nohata, N.; Uchida, A.; Kato, M.; Arai, T.; Moriya, S.; Mizuno, K.; Kojima, S.; Yamazaki, K.; Naya, Y.; et al. Replisome genes regulation by antitumor miR-101-5p in clear cell renal cell carcinoma. *Cancer Sci.* **2020**. [CrossRef]
9. Zhang, J.; Bellani, M.A.; James, R.C.; Pokharel, D.; Zhang, Y.; Reynolds, J.J.; McNee, G.S.; Jackson, A.P.; Stewart, G.S.; Seidman, M.M. DONSON and FANCM associate with different replisomes distinguished by replication timing and chromatin domain. *Nat. Commun.* **2020**, *11*, 3951. [CrossRef]
10. Reynolds, J.J.; Bicknell, L.S.; Carroll, P.; Higgs, M.R.; Shaheen, R.; Murray, J.E.; Papadopoulos, D.K.; Leitch, A.; Murina, O.; Tarnauskaitė, Ž.; et al. Mutations in DONSON disrupt replication fork stability and cause microcephalic dwarfism. *Nat. Genet.* **2017**, *49*, 537–549. [CrossRef]
11. Fuchs, F.; Pau, G.; Kranz, D.; Sklyar, O.; Budjan, C.; Steinbrink, S.; Horn, T.; Pedal, A.; Huber, W.; Boutros, M. Clustering phenotype populations by genome-wide RNAi and multiparametric imaging. *Mol. Syst. Biol.* **2010**, *6*, 370. [CrossRef] [PubMed]
12. Hanahan, D.; Weinberg, R.A. Hallmarks of Cancer: The Next Generation. *Cell* **2011**, *144*, 646–674. [CrossRef] [PubMed]
13. Epstein, J.I.; Egevad, L.; Amin, M.B.; Delahunt, B.; Srigley, J.R.; Humphrey, P.A. Grading Committee The 2014 International Society of Urological Pathology (ISUP) Consensus Conference on Gleason Grading of Prostatic Carcinoma: Definition of Grading Patterns and Proposal for a New Grading System. *Am. J. Surg. Pathol.* **2016**, *40*, 244–252. [CrossRef] [PubMed]
14. Taylor, B.S.; Schultz, N.; Hieronymus, H.; Gopalan, A.; Xiao, Y.; Carver, B.S.; Arora, V.K.; Kaushik, P.; Cerami, E.; Reva, B.; et al. Integrative Genomic Profiling of Human Prostate Cancer. *Cancer Cell* **2010**, *18*, 11–22. [CrossRef] [PubMed]
15. Chandran, U.R.; Ma, C.; Dhir, R.; Bisceglia, M.; Lyons-Weiler, M.; Liang, W.; Michalopoulos, G.; Becich, M.; Monzon, F.A. Gene expression profiles of prostate cancer reveal involvement of multiple molecular pathways in the metastatic process. *BMC Cancer* **2007**, *7*, 64. [CrossRef] [PubMed]
16. Chandran, U.R.; Dhir, R.; Ma, C.; Michalopoulos, G.; Becich, M.; Gilbertson, J. Differences in gene expression in prostate cancer, normal appearing prostate tissue adjacent to cancer and prostate tissue from cancer free organ donors. *BMC Cancer* **2005**, *5*, 45. [CrossRef] [PubMed]
17. Yu, Y.P.; Landsittel, D.; Jing, L.; Nelson, J.; Ren, B.; Liu, L.; McDonald, C.; Thomas, R.; Dhir, R.; Finkelstein, S.; et al. Gene expression alterations in prostate cancer predicting tumor aggression and preceding development of malignancy. *J. Clin. Oncol. Off. J. Am. Soc. Clin. Oncol.* **2004**, *22*, 2790–2799. [CrossRef]
18. Inwald, E.C.; Klinkhammer-Schalke, M.; Hofstädter, F.; Zeman, F.; Koller, M.; Gerstenhauer, M.; Ortmann, O. Ki-67 is a prognostic parameter in breast cancer patients: Results of a large population-based cohort of a cancer registry. *Breast Cancer Res. Treat.* **2013**, *139*, 539–552. [CrossRef]
19. Hammarsten, P.; Josefsson, A.; Thysell, E.; Lundholm, M.; Hägglöf, C.; Iglesias-Gato, D.; Flores-Morales, A.; Stattin, P.; Egevad, L.; Granfors, T.; et al. Immunoreactivity for prostate specific antigen and Ki67 differentiates subgroups of prostate cancer related to outcome. *Mod. Pathol.* **2019**, *32*, 1310–1319. [CrossRef]

20. Uhlén, M.; Fagerberg, L.; Hallström, B.M.; Lindskog, C.; Oksvold, P.; Mardinoglu, A.; Sivertsson, Å.; Kampf, C.; Sjöstedt, E.; Asplund, A.; et al. Tissue-based map of the human proteome. *Science* **2015**, *347*, 1260419. [CrossRef]
21. Uhlén, M.; Björling, E.; Agaton, C.; Szigyarto, C.A.-K.; Amini, B.; Andersen, E.; Andersson, A.-C.; Angelidou, P.; Asplund, A.; Asplund, C.; et al. A human protein atlas for normal and cancer tissues based on antibody proteomics. *Mol. Cell. Proteom. MCP* **2005**, *4*, 1920–1932. [CrossRef] [PubMed]
22. Donovan, M.J.; Hamann, S.; Clayton, M.; Khan, F.M.; Sapir, M.; Bayer-Zubek, V.; Fernandez, G.; Mesa-Tejada, R.; Teverovskiy, M.; Reuter, V.E.; et al. Systems pathology approach for the prediction of prostate cancer progression after radical prostatectomy. *J. Clin. Oncol. Off. J. Am. Soc. Clin. Oncol.* **2008**, *26*, 3923–3929. [CrossRef] [PubMed]
23. Mang, J.; Korzeniewski, N.; Dietrich, D.; Sailer, V.; Tolstov, Y.; Searcy, S.; von Hardenberg, J.; Perner, S.; Kristiansen, G.; Marx, A.; et al. Prognostic Significance and Functional Role of CEP57 in Prostate Cancer. *Transl. Oncol.* **2015**, *8*, 487–496. [CrossRef]
24. Natsume, T.; Tanaka, T.U. Spatial regulation and organization of DNA replication within the nucleus. *Chromosome Res.* **2010**, *18*, 7–17. [CrossRef] [PubMed]
25. Hu, R.; Denmeade, S.R.; Luo, J. Molecular processes leading to aberrant androgen receptor signaling and castration resistance in prostate cancer. *Expert Rev. Endocrinol. Metab.* **2010**, *5*, 753–764. [CrossRef]
26. Rai, R.; Gu, P.; Broton, C.; Kumar-Sinha, C.; Chen, Y.; Chang, S. The Replisome Mediates A-NHEJ Repair of Telomeres Lacking POT1-TPP1 Independently of MRN Function. *Cell Rep.* **2019**, *29*, 3708–3725.e5. [CrossRef]
27. Stein, J.; Majores, M.; Rohde, M.; Lim, S.; Schneider, S.; Krappe, E.; Ellinger, J.; Dietel, M.; Stephan, C.; Jung, K.; et al. KDM5C Is Overexpressed in Prostate Cancer and Is a Prognostic Marker for Prostate-Specific Antigen-Relapse Following Radical Prostatectomy. *Am. J. Pathol.* **2014**, *184*, 2430–2437. [CrossRef]
28. Gevensleben, H.; Dietrich, D.; Golletz, C.; Steiner, S.; Jung, M.; Thiesler, T.; Majores, M.; Stein, J.; Uhl, B.; Muller, S.; et al. The Immune Checkpoint Regulator PD-L1 Is Highly Expressed in Aggressive Primary Prostate Cancer. *Clin. Cancer Res.* **2016**, *22*, 1969–1977. [CrossRef]
29. Klümper, N.; Syring, I.; Offermann, A.; Shaikhibrahim, Z.; Vogel, W.; Müller, S.C.; Ellinger, J.; Strauß, A.; Radzun, H.J.; Ströbel, P.; et al. Differential expression of Mediator complex subunit MED15 in testicular germ cell tumors. *Diagn. Pathol.* **2015**, *10*, 165. [CrossRef]
30. Klümper, N.; Syring, I.; Vogel, W.; Schmidt, D.; Müller, S.C.; Ellinger, J.; Shaikhibrahim, Z.; Brägelmann, J.; Perner, S. Mediator Complex Subunit MED1 Protein Expression Is Decreased during Bladder Cancer Progression. *Front. Med.* **2017**, *4*, 30. [CrossRef]
31. Blajan, I.; Miersch, H.; Schmidt, D.; Kristiansen, G.; Perner, S.; Ritter, M.; Ellinger, J.; Klümper, N. Comprehensive Analysis of the ATP-binding Cassette Subfamily B Across Renal Cancers Identifies ABCB8 Overexpression in Phenotypically Aggressive Clear Cell Renal Cell Carcinoma. *Eur. Urol. Focus* **2020**. [CrossRef] [PubMed]
32. Bankhead, P.; Loughrey, M.B.; Fernández, J.A.; Dombrowski, Y.; McArt, D.G.; Dunne, P.D.; McQuaid, S.; Gray, R.T.; Murray, L.J.; Coleman, H.G.; et al. QuPath: Open source software for digital pathology image analysis. *Sci. Rep.* **2017**, *7*. [CrossRef] [PubMed]

7

Differential Expression and Clinicopathological Significance of HER2, Indoleamine 2,3-Dioxygenase and PD-L1 in Urothelial Carcinoma of the Bladder

Donghyun Kim [1,2], Jin Man Kim [1,2], Jun-Sang Kim [3,4], Sup Kim [4,*] and Kyung-Hee Kim [1,2,5,*]

1 Department of Pathology, Chungnam National University School of Medicine, 266 Munhwa Street, Daejeon 35015, Korea; duras3516@cnuh.co.kr (D.K.); jinmank@cnu.ac.kr (J.M.K.)
2 Department of Pathology, Chungnam National University Hospital, 282 Munwha-ro, Daejeon 35015, Korea
3 Department of Radiation Oncology, Chungnam National University School of Medicine, 288 Munhwa Street, Daejeon 35015, Korea; k423j@cnu.ac.kr
4 Department of Radiation Oncology, Chungnam National University Hospital, 282 Munwha-ro, Daejeon 35015, Korea
5 Department of Pathology, Chungnam National University Sejong Hospital, 20 Bodeum 7-ro, Sejong-si 30099, Korea
* Correspondence: supkim@cnuh.co.kr (S.K.); phone330@cnu.ac.kr (K.-H.K.)

Abstract: Purpose: Evasion of the immune system by cancer cells allows for the progression of tumors. Antitumor immunotherapy has shown remarkable effects in a diverse range of cancers. The aim of this study was to determine the clinicopathological significance of human epidermal growth factor receptor 2 (HER2), indoleamine 2,3-dioxygenase (IDO), and programmed death ligand-1 (PD-L1) expression in urothelial carcinoma of the bladder (UCB). Materials and Methods: We retrospectively studied 97 patients with UCB. We performed an immunohistochemical study to measure the expression levels of HER2, IDO, and PD-L1 in UCB tissue from these 97 patients. Results: In all 97 cases, the PD-L1 expression of tumor-infiltrating immune cells (ICs) was significantly correlated with higher pathologic tumor stage (pT). In pT2–pT4 cases (n = 69), higher levels of HER2 and IDO expression in invasive tumor cells (TCs) were associated with shorter periods of disease-free survival (DFS). Conclusion: These results imply that the expression of PD-L1 in ICs of the UCB microenvironment is associated with cancer invasion and the expression of HER2 or IDO in the invasive cancer cell and suggestive of the potential for cancer recurrence. We suggest that the expression levels of IDO, HER2, and PD-L1 could be useful as targets in the development of combined cancer immunotherapeutic strategies.

Keywords: human epidermal growth factor receptor 2; indoleamine 2,3-dioxygenase; programmed death ligand-1; urothelial carcinoma; urinary bladder; immunotherapy

---

1. Introduction

Urothelial carcinoma of the bladder (UCB) remains one of the most common malignant cancers of the genitourinary tract [1]. Among UCB patients, approximately 30% will have muscle invasion at diagnosis, show rapid progression to metastatic disease, and succumb to their disease [2]. Although there are several different treatment regimens, very poor treatment outcomes have been reported in locally advanced and metastatic UCB patients, and this trend has remained unchanged in the last few decades [3,4]. Therefore, further studies are required to better understand the molecular mechanisms of tumor aggressiveness in UCB.

One barrier limiting the efficacy of classic cancer therapies is the interactions of cancer cells with their microenvironment, which ultimately determine whether the primary tumor is eradicated, metastasizes, or establishes dormant micrometastases [5]. Furthermore, the tumor microenvironment can also determine treatment outcome and resistance [6]. Thus, future anticancer treatment strategies should not only act directly on the proliferative processes of transformed cells but also interrupt the crosstalk circuits established by tumor cells with the host microenvironment [7].

Tumor immunogenicity is simply defined as the ability to induce adaptive immune responses [6]. Although most tumors carry particular substances which can induce an immune response, such as antigens or epitopes, the immunogenicity of cancer varies greatly between cancer types. It has been reported that tumor immunogenicity relies on its own antigenicity and several immunomodulatory mechanisms that render tumor cells less sensitive to immune system attack, or create a highly immunosuppressive tumor microenvironment [8]. Classic cancer therapies, such as chemotherapy and radiotherapy, reduce the tumor burden by killing cancer cells. Furthermore, during apoptosis and necrosis, antigens and damage-associated molecular patterns (DAMPs) stimulate an antitumor immune response which induces immunogenic cell death [9,10]. However, cancer cells can escape immune surveillance and progress through modulating immune checkpoint molecules that suppress antitumor immune responses [8].

Considering their high immunogenicity, the expression levels of immune checkpoint-related proteins have been measured and linked to the clinicopathological features and treatment outcomes in UCB. Many studies have reported that expression of immune checkpoint-related proteins, such as programmed cell death 1 (PD-1)/programmed death ligand-1 (PD-L1) and indoleamine 2,3-dioxygenase (IDO) show prognostic significance in UCB [11–13]. Additionally, various cancers have responded to treatment with immune checkpoint inhibitors, including UCB [14].

In breast cancer, Filippo et al. highlighted the role of innate and adaptive immune responses in HER2-targeted drugs [15]. This article has prompted investigations into the interaction of immune checkpoint proteins with HER2 targeted therapies. Recently, human epidermal growth factor receptor 2 (HER2) signals have been found to potentially regulate the infiltration of tumor microenvironment immune cells, and to have a role in the expression of PD-L1 in breast and gastric cancers [16,17]. Similarly, increased IDO expression was observed in a subset of HER2+ breast tumors (43.1%), which could be used to develop a combination treatment regimen [18]. These results suggest that immune-escape genes could be used to develop a combination treatment regimen in HER2 overexpression UCB patients. However, the clinical significance of immune checkpoint-related molecules in the context of HER2-positive and -negative UCB have not yet been fully evaluated.

We hypothesized that information on the expression of HER2 and immune-escape genes could be useful in the development of therapeutic strategies. This study aimed to evaluate the expression levels of HER2 and immune-escape genes by immunohistochemistry (IHC) in 97 cases of UCB. Therefore, we first evaluated the influence of immune cell infiltration on UCB survival using the Tumor IMmune Estimation Resource (TIMER) database. Then, to identify immunomodulatory genes, correlations between CD8+ T cell infiltration and candidate genes were analyzed by TIMER. Finally, we evaluated expression levels of HER2, IDO, and PD-L1 by immunohistochemistry (IHC) in 97 cases of UCB. The levels of these three protein expressions were correlated with various clinicopathological characteristics, including patient survival.

2. Patients and Methods

2.1. Patients and Tissue Samples

This study was approved by the Institutional Review Board of Chungnam National University Hospital (CNUH 2019-10-041). All formalin-fixed paraffin-embedded (FFPE) tissue samples for IHC and clinical data were obtained from the National Biobank of Korea at Chungnam National University Hospital. The requirement for informed consent for the retrospective comparison study was waived because the study was based on immunohistochemical analysis using FFPE tissue.

We conducted a review of the records of 97 patients with UCB between 1999 and 2014 at Chungnam National University Hospital in Daejeon, South Korea. The inclusion criteria were that the FFPE UCB tissues were available, and that the follow-up clinical data were sufficiently detailed. The exclusion criteria were as follows: (1) patients had a previous history of other cancers; (2) patients had received previous curative resection for any urinary tract tumor lesion; (3) patients had received preoperative chemotherapy or radiation therapy; or (4) patients had received any molecular targeted therapy. The tumor, node, and metastasis (TNM) staging and histologic grading for UCB were determined at the time of tumor resection, and were based on the 8th edition of the American Joint Committee on Cancer (AJCC) staging system [19].

The 97 UCB cases included 4 cases of noninvasive papillary urothelial carcinoma, 24 cases of pT1, 40 cases of pT2, 26 cases of pT3, and 3 cases of pT4. The 28 patients who underwent transurethral resection of the bladder (TUR-B) were in the pathologic tumor stage (pT) pTa–pT1; the 69 patients who underwent total or partial cystectomy were pT2–pT4. The histologic type of all 97 cases was conventional urothelial carcinoma. For the 69 cases of pT2–pT4, data were collected regarding their disease-free survival (DFS) and overall survival (OS) periods. Among the 69 cases, 29 patients underwent post-operative radiotherapy (PORT). DFS was determined as the time interval between the date of initial surgical resection and the date of UCB recurrence or metastasis. UCB recurrence or metastasis was determined via imaging and/or histological analysis. OS was defined as from the time of initial surgical resection to the date of death due to any cause. Without confirmation of death, recurrence, or metastasis, OS or DFS time was recorded based on the last known date that the patient was alive. We used representative FFPE whole-tissue samples of 97 UCB cases for immunohistochemistry (IHC).

2.2. *Immunohistochemical Staining Analysis*

Immunohistochemical staining of the FFPE tissue sample of UCB was conducted as previously described [20]. Target Retrieval Solution, pH 9 (catalog #S2368, Dako, Glostrup, Denmark), was used for antigen revitalization. The tissue sections were incubated for 30 min at room temperature with the following primary antibodies: rabbit polyclonal anti-human c-erbB-2 oncoprotein (1:200, catalog #A0485, Dako, Glostrup, Denmark), rabbit polyclonal anti-PD-L1 antibody (1:200, catalog #GTX104763, CD274 molecule, GeneTex, Irvine, CA, USA), mouse monoclonal anti-indoleamine 2,3-dioxygenase antibody, clone 10.1 (1:100, catalog #MAB5412, MERCK, Bellanca, MA, USA), CD8 (Ready-to-Use, catalog #IR623, Dako, Glostrup, Denmark), and CD43 (Ready-to-Use, catalog #IR636, Dako, Glostrup, Denmark).

We only scored HER2, IDO, and PD-L1 IHC stains for invasive urothelial carcinoma cells of 93 invasive UCB cases, while four cases of noninvasive papillary urothelial carcinoma were evaluated for intraepithelial dysplastic urothelial cells. We analyzed the cytoplasmic or cytoplasmic membrane expression of HER2 using the modified DAKO HercepTest ™ Interpretation Manual—Breast Cancer Row version [21] (Staining scored 0, 1+, 2+ and 3+). Staining of 2+ or 3+ was regarded as high expression of HER2. The PD-L1 IHC staining was interpreted using the PD-L1 IHC 22C3 pharmDx Interpretation Manual—Urothelial Carcinoma [22] and VENTANA PD-L1 (SP142) Assay Interpretation Guide for Urothelial Carcinoma [23]. Any convincing partial or complete linear cytoplasmic membrane staining of viable tumor cells (TCs) exceeding 1% of the tumor cell proportion was defined as high expression of TC. Presence of discernible PD-L1, CD43, and CD8 staining of any intensity in the tumor-infiltrating immune cells (ICs) covering ≥1% of the tumor area was regarded as high expression of ICs. For CD43 and CD8, we only scored IHC staining of tumor microenvironment ICs in the muscularis propria of 61 cystectomized UCB cases among 67 cases of pT2–pT4. IDO cytoplasmic expression in TCs was scored using the method described by Allred et al. (score 0–8) [24]. A high expression of IDO was regarded as a median score or above (score ≥5). The results were examined separately and scored by Kim, K-H, and Kim, J-M, who were blinded to the patients' clinicopathological details. Any discrepancies in the scores were discussed to obtain a consensus.

2.3. TIMER Database Analysis

TIMER is a comprehensive resource for systematic analysis of immune infiltrates across diverse cancer types (https://cistrome.shinyapps.io/timer/) [25]. TIMER applies a deconvolution previously published statistical method to infer the abundance of tumor-infiltrating immune cells (TIICs) from gene expression profiles [26]. We investigated the relationship between tumor-infiltrating immune cells and UCB survival outcomes. Additionally, we analyzed the correlation of PDL1, IDO, CTLA4, CCL1, CCL2, and CCR2 expression with the abundance of CD8+ T cells.

2.4. Statistical Analyses

The correlations of the clinicopathological parameters with expressions of HER2, IDO, and PD-L1 were evaluated using Pearson's chi-square test and Fisher's exact test. The associations between HER2, IDO, PD-L1, CD43 and CD8 proteins were examined by Spearman rank correlation coefficients. Postoperative OS and DFS were determined using Kaplan–Meier survival curves and a log-rank test. The Cox proportional hazards model was applied for univariate and multivariate survival analyses. The mean values of absolute lymphocyte count (ALC), absolute neutrophil count (ANC), and neutrophil to lymphocyte ratio (NLR) were compared for the subgroups with HER2, IDO, PD-L1 (TCs), and PD-L1 (ICs) expression using an unpaired Student's t-test. Statistical significance was set at $p < 0.05$ (SPSS v.24; SPSS Inc., Chicago, IL, USA).

3. Results

3.1. Association of Immune Cell Infiltration with Survival and Expression of Immune Escape Genes

Even if there is evidence for the action of various immune cell populations in bladder cancer, a comprehensive landscape of the immune response to UCB and its driving forces is still lacking. Therefore, we tried to identify the correlation between immune cell infiltration of this cancer and survival by using the TIMER (Tumor IMmune Estimation Resource) database. In UCB, only the immune infiltrating level of CD8+ T cells was negatively correlated with survival (Figure S1). These results are in line with the tumorcidial function of CD8+ T in immune cells, which can be mitigated by the immune escape mechanism [27].

It was reported that various molecules may be involved in tumor-induced immune tolerance in UCB [28,29]. Therefore, we evaluated the correlation between CD8+ T cell infiltration of UCB and these molecules by using TIMER. Among various molecules, PD-L1 and IDO1 expression are most highly correlated with CD8+ T cell infiltration in UCB (Table S1).

3.2. Association of Clinicopathological Characteristics with Expression of HER2, IDO and PD-L1

The 97 UCB cases were evaluated using IHC to determine HER2, IDO, and PD-L1 levels. The clinicopathological characteristics of the 97 UCB patients associated with expressions of HER2, IDO, and PD-L1 are presented in Table 1. Most non-neoplastic urothelial epithelial cells or noninvasive urothelial carcinoma cells showed no expression of PD-L1, while HER2 and IDO were generally expressed with mild to moderate intensity in a large majority of reactive urothelial cells or noninvasive intraepithelial urothelial carcinoma cells, while there was no expression of IDO in normal urothelial epithelia. Invasive UCB cancer cells in lamina propria showed a relatively decreased expression of HER2 or IDO in comparison to the expression of reactive or dysplastic intraepithelial urothelial cells (Figure 1). Invasive UCB was scored using IHC stains of deeper invasive cancer lesions, except for intraepithelial lesion. However, the noninvasive papillary urothelial carcinomas were evaluated for intraepithelial dysplastic urothelial cells. Expression of HER2 or IDO in the 97 cases of UCB showed trends of decreased expression in pT2–pT4 compared to pTa–pT1 ($p = 0.055$ and $p = 0.0007$). However, PD-L1 expression of ICs was higher in pT2–pT4 than in pTa–pT1 ($p = 0.001$). HER2 expression in TCs was marginally associated with ALC /μL ($p = 0.069$). IDO expression in TCs was positively correlated with ALC /μL ($p = 0.030$) and was negatively correlated with ANC /μL ($p = 0.007$) and NLR ($p = 0.050$).

PD-L1 expression in ICs was positively correlated with ANC /μL (p = 0.041) and NLR (p = 0.063) (Table S2).

Table 1. Correlations of HER2, IDO, and PD-L1 expressions with clinicopathological factors in 97 patients with urothelial carcinoma of the bladder.

Variable	No.	HER2			IDO			PD-L1 (TCs)			PD-L1 (ICs)		
		Low	High	p *	Low	High	p *	Low	High	p *	Low	High	p *
Gender		$N = 46$	$N = 51$	**0.605**	$N = 45$	$N = 52$	**0.676**	$N = 52$	$N = 45$	**0.102**	$N = 48$	$N = 49$	**0.760**
Male	78	38	40		37	41		45	33		38	40	
Female	19	8	11		8	11		7	12		10	9	
Age (years)				0.087			0.164			0.900			0.732
≤65	36	13	23		20	16		19	17		17	19	
>65	61	33	28		25	36		33	28		31	30	
Grade				1.000			0.029			1.000			0.436
low	6	3	3		0	6		3	3		4	2	
high	91	43	48		45	46		49	42		44	47	
Tumor stage				0.055			0.007			0.179			0.001
pTa–pT1	28	9	19		7	21		18	10		21	7	
pT2–pT4	69	37	32		38	31		34	35		27	42	

* Pearson's chi-square test or Fisher's exact test.

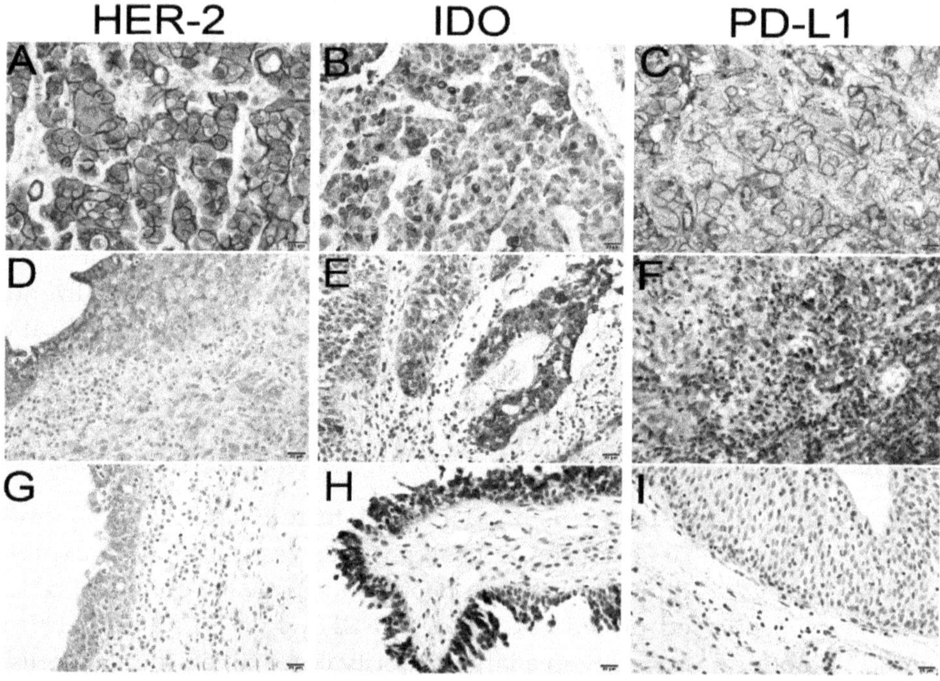

Figure 1. Representative images of HER2, IDO, and PD-L1 immunohistochemical staining in urothelial carcinoma of the bladder (UCB). (**A–C**) Invasive cancer cells with strongly positive expressions of HER2, IDO, and PD-L1. (**D**) Intermediate positive expression of HER2 in low-grade noninvasive urothelial tumor (left upper) and very weakly positive expression of HER2 in invasive cancer cells (right lower). (**E**) Intermediate positive expression of IDO in a low-grade noninvasive urothelial tumor (left) and strongly positive expression of IDO in a high-grade urothelial tumor (right). (**F**) Strongly positive expression of PD-L1 in intra-tumoral immune cells. (**G**) Weakly positive expression of HER2 in reactive urothelial epithelium. (**H**) Strongly positive in situ expression of IDO in urothelial carcinoma. (**I**) Negative expression of PD-L1 in reactive urothelium (scale bar = 20 μm).

3.3. Correlation Between Expression of HER2, IDO, PD-L1, CD43 and CD8 Measured in Tumor Cells or Immune Cells

The correlation between expression of the five proteins is presented in Table 2. CD43 is one of the major glycoproteins of thymocytes and T lymphocytes, suggesting a negative regulatory role in adaptive immune reactions as one of the positive markers of myeloid-derived suppressor cell phenotyping. The inverse correlation between PD-L1 expression in ICs and IDO expression in TCs was observed ($p = 0.010$). HER2 expression in TC was marginally associated with IDO expression in TCs ($p = 0.058$). There was significant positive correlation between the expression of PD-L1, CD43 and CD8 in ICs. There was a tendency to have a negative feedback phenomenon between the expression of IDO and HER2 in TC and the expression of PD-L1, CD43, and CD8 in ICs.

Table 2. Correlations between HER2, IDO, PD-L1, CD43, and CD8 expression according to immunohistochemical staining of urothelial carcinoma of the bladder.

Spearman's rho		HER2 (TCs)	IDO (TCs)	PD-L1 (TCs)	PD-L1 (ICs)	CD43 (ICs)	CD8 (ICs)
HER2 (TCs)	Correlation coefficient	1.000	0.193	−0.110	−0.155	−0.091	−0.021
	Sig. (2-tailed) *	-	0.058	0.283	0.129	0.485	0.875
	No.	97	97	97	97	61	61
IDO (TCs)	Correlation coefficient	0.193	1.000	−0.171	−0.259 *	−0.247	−0.126
	Sig. (2-tailed) *	0.058	-	0.094	0.010	0.055	0.334
	No.	97	97	97	97	61	61
PD-L1 (TCs)	Correlation coefficient	−0.110	−0.171	1.000	0.383 **	0.242	0.175
	Sig. (2-tailed) *	0.283	0.094	-	0.000	0.060	0.177
	No.	97	97	97	97	61	61
PD-L1 (ICs)	Correlation coefficient	−0.155	−0.259 *	0.383 **	1.000	0.429 **	0.470 **
	Sig. (2-tailed) *	0.129	0.010	0.000	-	0.001	0.000
	No.	97	97	97	97	61	61
CD43 (ICs)	Correlation coefficient	−0.091	−0.247	0.242	0.429 **	1.000	0.608 **
	Sig. (2-tailed) *	0.485	0.055	0.060	0.001	-	0.000
	No.	61	61	61	61	61	61
CD8 (ICs)	Correlation coefficient	−0.021	−0.126	0.175	0.470 **	0.608 **	1.000
	Sig. (2-tailed) *	0.875	0.334	0.177	0.000	0.000	-
	No.	61	61	61	61	61	61

**, Correlation is significant at the 0.01 level (2-tailed); *, Correlation is significant at the 0.05 level (2-tailed); TC, tumor cell; IC, immune cell.

It has been observed that expression of CD43 and CD8 in tumor microenvironment ICs is generally predominant in the lamina propria rather than the muscle layer. Since CD8 and CD43 expression showed various degrees according to the depth of tumor infiltration, intra-tumoral or contiguous peritumoral ICs in the muscularis propria and deeper layer were evaluated in 61 cases of pT2–pT4 (Figure 2).

3.4. Expression of HER2 or IDO May Predict Shorter Disease-Free Survival Period in 69 Cases of pT2–pT4

In pT2–pT4 cases ($n = 69$), we found that expression of HER2 or IDO in TCs was associated with a shorter DFS in both univariate Cox regression analysis ($p = 0.028$ and $p = 0.048$, respectively) (Table 3) and Kaplan–Meier survival curves ($p = 0.022$ and $p = 0.040$, respectively) (Figure 3). The expression of HER2 in TCs was also associated with shorter OS and DFS periods according to multivariate Cox regression analysis for HER2 expression, IDO expression, gender, age, pathologic tumor stage, and radiation therapy after surgery ($p = 0.031$ and $p = 0.019$, respectively) (Table 4). The PD-L1 expression in TCs or ICs showed no correlation with survival outcome (Table 3 and Figure 3), even though the PD-L1 expression of ICs was higher in pT2–pT4 than in pTa–pT1 ($p = 0.001$). The expression of CD43 and CD8 in ICs showed no correlation with survival outcome. In 29 cases of pT2–pT4 with radiation therapy after surgery, the expression of HER2 or IDO in TCs showed an association with shorter DFS in Kaplan–Meier survival curves ($p = 0.061$ and $p = 0.033$) (Figure 4).

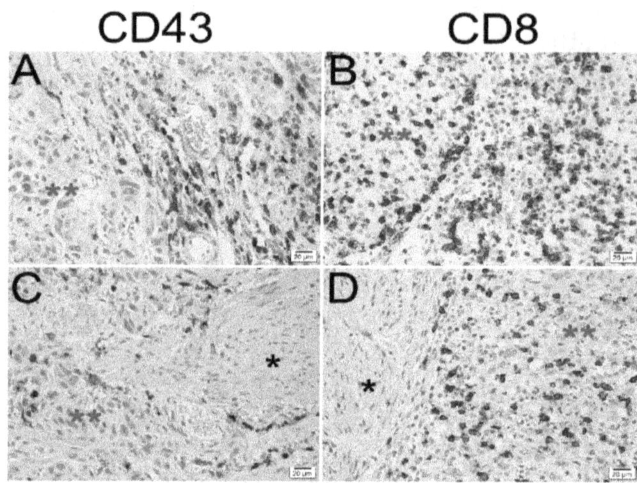

Figure 2. Representative images of CD43 and CD8 immunohistochemical staining in urothelial carcinoma of the bladder (UCB). Positive expression of CD43 and CD8 in intra-tumoral or contiguous peritumoral immune cells of lamina propria invasion (**A**,**B**) and muscularis propria (**C**,**D**) (scale bar = 20 μm; *, muscularis propria; and **, tumor cells).

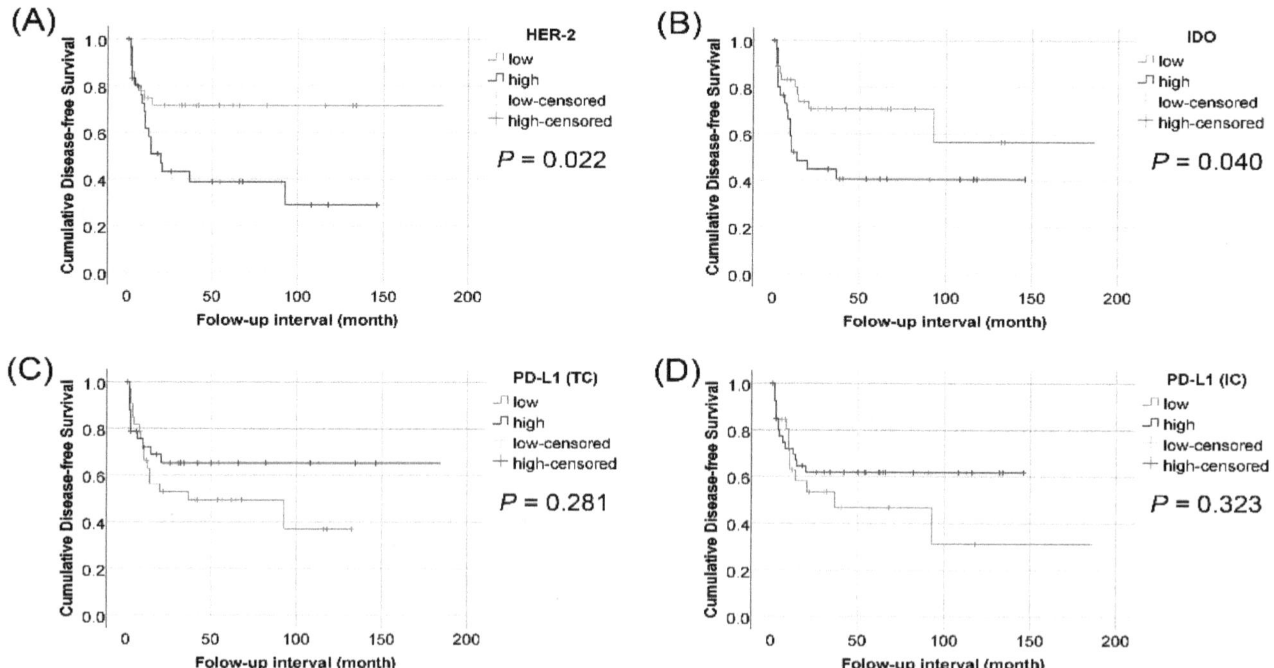

Figure 3. Kaplan–Meier survival curves of disease-free survival in 69 patients with pathologic tumor stage pT2–pT4 urothelial carcinoma of the bladder according to expression of HER2 in tumor cells, IDO in tumor cells, PD-L1 in tumor cells, and PD-L1 in immune cells. (**A**) HER2; (**B**) IDO; (**C**) PD-L1 (TCs); (**D**) PD-L1 (ICs)).

Table 3. Univariate analysis of overall survival and disease-free survival in 69 patients with pathologic tumor stage pT2–pT4 urothelial carcinoma of the bladder.

	Overall Survival			Disease-free Survival		
	P *	**HR**	**95% CI**	***P*** *	**HR**	**95% CI**
HER2 expression (TCs)	0.143			0.028		
Low		1 (reference)			1 (reference)	
High		1.792	0.822–3.907		2.381	1.097–5.169
IDO expression (TCs)	0.683			0.048		
Low		1 (reference)			1 (reference)	
High		0.850	0.390–1.852		2.158	1.007–4.622
PD-L1 expression (TCs)	0.854			0.291		
Low		1 (reference)			1 (reference)	
High		1.075	0.498–2.320		0.664	0.311–1.420
PD-L1 expression (ICs)	0.741			0.333		
Low		1 (reference)			1 (reference)	
High		1.146	0.510–2.577		0.692	0.329–1.458
Gender	0.360			0.164		
Male		1 (reference)			1 (reference)	
Female		0.605	0.206–1.774		0.425	0.128–1.417
Age (years)	0.357			0.922		
≤65		1 (reference)			1 (reference)	
>65		1.481	0.643–3.413		0.962	0.444–2.085
Tumor stage	0.016			0.804		
pT2		1 (reference)			1 (reference)	
pT3–pT4		2.639	1.196–5.824		1.100	0.520–2.326
Radiation therapy after surgery	0.395			0.716		
No		1 (reference)			1 (reference)	
Yes		0.706	0.316–1.576		0.870	0.410–1.844

* univariate Cox regression analysis; HR, hazard ratio; CI, confidence interval; TC, tumor cell; IC, immune cell.

Table 4. Multivariate analysis of overall survival and disease-free survival in 69 patients with pathologic tumor stage pT2–pT4 urothelial carcinoma of the bladder.

	Overall Survival			Disease-free Survival		
	P	**HR**	**95% CI**	***P***	**HR**	**95% CI**
HER2 expression (TCs)	0.031			0.019		
Low		1 (reference)			1 (reference)	
High		2.501	1.090–5.743		2.729	0.076–6.332
IDO expression (TCs)	0.545			0.101		
Low		1 (reference)			1 (reference)	
High		0.772	0.334–1.786		1.988	0.876–4.514
Gender	0.350			0.054		
Male		1 (reference)			1 (reference)	
Female		0.576	0.181–1.833		0.283	0.078–1.024

Table 4. *Cont.*

	Overall Survival			Disease-free Survival		
	P	HR	95% CI	*P*	HR	95% CI
Age (years)	0.107			0.858		
≤65		1 (reference)			1 (reference)	
>65		2.036	0.858–4.833		1.079	0.470–2.476
Tumor stage	0.045			0.886		
pT2		1 (reference)			1 (reference)	
pT3–pT4		2.424	1.020–5.760		0.942	0.419–2.118
Radiation therapy after surgery	0.744			0.505		
No		1 (reference)			1 (reference)	
Yes		0.867	0.369–2.039		0.766	0.350–1.675

* multivariate Cox regression analysis; HR, hazard ratio; CI, confidence interval; TC, tumor cell; IC, immune cell.

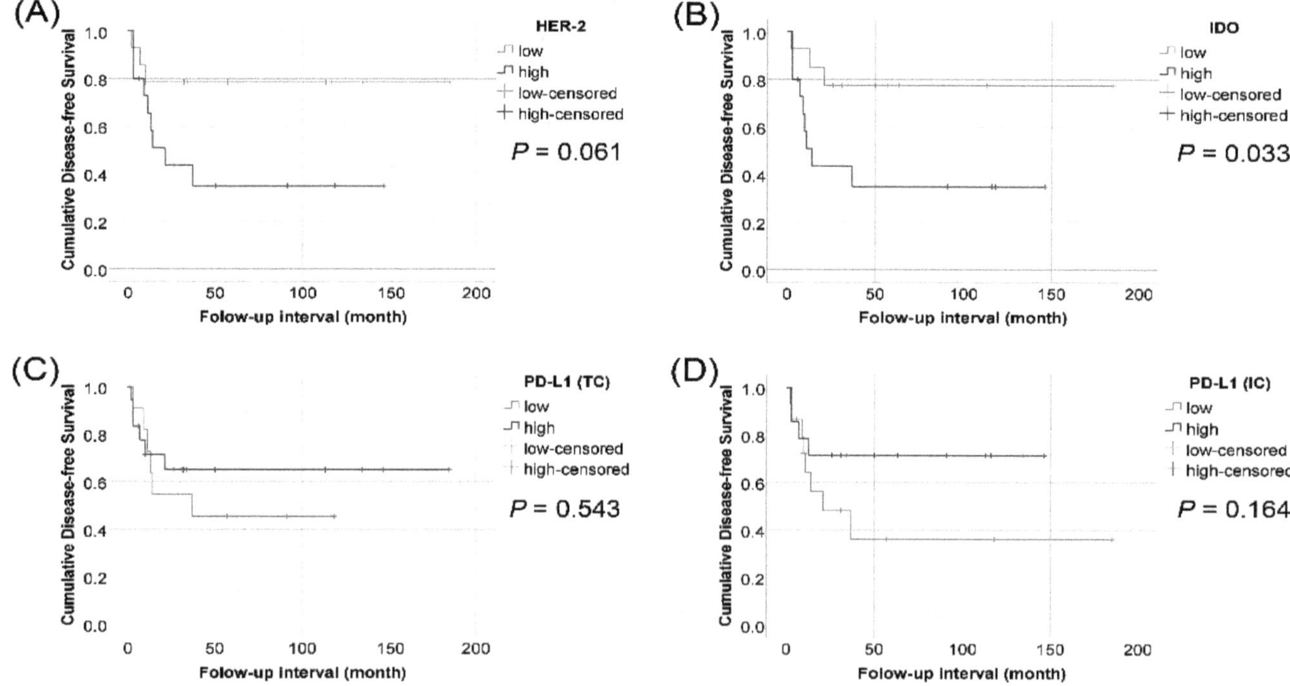

Figure 4. Kaplan–Meier survival curves of disease-free survival in 29 cases with post-operative radiotherapy among 69 patients of pathologic tumor stage pT2–pT4 urothelial carcinoma of the bladder, according to expression of HER2 in tumor cells, IDO in tumor cells, PD-L1 in tumor cells, and PD-L1 in immune cells. (**A**) HER2; (**B**) IDO; (**C**) PD-L1 (TCs); (**D**) PD-L1 (ICs)).

4. Discussion

In this study, we evaluated the expression of HER2, IDO, and PD-L1 in 97 UCB cases. The three proteins showed a correlation with tumor progression or patient outcome, although they did not show the same trends for clinicopathological correlations. We demonstrated that PD-L1 expression in ICs was significantly higher in pT2–pT4 than in pTa–pT1. Increased HER2 and IDO levels in TCs of 69 pT2–pT4 cases were positively correlated with a shorter DFS period, and could be considered potential factors in poor disease outcomes.

The roles of HER2 and IDO protein in cancer initiation or progression are still poorly understood. The consistent association between the effects of anti-HER2 therapies and immune infiltration has been reported in breast cancer and supports that an anti-tumor immune response can modulate the effect of anti-HER2 therapy [30,31]. In our study, the invasive UCB cancer cells showed a relatively reduced expression of HER2 or IDO in comparison to the expression of reactive or dysplastic intraepithelial urothelial cells. In pTa–pT1 UCBs, the expression of HER2 and IDO increased relative to that of pT2–pT4, apart from that, in pT2–pT4 cases, increased expressions of the two proteins are associated with reduced DFS expression. The altered expression of IDO or HER2 could be interpreted to be a different phase or play a different role for cancer immunoediting to the immune response against noninvasive UCB and invasive UCB [30,32,33]. Our data show a significant positive correlation between the expression of PD-L1, CD43 and CD8 in ICs. It has been observed that there is higher expression of CD43 and CD8 in lamina propria invasion in comparison to muscularis propria invasion. Moreover, there was a tendency to have a reverse correlation between the expression of IDO and HER2 in TCs and the expression of PD-L1, CD43 and CD8 in ICs. Cancer immunoediting describes a complex mechanism between ICs and TCs and has three phases: elimination, equilibrium and escape [34]. In the final escape phase, the expression of IDO in cancer cells inhibits the host immune protection. Paradoxically, IDO is elevated upon various immune molecules of adaptive or innate or tolerogenic immune cells. We speculate that elevated levels of IDO and HER2 in TC may reflect a tumor microenvironment immune reaction. And those immune-evasive transformed cancer cells may reduce IDO expression after down-regulation of immune response with a negative feedback mechanism [30,33,35]. It is predicted that in early cancer development, the expression of IDO or HER2 is upregulated in the majority of cancer cells stimulated by various immune molecules, including IFN-γ, IL-10, IL-27, CTLA4, TGF-β, cyclooxygenase-2 and prostaglandin E2, which are regulated by tumor antigen level or tolerogenic tumor microenvironment [33]. In advanced invasive cancer, the two proteins could be continuously expressed in a relatively reduced number of poorly immunogenic and immune evasive transformed cancer cells, which can lead to a poor prognosis [34]. Therefore, a spatial and periodic variety of cancer immunoediting phase could be in the same tumor mass.

In UCB, HER2 expression status has been evaluated since 1990, when overexpression of HER2 protein was first reported [36]. One study of high-grade UCB (pT2–pT4) ranked the *HER2* gene amplification as the third most significant in terms of associated genetic mutations [37]. Although the first study on the relationship of HER2 expression with clinical outcomes is confounding, a meta-analysis has indicated that its expression is associated with tumor grade, lymph node metastasis, and poor prognosis in UCB [38]. Even so, recent studies have not produced encouraging results for HER2 targeted therapy as a strategy against UCB [39–41]. The major scientific reasons for the failure of HER2 targeted therapy are a lack of standardization of HER2 testing and co-expression of other immunomodulatory molecules [42]. To overcome the poor results achieved thus far with anti-HER2 therapy, it is necessary to identify correlations between HER2 and immune checkpoint proteins in UCB. Our study reported that HER2 expression is marginally associated with IDO expression. To the best of our knowledge, this is the first study to correlate HER2 and immunosuppressive molecules in UCB.

Anti-HER2 therapy has revolutionized the treatment of malignant tumors, especially overexpressing breast cancer. Furthermore, with increasing concentrations of anticancer immunotherapy, the connection between HER2 expression and antitumor immunity has emerged as a possible target for combined oncological treatment. The whole-transcriptome profiling of HER2-positive breast carcinomas has revealed a remarkable enrichment in immune pathways [43]. HER2-positive trastuzumab-sensitive breast carcinomas have shown positive associations with chemokines involved in immune cell infiltration of the tumor microenvironment and the expression of PD-1 ligands in tumor cells [16,44]. HER2 expression has recently been found to suppress antiviral defenses and antitumor immunity as a result of HER2 signaling through its intracellular domain, which interferes with cyclic GMP-AMP synthase-stimulator of interferon genes (cGAS-STING) pathway and prevents cancer cell death [45]. Therefore, innate and adaptive immune system responses are increasingly being acknowledged as important regulators of the effects of HER2 targeted therapy [46,47]. Based on previous research, in this study HER2 expression was scored in the cytoplasm as well as the cytoplasmic membrane to include the immune systemic function of the intracellular domain of HER2 signaling. Considering the role of HER2 protein in interfering with antitumor immunity in the cytoplasm, the indications for HER2 targeted therapy are not limited to the cytoplasmic membrane expression of HER2 and we expect that they may also be extended to HER2 protein expression in the cytoplasm of cancer cells.

IDO, also referred to as IDO1, is one of the cytosolic enzymes that catalyzes the initial and rate-limiting steps of tryptophan to kynurenine [33,48]. IDO has been described as having immunosuppressive functions on host immune surveillance of tumor cells, with a focus on its potential immunotherapeutic targets [49]. The role of IDO has been implicated in immune tolerance related to the suppression of T-cell responses such as fetal tolerance, tumor resistance, chronic infections, and autoimmune diseases [50]. One study delineated the action of kynurenine to promote apoptosis in murine bone marrow-derived neutrophils, providing a possible mechanism for increased neutrophil accumulation in IDO-deficient mice [51]. Our results show that IDO expression is correlated with increased ALC and decreased ANC. These findings support previous studies on the immunomodulatory functions of IDO, although its effects or mechanisms in tumor progression remain unclear. IDO expression in TCs showed a negative correlation with ANC and positive correlation with ALC, while the PD-L1 expression in ICs was positively correlated with ANC in the 97 UCB cases.

Recently, phase II and preliminary phase III studies have shown that the application of a PD-L1 inhibitor in metastatic platinum-refractory NSCLC and urothelial cancer resulted in a significant improvement in the response rate and median overall survival [52]. Furthermore, PD-L1 tumor expression has emerged as a biomarker for patient stratification in immunotherapy targeting for the PD-L1/PD-1 pathway, particularly for NSCLC [53]. However, the prognostic impact of this molecule in tumor tissue is still controversial in various cancers, such as NSCLC and head and neck squamous cell carcinoma, because of the high discrepancies between PD-L1 expression and treatment outcomes [54,55]. Some studies have emphasized the significance of a comprehensive evaluation of PD-L1 expression on tumor and immune cells because its expression in immune cells, but not tumor cells, is a favorable prognostic factor for NSCLC and HNSCC [55–57]. However, our results show that PD-L1 expression in ICs is a significant poor prognostic factor in UCB.

Radiotherapy induces a host immune response by exposing tumor-specific antigens that make tumor cells detectable by the immune system, promoting the priming and activation of cytotoxic T cells [58]. Furthermore, radiation may have an impact on the tumor microenvironment by facilitating the recruitment and infiltration of immune cells [58–60]. Although radiotherapy acts as an in-situ tumor vaccine, it may be insufficient to sustain long-term antitumor immunity, resulting in later relapse [61]. Therefore, there are many studies identifying correlations between molecular regulators of tumor immune escapes and radio-resistance. PD-L1 positive cancer cells have been demonstrated to have a radio-resistant phenotype, inhibiting T cell signaling and T cell-mediated immunogenic cell death [62]. HER2 activation is a potential mechanism that may compromise the outcome of radiotherapy [63,64]. Additionally, in vitro and in vivo experiments blocking PD-L1 and IDO alongside radiation have successfully overcome rebound immune suppression [65,66]. Similarly, our data reveal that the expression of HER2 and IDO are significantly associated with DFS in UCB treated with radiotherapy after surgery (Figure 4).

5. Conclusions

The present study is the first to measure the expression levels of IDO, HER2, and PD-L1 and to analyze the correlation between these three proteins and clinicopathological values in UCB. The expression of IDO and HER2 in TCs and PD-L1 in ICs were positively correlated with poor prognostic factors in pT2–pT4 cases, including shorter DFS and OS periods or higher tumor stage. Our results suggest that the expression of IDO, HER2, and PD-L1 are useful as predictive prognostic factors and could potentially be utilized for the development of combined cancer immunotherapeutic strategies.

Author Contributions: Conceptualization, K.-H.K.; Data curation, K.-H.K., D.K. and S.K.; Funding acquisition, K.-H.K. and S.K.; Investigation, K.-H.K., D.K. and S.K.; Methodology, S.K. and K.-H.K.; Project administration, K.-H.K.; Resources, J.-S.K., J.M.K., S.K. and K.-H.K.; Supervision, K.-H.K.; Validation, S.K. and J.M.K.; Writing–original draft, S.K. and K.-H.K.; Writing–review & editing, D.K., J.M.K., J.-S.K., S.K. and K.-H.K. All authors have read and agreed to the published version of the manuscript.

References

1. Siegel, R.; Naishadham, D.; Jemal, A. Cancer statistics, 2012. *CA Cancer J. Clin.* **2012**, *62*, 10–29. [CrossRef] [PubMed]
2. Kirkali, Z.; Chan, T.; Manoharan, M.; Algaba, F.; Busch, C.; Cheng, L.; Kiemeney, L.; Kriegmair, M.; Montironi, R.; Murphy, W.M.; et al. Bladder cancer: Epidemiology, staging and grading, and diagnosis. *Urology* **2005**, *66*, 4–34. [CrossRef] [PubMed]
3. Porter, M.P.; Kerrigan, M.C.; Donato, B.M.; Ramsey, S.D. Patterns of use of systemic chemotherapy for Medicare beneficiaries with urothelial bladder cancer. *Urol. Oncol.* **2011**, *29*, 252–258. [CrossRef] [PubMed]
4. Meeks, J.J.; Bellmunt, J.; Bochner, B.H.; Clarke, N.W.; Daneshmand, S.; Galsky, M.D.; Hahn, N.M.; Lerner, S.P.; Mason, M.; Powles, T.; et al. A systematic review of neoadjuvant and adjuvant chemotherapy for muscle-invasive bladder cancer. *Eur. Urol.* **2012**, *62*, 523–533. [CrossRef] [PubMed]
5. Helmy, K.Y.; Patel, S.A.; Nahas, G.R.; Rameshwar, P. Cancer immunotherapy: Accomplishments to date and future promise. *Ther. Deliv.* **2013**, *4*, 1307–1320. [CrossRef] [PubMed]
6. Salmon, H.; Remark, R.; Gnjatic, S.; Merad, M. Host tissue determinants of tumour immunity. *Nat. Rev. Cancer* **2019**, *19*, 215–227. [CrossRef]
7. Box, C.; Rogers, S.J.; Mendiola, M.; Eccles, S.A. Tumour-microenvironmental interactions: Paths to progression and targets for treatment. *Semin. Cancer Biol.* **2010**, *20*, 128–138. [CrossRef]
8. Blankenstein, T.; Coulie, P.G.; Gilboa, E.; Jaffee, E.M. The determinants of tumour immunogenicity. *Nat. Rev. Cancer* **2012**, *12*, 307–313. [CrossRef]
9. Kroemer, G.; Galluzzi, L.; Kepp, O.; Zitvogel, L. Immunogenic cell death in cancer therapy. *Annu. Rev. Immunol.* **2013**, *31*, 51–72. [CrossRef] [PubMed]
10. Krysko, D.V.; Garg, A.D.; Kaczmarek, A.; Krysko, O.; Agostinis, P.; Vandenabeele, P. Immunogenic cell death and DAMPs in cancer therapy. *Nat. Rev. Cancer* **2012**, *12*, 860–875. [CrossRef]
11. Huang, Y.; Zhang, S.D.; McCrudden, C.; Chan, K.W.; Lin, Y.; Kwok, H.F. The prognostic significance of PD-L1 in bladder cancer. *Oncol. Rep.* **2015**, *33*, 3075–3084. [CrossRef] [PubMed]
12. Hudolin, T.; Mengus, C.; Coulot, J.; Kastelan, Z.; El-Saleh, A.; Spagnoli, G.C. Expression of Indoleamine 2,3-Dioxygenase Gene Is a Feature of Poorly Differentiated Non-muscle-invasive Urothelial Cell Bladder Carcinomas. *Anticancer Res.* **2017**, *37*, 1375–1380. [CrossRef] [PubMed]
13. Yang, C.; Zhou, Y.; Zhang, L.; Jin, C.; Li, M.; Ye, L. Expression and function analysis of indoleamine 2 and 3-dioxygenase in bladder urothelial carcinoma. *Int. J. Clin. Exp. Pathol.* **2015**, *8*, 1768–1775. [PubMed]
14. Chism, D.D. Urothelial Carcinoma of the Bladder and the Rise of Immunotherapy. *J. Natl. Compr. Canc. Netw.* **2017**, *15*, 1277–1284. [CrossRef]
15. Bellati, F.; Napoletano, C.; Ruscito, I.; Liberati, M.; Panici, P.B.; Nuti, M. Cellular adaptive immune system plays a crucial role in trastuzumab clinical efficacy. *J. Clin. Oncol.* **2010**, *28*, e369–e370. [CrossRef]
16. Triulzi, T.; Forte, L.; Regondi, V.; Di Modica, M.; Ghirelli, C.; Carcangiu, M.L.; Sfondrini, L.; Balsari, A.; Tagliabue, E. HER2 signaling regulates the tumor immune microenvironment and trastuzumab efficacy. *Oncoimmunology* **2019**, *8*, e1512942. [CrossRef]
17. Suh, K.J.; Sung, J.H.; Kim, J.W.; Han, S.H.; Lee, H.S.; Min, A.; Kang, M.H.; Kim, J.E.; Kim, J.W.; Kim, S.H.; et al. EGFR or HER2 inhibition modulates the tumor microenvironment by suppression of PD-L1 and cytokines release. *Oncotarget* **2017**, *8*, 63901–63910. [CrossRef]
18. Soliman, H.; Rawal, B.; Fulp, J.; Lee, J.H.; Lopez, A.; Bui, M.M.; Khalil, F.; Antonia, S.; Yfantis, H.G.; Lee, D.H.; et al. Analysis of indoleamine 2-3 dioxygenase (IDO1) expression in breast cancer tissue by immunohistochemistry. *Cancer Immunol. Immunother.* **2013**, *62*, 829–837. [CrossRef]
19. Amin, M.; Edge, S.; Greene, F.; Byrd, D.R.; Brookland, R.K.; Washington, M.K. *AJCC Cancer Staging Manual*, 8th ed.; Springer: Chicago, IL, USA, 2017.

20. Yeo, M.K.; Kim, J.M.; Suh, K.S.; Kim, S.H.; Lee, O.J.; Kim, K.H. Decreased Expression of the Polarity Regulatory PAR Complex Predicts Poor Prognosis of the Patients with Colorectal Adenocarcinoma. *Transl. Oncol.* **2018**, *11*, 109–115. [CrossRef]
21. HercepTest™, Interpretation Manual Breast Cancer. Available online: https://www.agilent.com/cs/library/usermanuals/public/28630_herceptest_interpretation_manual-breast_ihc_row.pdf (accessed on 26 April 2020).
22. PD-L1 IHC 22C3 pharmDx Interpretation Manual—Urothelial Carcinoma. Available online: https://www.agilent.com/cs/library/usermanuals/public/29276_22C3_pharmdx_uc_interpretation_manual_us.pdf (accessed on 26 April 2020).
23. VENTANA PD-L1 (SP142) Assay. Available online: https://www.accessdata.fda.gov/cdrh_docs/pdf16/P160002c.pdf (accessed on 26 April 2020).
24. Allred, D.C.; Harvey, J.M.; Berardo, M.; Clark, G.M. Prognostic and predictive factors in breast cancer by immunohistochemical analysis. *Mod. Pathol.* **1998**, *11*, 155–168.
25. Li, T.; Fan, J.; Wang, B.; Traugh, N.; Chen, Q.; Liu, J.S.; Li, B.; Liu, X.S. TIMER: A Web Server for Comprehensive Analysis of Tumor-Infiltrating Immune Cells. *Cancer Res.* **2017**, *77*, e108–e110. [CrossRef] [PubMed]
26. Li, B.; Severson, E.; Pignon, J.C.; Zhao, H.; Li, T.; Novak, J.; Jiang, P.; Shen, H.; Aster, J.C.; Rodig, S.; et al. Comprehensive analyses of tumor immunity: Implications for cancer immunotherapy. *Genome Biol.* **2016**, *17*, 174. [CrossRef]
27. Rabinovich, G.A.; Gabrilovich, D.; Sotomayor, E.M. Immunosuppressive strategies that are mediated by tumor cells. *Annu. Rev. Immunol.* **2007**, *25*, 267–296. [CrossRef] [PubMed]
28. Crispen, P.L.; Kusmartsev, S. Mechanisms of immune evasion in bladder cancer. *Cancer Immunol. Immunother.* **2020**, *69*, 3–14. [CrossRef] [PubMed]
29. Liu, M.; Wang, X.; Wang, L.; Ma, X.; Gong, Z.; Zhang, S.; Li, Y. Targeting the IDO1 pathway in cancer: From bench to bedside. *J. Hematol. Oncol.* **2018**, *11*, 100. [CrossRef] [PubMed]
30. Teng, M.W.; Galon, J.; Fridman, W.H.; Smyth, M.J. From mice to humans: Developments in cancer immunoediting. *J. Clin. Investig.* **2015**, *125*, 3338–3346. [CrossRef] [PubMed]
31. Bianchini, G.; Gianni, L. The immune system and response to HER2-targeted treatment in breast cancer. *Lancet Oncol.* **2014**, *15*, e58–e68. [CrossRef]
32. Kim, R.; Emi, M.; Tanabe, K. Cancer immunoediting from immune surveillance to immune escape. *Immunology* **2007**, *121*, 1–14. [CrossRef]
33. Hornyak, L.; Dobos, N.; Koncz, G.; Karanyi, Z.; Pall, D.; Szabo, Z.; Halmos, G.; Szekvolgyi, L. The Role of Indoleamine-2,3-Dioxygenase in Cancer Development, Diagnostics, and Therapy. *Front. Immunol.* **2018**, *9*, 151. [CrossRef]
34. Schreiber, R.D.; Old, L.J.; Smyth, M.J. Cancer immunoediting: Integrating immunity's roles in cancer suppression and promotion. *Science* **2011**, *331*, 1565–1570. [CrossRef]
35. Spranger, S.; Spaapen, R.M.; Zha, Y.; Williams, J.; Meng, Y.; Ha, T.T.; Gajewski, T.F. Up-regulation of PD-L1, IDO, and T(regs) in the melanoma tumor microenvironment is driven by CD8(+) T cells. *Sci. Transl. Med.* **2013**, *5*, 200ra116. [CrossRef]
36. Wright, C.; Mellon, K.; Neal, D.E.; Johnston, P.; Corbett, I.P.; Horne, C.H. Expression of c-erbB-2 protein product in bladder cancer. *Br. J. Cancer* **1990**, *62*, 764–765. [CrossRef] [PubMed]
37. Cancer Genome Atlas Research Network. Comprehensive molecular characterization of urothelial bladder carcinoma. *Nature* **2014**, *507*, 315–322. [CrossRef] [PubMed]
38. Zhao, J.; Xu, W.; Zhang, Z.; Song, R.; Zeng, S.; Sun, Y.; Xu, C. Prognostic role of HER2 expression in bladder cancer: A systematic review and meta-analysis. *Int. Urol. Nephrol.* **2015**, *47*, 87–94. [CrossRef] [PubMed]
39. Oudard, S.; Culine, S.; Vano, Y.; Goldwasser, F.; Theodore, C.; Nguyen, T.; Voog, E.; Banu, E.; Vieillefond, A.; Priou, F.; et al. Multicentre randomised phase II trial of gemcitabine+platinum, with or without trastuzumab, in advanced or metastatic urothelial carcinoma overexpressing Her2. *Eur. J. Cancer* **2015**, *51*, 45–54. [CrossRef] [PubMed]
40. Wulfing, C.; Machiels, J.P.; Richel, D.J.; Grimm, M.O.; Treiber, U.; De Groot, M.R.; Beuzeboc, P.; Parikh, R.; Petavy, F.; El-Hariry, I.A. A single-arm, multicenter, open-label phase 2 study of lapatinib as the second-line treatment of patients with locally advanced or metastatic transitional cell carcinoma. *Cancer* **2009**, *115*, 2881–2890. [CrossRef]

41. Powles, T.; Huddart, R.A.; Elliott, T.; Sarker, S.J.; Ackerman, C.; Jones, R.; Hussain, S.; Crabb, S.; Jagdev, S.; Chester, J.; et al. Phase III, Double-Blind, Randomized Trial That Compared Maintenance Lapatinib Versus Placebo After First-Line Chemotherapy in Patients with Human Epidermal Growth Factor Receptor 1/2-Positive Metastatic Bladder Cancer. *J. Clin. Oncol.* **2017**, *35*, 48–55. [CrossRef]
42. Koshkin, V.S.; O'Donnell, P.; Yu, E.Y.; Grivas, P. Systematic Review: Targeting HER2 in Bladder Cancer. *Bladder Cancer* **2019**, *5*, 1–12. [CrossRef]
43. Triulzi, T.; De Cecco, L.; Sandri, M.; Prat, A.; Giussani, M.; Paolini, B.; Carcangiu, M.L.; Canevari, S.; Bottini, A.; Balsari, A.; et al. Whole-transcriptome analysis links trastuzumab sensitivity of breast tumors to both HER2 dependence and immune cell infiltration. *Oncotarget* **2015**, *6*, 28173–28182. [CrossRef]
44. Gil Del Alcazar, C.R.; Huh, S.J.; Ekram, M.B.; Trinh, A.; Liu, L.L.; Beca, F.; Zi, X.; Kwak, M.; Bergholtz, H.; Su, Y.; et al. Immune Escape in Breast Cancer During In Situ to Invasive Carcinoma Transition. *Cancer Discov.* **2017**, *7*, 1098–1115. [CrossRef]
45. Wu, S.; Zhang, Q.; Zhang, F.; Meng, F.; Liu, S.; Zhou, R.; Wu, Q.; Li, X.; Shen, L.; Huang, J.; et al. HER2 recruits AKT1 to disrupt STING signalling and suppress antiviral defence and antitumour immunity. *Nat. Cell Biol.* **2019**, *21*, 1027–1040. [CrossRef]
46. Verma, S.; Miles, D.; Gianni, L.; Krop, I.E.; Welslau, M.; Baselga, J.; Pegram, M.; Oh, D.Y.; Dieras, V.; Guardino, E.; et al. Trastuzumab emtansine for HER2-positive advanced breast cancer. *N. Engl. J. Med.* **2012**, *367*, 1783–1791. [CrossRef] [PubMed]
47. Ferris, R.L.; Jaffee, E.M.; Ferrone, S. Tumor antigen-targeted, monoclonal antibody-based immunotherapy: Clinical response, cellular immunity, and immunoescape. *J. Clin. Oncol.* **2010**, *28*, 4390–4399. [CrossRef] [PubMed]
48. Brochez, L.; Chevolet, I.; Kruse, V. The rationale of indoleamine 2,3-dioxygenase inhibition for cancer therapy. *Eur. J. Cancer* **2017**, *76*, 167–182. [CrossRef] [PubMed]
49. Zhu, M.M.T.; Dancsok, A.R.; Nielsen, T.O. Indoleamine Dioxygenase Inhibitors: Clinical Rationale and Current Development. *Curr. Oncol. Rep.* **2019**, *21*, 2. [CrossRef]
50. Mellor, A.L.; Munn, D.H. IDO expression by dendritic cells: Tolerance and tryptophan catabolism. *Nat. Rev. Immunol.* **2004**, *4*, 762–774. [CrossRef]
51. El-Zaatari, M.; Chang, Y.M.; Zhang, M.; Franz, M.; Shreiner, A.; McDermott, A.J.; van der Sluijs, K.F.; Lutter, R.; Grasberger, H.; Kamada, N.; et al. Tryptophan catabolism restricts IFN-gamma-expressing neutrophils and Clostridium difficile immunopathology. *J. Immunol.* **2014**, *193*, 807–816. [CrossRef]
52. Krishnamurthy, A.; Jimeno, A. Atezolizumab: A novel PD-L1 inhibitor in cancer therapy with a focus in bladder and non-small cell lung cancers. *Drugs Today* **2017**, *53*, 217–237. [CrossRef]
53. Brody, R.; Zhang, Y.; Ballas, M.; Siddiqui, M.K.; Gupta, P.; Barker, C.; Midha, A.; Walker, J. PD-L1 expression in advanced NSCLC: Insights into risk stratification and treatment selection from a systematic literature review. *Lung Cancer* **2017**, *112*, 200–215. [CrossRef]
54. Takada, K.; Okamoto, T.; Toyokawa, G.; Kozuma, Y.; Matsubara, T.; Haratake, N.; Akamine, T.; Takamori, S.; Katsura, M.; Shoji, F.; et al. The expression of PD-L1 protein as a prognostic factor in lung squamous cell carcinoma. *Lung Cancer* **2017**, *104*, 7–15. [CrossRef]
55. Kim, H.R.; Ha, S.J.; Hong, M.H.; Heo, S.J.; Koh, Y.W.; Choi, E.C.; Kim, E.K.; Pyo, K.H.; Jung, I.; Seo, D.; et al. PD-L1 expression on immune cells, but not on tumor cells, is a favorable prognostic factor for head and neck cancer patients. *Sci. Rep.* **2016**, *6*, 36956. [CrossRef] [PubMed]
56. Bocanegra, A.; Fernandez-Hinojal, G.; Zuazo-Ibarra, M.; Arasanz, H.; Garcia-Granda, M.J.; Hernandez, C.; Ibanez, M.; Hernandez-Marin, B.; Martinez-Aguillo, M.; Lecumberri, M.J.; et al. PD-L1 Expression in Systemic Immune Cell Populations as a Potential Predictive Biomarker of Responses to PD-L1/PD-1 Blockade Therapy in Lung Cancer. *Int. J. Mol. Sci.* **2019**, *20*, 1631. [CrossRef] [PubMed]
57. Birtalan, E.; Danos, K.; Gurbi, B.; Brauswetter, D.; Halasz, J.; Kalocsane Piurko, V.; Acs, B.; Antal, B.; Mihalyi, R.; Pato, A.; et al. Expression of PD-L1 on Immune Cells Shows Better Prognosis in Laryngeal, Oropharygeal, and Hypopharyngeal Cancer. *Appl. Immunohistochem. Mol. Morphol.* **2018**, *26*, e79–e85. [CrossRef] [PubMed]
58. Formenti, S.C.; Demaria, S. Combining radiotherapy and cancer immunotherapy: A paradigm shift. *J. Natl. Cancer Inst.* **2013**, *105*, 256–265. [CrossRef] [PubMed]

59. McBride, W.H.; Chiang, C.S.; Olson, J.L.; Wang, C.C.; Hong, J.H.; Pajonk, F.; Dougherty, G.J.; Iwamoto, K.S.; Pervan, M.; Liao, Y.P. A sense of danger from radiation. *Radiat. Res.* **2004**, *162*, 1–19. [CrossRef]
60. Haikerwal, S.J.; Hagekyriakou, J.; MacManus, M.; Martin, O.A.; Haynes, N.M. Building immunity to cancer with radiation therapy. *Cancer Lett.* **2015**, *368*, 198–208. [CrossRef]
61. Wennerberg, E.; Lhuillier, C.; Vanpouille-Box, C.; Pilones, K.A.; Garcia-Martinez, E.; Rudqvist, N.P.; Formenti, S.C.; Demaria, S. Barriers to Radiation-Induced In Situ Tumor Vaccination. *Front. Immunol.* **2017**, *8*, 229. [CrossRef]
62. Lyu, X.; Zhang, M.; Li, G.; Jiang, Y.; Qiao, Q. PD-1 and PD-L1 Expression Predicts Radiosensitivity and Clinical Outcomes in Head and Neck Cancer and is Associated with HPV Infection. *J. Cancer* **2019**, *10*, 937–948. [CrossRef]
63. Duru, N.; Fan, M.; Candas, D.; Menaa, C.; Liu, H.C.; Nantajit, D.; Wen, Y.; Xiao, K.; Eldridge, A.; Chromy, B.A.; et al. HER2-associated radioresistance of breast cancer stem cells isolated from HER2-negative breast cancer cells. *Clin. Cancer Res.* **2012**, *18*, 6634–6647. [CrossRef]
64. Cao, N.; Li, S.; Wang, Z.; Ahmed, K.M.; Degnan, M.E.; Fan, M.; Dynlacht, J.R.; Li, J.J. NF-kappaB-mediated HER2 overexpression in radiation-adaptive resistance. *Radiat. Res.* **2009**, *171*, 9–21. [CrossRef]
65. Liu, M.; Li, Z.; Yao, W.; Zeng, X.; Wang, L.; Cheng, J.; Ma, B.; Zhang, R.; Min, W.; Wang, H. IDO inhibitor synergized with radiotherapy to delay tumor growth by reversing T cell exhaustion. *Mol. Med. Rep.* **2020**, *21*, 445–453. [CrossRef]
66. Ladomersky, E.; Zhai, L.; Lenzen, A.; Lauing, K.L.; Qian, J.; Scholtens, D.M.; Gritsina, G.; Sun, X.; Liu, Y.; Yu, F.; et al. IDO1 Inhibition Synergizes with Radiation and PD-1 Blockade to Durably Increase Survival Against Advanced Glioblastoma. *Clin. Cancer Res.* **2018**, *24*, 2559–2573. [CrossRef]

Epidemiological Characteristics and Survival in Patients with De Novo Metastatic Prostate Cancer

Carlo Cattrini [1,2,*], Davide Soldato [1,3], Alessandra Rubagotti [3,4], Linda Zinoli [3], Elisa Zanardi [1,3], Paola Barboro [3], Carlo Messina [5], Elena Castro [6], David Olmos [2] and Francesco Boccardo [1,3]

1 Department of Internal Medicine and Medical Specialties (DIMI), School of Medicine, University of Genoa, 16132 Genoa, Italy; davide.soldato@gmail.com (D.S.); elisa.zanardi@unige.it (E.Z.); fboccardo@unige.it (F.B.)
2 Prostate Cancer Clinical Research Unit, Spanish National Cancer Research Centre (CNIO), 28029 Madrid, Spain; dolmos@cnio.es
3 Academic Unit of Medical Oncology, IRCCS Ospedale Policlinico San Martino, 16132 Genoa, Italy; alessandra.rubagotti@unige.it (A.R.); datamanager.omb@unige.it (L.Z.); paola.barboro@hsanmartino.it (P.B.)
4 Department of Health Sciences (DISSAL), School of Medicine, University of Genoa, 16132 Genoa, Italy
5 Department of Medical Oncology, Santa Chiara Hospital, 38122 Trento, Italy; carlo.messina@apss.tn.it
6 CNIO-IBIMA Genitourinary Cancer Unit, Hospitales Universitarios Virgen de la Victoria y Regional de Málaga, Instituto de Investigación Biomédica de Málaga, 29010 Malaga, Spain; ecastro@ext.cnio.es
* Correspondence: ccattrini@cnio.es

Simple Summary: In randomized trials, both chemotherapy and androgen-receptor signaling inhibitors provided significant survival benefits in patients with metastatic prostate cancer (mPCa). However, it is largely unknown to what extent these therapeutic advances have impacted the general, real-world survival of patients with de novo mPCa. Here, we analyzed more than 26,000 patients included in the U.S. Surveillance, Epidemiology, and End Results (SEER) database to describe potential recent improvements in overall and cancer-specific survival. We found that patients diagnosed in the latest years showed a modest reduction in the risk of death and cancer-specific death, compared with those diagnosed in 2000–2003 and 2004–2010. Although our analysis was not adjusted for many confounders, the overall population of patients diagnosed in 2011–2014 only showed a survival gain of 4 months. Patients' ineligibility or refusal of anticancer treatments, insurance issues, intrinsic disease aggressiveness, or prior unavailability of drugs in a hormone-sensitive setting might contribute to these disappointing results.

Abstract: The real-world outcomes of patients with metastatic prostate cancer (mPCa) are largely unexplored. We investigated the trends in overall survival (OS) and cancer-specific survival (CSS) in patients with de novo mPCa according to distinct time periods. The U.S. Surveillance, Epidemiology, and End Results (SEER) Research Data (2000–2017) were analyzed using the SEER*Stat software. The Kaplan– Meier method and Cox regression were used. Patients with de novo mPCa were allocated to three cohorts based on the year of diagnosis: A (2000–2003), B (2004–2010), and C (2011–2014). The maximum follow-up was fixed to 5 years. Overall, 26,434 patients were included. Age, race, and metastatic stage (M1) significantly affected OS and CSS. After adjustment for age and race, patients in Cohort C showed a 9% reduced risk of death (hazard ratio (HR): 0.91 (95% confidence interval [CI] 0.87–0.95), $p < 0.001$) and an 8% reduced risk of cancer-specific death (HR: 0.92 (95% CI 0.88–0.96), $p < 0.001$) compared with those in Cohort A. After adjustment for age, race, and metastatic stage, patients in Cohort C showed an improvement in OS and CSS compared with Cohort B (HR: 0.94 (95% CI 0.91–0.97), $p = 0.001$; HR: 0.89 (95% CI 0.85–0.92), $p < 0.001$). Patients with M1c disease had a more pronounced improvement in OS and CSS compared with the other stages. No differences were found between Cohorts B and C. In conclusion, the real-world survival of de novo mPCa remains poor, with a median OS and CSS improvement of only 4 months in the latest years.

Keywords: prostatic neoplasms/mortality; prostatic neoplasms/epidemiology; SEER Program

1. Introduction

The treatment landscape of metastatic prostate cancer (mPCa) has completely changed over the last decades. In 2004, docetaxel was the first drug to demonstrate an overall survival (OS) benefit of 2.4 months in mPCa, compared with mitoxantrone, and was approved for the treatment of men with metastatic castration-resistant prostate cancer (mCRPC) [1]. Cabazitaxel showed a similar OS increase compared with mitoxantrone and became a second-line treatment option for mCRPC in 2010 [2]. Subsequently, abiraterone acetate and enzalutamide were approved in both post-docetaxel [3,4] (2011–2012) and pre-docetaxel mCRPC [5,6] (2013–2014), reporting OS advantages between 4.0 and 4.8 months compared with placebo (Figure 1). Docetaxel was also introduced for the hormone-sensitive phase of mPCa (mHSPC) in 2015 [7]. Several androgen-receptor signaling inhibitors (ARSi)—abiraterone, enzalutamide, and apalutamide—were then approved for the treatment of mHSPC [8].

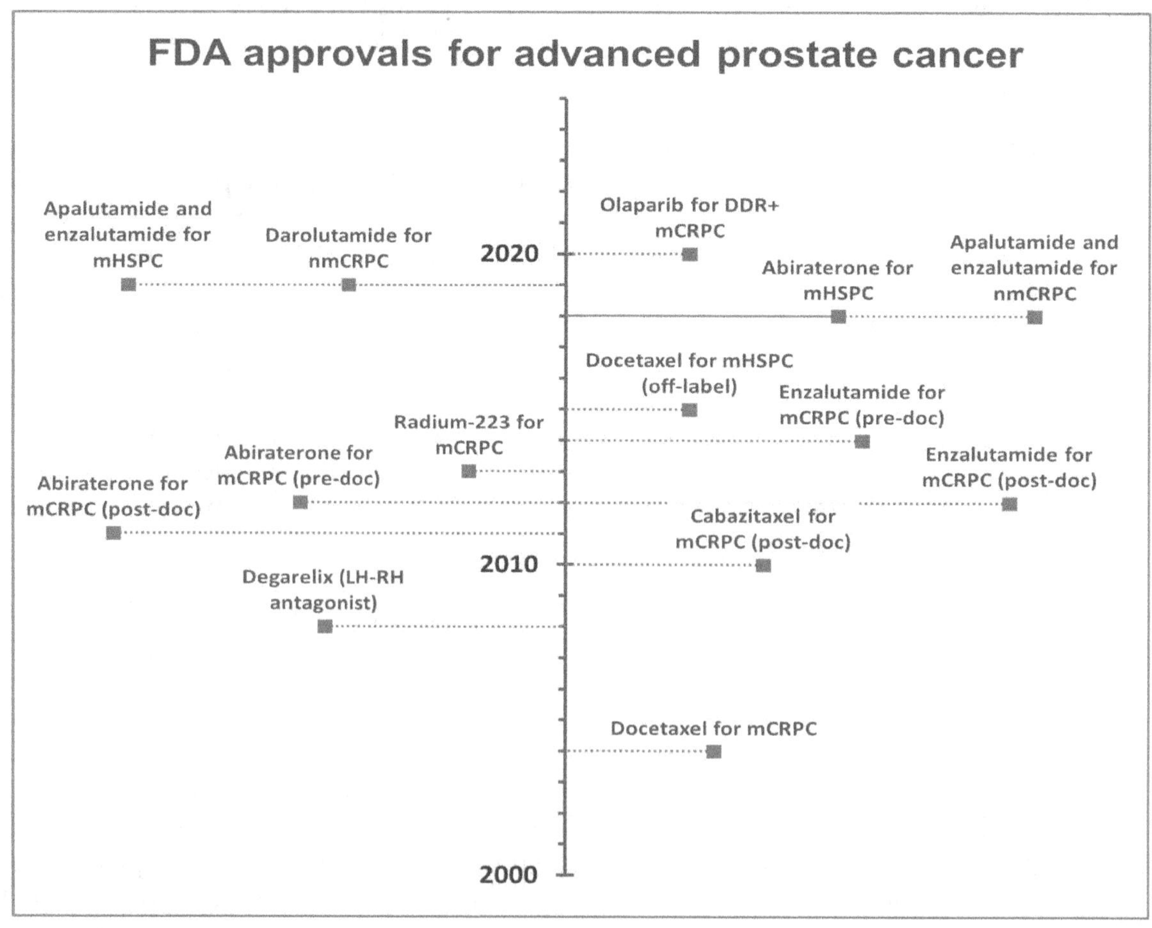

Figure 1. Regulatory timeline of approvals in advanced prostate cancer therapies. DDR+: DNA damage response genes mutated; mHSPC: metastatic hormone-sensitive prostate cancer; mCRPC: metastatic castration-resistant prostate cancer; nmCRPC: nonmetastatic castration-resistant prostate cancer; post-doc: post-docetaxel; pre-doc: pre-docetaxel.

Although the aforementioned randomized trials showed significant survival improvements in the first- and second-line of mCRPC, the real-world survival benefit in the population of patients outside of clinical trials is largely unexplored. The ideal population of patients enrolled in clinical trials might overestimate the true benefit induced by approved drugs in the general population of patients with newly diagnosed mPCa. For example, not all patients can receive chemotherapy. Although no specific advice is included in the U.S. National Comprehensive Cancer Network guidelines, the European Association of Urology guidelines recommend that docetaxel should be only offered to mHSPC patients who are fit enough for chemotherapy [9]. Of note, the STAMPEDE trial of docetaxel in mHSPC only included patients fit for chemotherapy and without significant cardiovascular history. Many patients with mPCa in the real-world are elderly with many comorbidities, and they cannot receive chemotherapy [10]. In addition, patients with poor general conditions or poor performance status are often not suitable for aggressive anticancer therapies. Moreover, although some retrospective data have been reported [11], no randomized trial has ever assessed the long-term, cumulative benefit on survival that can derive from the temporal sequence of different treatment strategies. Finally, the U.S. insurance policies or limited access to healthcare services could contribute to producing a discrepancy between the expected survival gain and the real-world data [12].

Here, we investigated the survival trends and prognostic variables in patients with de novo mPCa included in the U.S. Surveillance, Epidemiology, and End Results (SEER) database. Given the introduction of chemotherapy in 2004 and of ARSi in 2011, we hypothesized that a significant difference in OS and cancer-specific survival (CSS) was detectable in patients diagnosed in three time periods: 2000–2003 (Cohort A), 2004–2010 (Cohort B), and 2011–2014 (Cohort C). Of note, our study should not be intended to provide data on the efficacy of the newer treatments, but to provide epidemiological results about the survival trends in patients with de novo mPCa diagnosed in the United States in the last two decades.

2. Results

2.1. Study Cohort

Our selection criteria identified 26,434 patients with de novo mPCa diagnosed between 2000 and 2014. Of these, 6047 were diagnosed between 2000 and 2003 (Cohort A), 11,815 between 2004 and 2010 (Cohort B), and 8572 between 2011 and 2014 (Cohort C). The main characteristics of the study population are summarized in Table 1. Overall, 68.3% of patients were ≥65 years. The percentage of patients younger than 75 years was higher in Cohort C compared to Cohorts B and A (64.8% vs. 61.1% vs. 58.3%, respectively). The majority of patients were white (62.7%), followed by black (19.4%) and Hispanic (11.6%). Metastatic classification (American Joint Committee on Cancer (AJCC), 6th edition) was available for Cohorts B and C. The majority of patients were M1b (72.7%), with a significant difference between Cohorts B (70.1%) and C (76.4%). The full contingency table with the comparison of baseline characteristics among the cohorts is available in Table S1. The median follow-up was 25, 26, and 29 months in Cohorts A, B, and C, respectively, with a median follow-up of censored patients of 60, 60, and 51 months.

2.2. Clinical Outcome and Prognostic Variables

In the 26,434 patients analyzed for OS, the median values for OS in Cohorts A, B, and C were 26 (95% confidence interval (CI) 25.0–27.0), 26 (95% CI 25.3–26.7), and 30 (95% CI 29.1–30.9) months (Figure 2A). In the 26,032 patients analyzed for CSS, the median values of CSS were 31 (95% CI 29.7–32.3), 31 (95% CI 30.1–31.9), and 35 months (95% CI 32.4–33.6) in Cohorts A, B, and C, respectively (Figure 2B). The detailed age-standardized 1- to 5-year OS and CSS are shown in Figure 3.

Table 1. Basal characteristics of patients.

Variables		Number of Patients (%)			
		Total	2000–2003	2004–2010	2011–2014
Age (years)	15–54	2087 (7.9)	474 (7.8)	970 (8.2)	643 (7.5)
	55–64	6323 (23.9)	1250 (20.7)	2857 (24.2)	2216 (25.9)
	65–74	7892 (29.9)	1804 (29.8)	3391 (28.7)	2697 (31.5)
	75–84	7099 (26.9)	1862 (30.8)	3268 (27.7)	1969 (23.0)
	≥85	3033 (11.5)	657 (10.9)	1329 (11.2)	1047 (12.2)
	Total	26,434 (100)	6047 (100)	11,815 (100)	8572 (100)
Race	White	16,513 (62.7)	3830 (63.5)	7361 (62.5)	5322 (62.3)
	Black	5111 (19.4)	1227 (20.3)	2279 (19.3)	1605 (18.8)
	Am. Indian/Alaska Native	170 (0.6)	31 (0.5)	76 (0.6)	63 (0.7)
	Asian or Pacific Islander	1484 (5.6)	329 (5.4)	680 (5.8)	475 (5.6)
	Hispanic	3066 (11.6)	614 (10.2)	1377 (11.7)	1075 (12.6)
	Total	26,344 (100)	6031 (100)	11,773 (100)	8540 (100)
Metastatic stage	M1a	1097 (5.6)	-	610 (5.3)	487 (5.9)
	M1b	14,301 (72.7)	-	8011 (70.1)	6290 (76.4)
	M1c	4265 (21.7)	-	2811 (24.6)	1454 (17.7)
	Total	19,663 (100)	-	11,432 (100)	8231 (100)

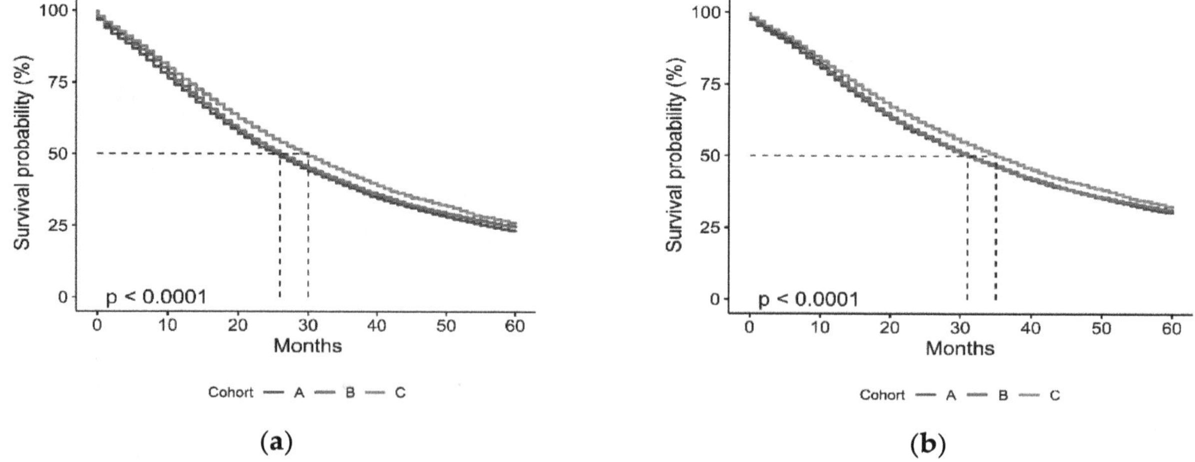

Figure 2. Kaplan–Meier estimations of overall survival (OS) (**a**) and cancer-specific survival (CSS) (**b**) according to cohort allocation. *p*-value from log-rank test.

Age, race, and metastatic stage (the latter was only analyzed in Cohorts B and C) were identified as significant prognostic factors at univariate analysis (data not shown) and were included in the multivariable models.

2.3. Multivariable Models

The multivariable models for OS and CSS showed a substantially increased risk of death according to age, with the highest risk in patients ≥85 (Tables 2 and 3). Black patients showed a slightly higher risk of death compared to white, whereas Asians/Pacific Islanders showed better outcomes compared to white. A 9% decreased risk of death and an 8% decreased risk of cancer-specific death were found in Cohort C compared with Cohort A (hazard ratio (HR): 0.91 (95% CI 0.87–0.95), $p < 0.001$ for OS; HR: 0.92 (95% CI 0.88–0.96), $p < 0.001$ for CSS), whereas no statistically significant differences in OS and CSS were found between Cohorts A and B. Exploratory multivariable models were also performed in Cohorts B and C to include the metastatic stage classification (AJCC, 6th edition), which was found to be associated with distinct OS and CSS outcomes (Tables S2 and S3). In these multivariable models, significant OS and CSS advantages were reported in Cohort C compared with Cohort B (HR: 0.94 (95% CI 0.91–0.97), $p = 0.001$ for OS; HR: 0.89 (95% CI 0.85–0.92), $p < 0.001$ for CSS). In the exploratory subgroup analysis comparing the OS and CSS of Cohort C with Cohort B, a significant interaction was found among the subgroups of the AJCC metastatic classification. More pronounced OS and CSS advantages in Cohort C were shown in M1c patients compared with patients with metastases that were limited to nodes or bone (M1c HR: 0.87 (95% CI 0.81–0.94), interaction $p = 0.014$ for OS; M1c HR: 0.81 (0.75–0.88), interaction $p = 0.015$ for CSS) (Table 4).

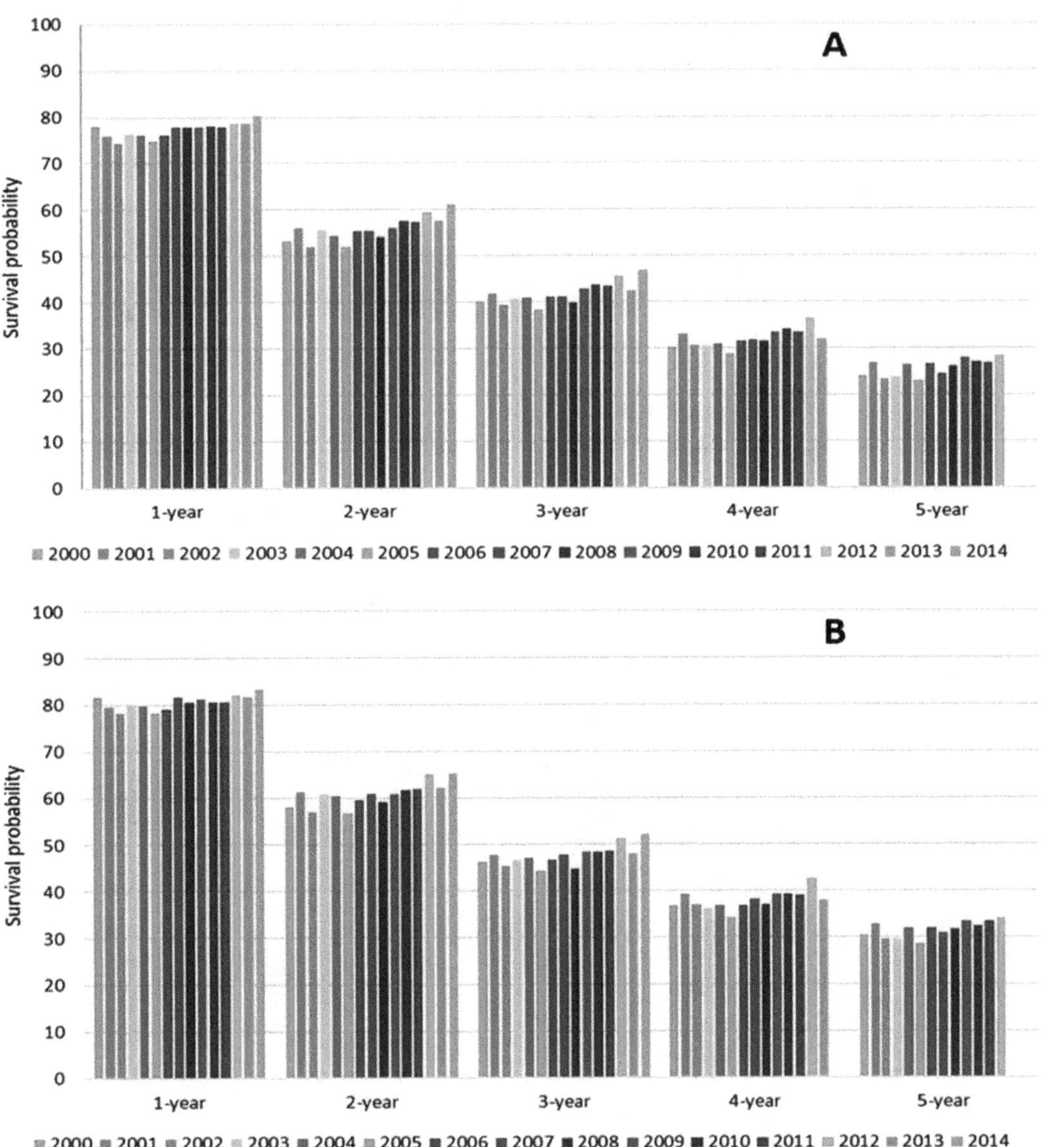

Figure 3. Age-standardized 1- to 5-year OS (**A**) and CSS (**B**) of patients according to year of diagnosis.

Table 2. Multivariable analysis for OS.

Variables		Number of Patients	HR	95% CI		p
				Lower	Upper	
Age (years)	15–54	2081				<0.001
	55–64	6300	0.98	0.92	1.04	0.515
	65–74	7857	1.03	0.97	1.09	0.286
	75–84	7078	1.42	1.34	1.50	<0.001
	≥85	3028	2.18	2.04	2.32	<0.001
Race	White	16,513				<0.001
	Black	5111	1.10	1.06	1.14	<0.001
	Am. Indian/Alaska Native	170	1.08	0.91	1.28	0.393
	Asian or Pacific Islander	1484	0.74	0.69	0.79	<0.001
	Hispanic	3066	0.94	0.90	0.98	0.010
Year of diagnosis	2000–2003 (Cohort A)	6031				<0.001
	2004–2010 (Cohort B)	11,773	0.97	0.94	1.01	0.145
	2011–2014 (Cohort C)	8540	0.91	0.87	0.95	<0.001

Table 3. Multivariable analysis for CSS.

Variables		Number of Patients	HR	95% CI		p
				Lower	Upper	
Age (years)	15–54	2049				<0.001
	55–64	6216	0.94	0.88	0.99	0.048
	65–74	7720	0.93	0.88	0.99	0.033
	75–84	6979	1.20	1.12	1.27	<0.001
	≥85	2987	1.74	1.62	1.87	<0.001
Race	White	16,376				<0.001
	Black	5053	1.09	1.04	1.13	<0.001
	Am. Indian/Alaska Native	167	1.01	0.83	1.23	0.922
	Asian or Pacific Islander	1423	0.73	0.67	0.78	<0.001
	Hispanic	2932	0.95	0.91	1.00	0.076
Year of diagnosis	2000–2003 (Cohort A)	5928				<0.001
	2004–2010 (Cohort B)	11,599	0.99	0.95	1.03	0.596
	2011–2014 (Cohort C)	8424	0.92	0.88	0.96	<0.001

Table 4. Subgroup analysis of OS and CSS between Cohorts C and B.

2011–2014 (Cohort C) vs. 2004–2010 (Cohort B)		Number of Patients	HR	95% CI		p
				Lower	Upper	
OS Metastatic Stage	M1a	1088	1.09	0.93	1.28	0.014 *
	M1b	14,250	0.96	0.92	0.99	
	M1c	4254	0.87	0.81	0.94	
All [1]		19,592	0.94	0.91	0.97	0.001
CSS Metastatic Stage	M1a	1069	1.01	0.85	1.20	0.015 *
	M1b	14,050	0.91	0.87	0.95	
	M1c	4189	0.81	0.75	0.88	
All [1]		19,308	0.89	0.85	0.92	<0.001

Multivariable models including age and race were used to compute the hazard ratios (HR) and their 95% confidence intervals (CI) for OS and CSS in the metastatic subgroups of patients diagnosed in 2011–2014 vs. 2004–2010. * p-value for interaction; [1] Multivariable model including age, race and metastatic stage for OS and CSS (Cohort C vs. Cohort B).

3. Discussion

Several randomized trials demonstrated that both chemotherapy and ARSi provided a significant survival benefit in mPCa [1–8]. However, the real-world survival outcomes of patients with de novo mPCa remain largely unexplored.

A recent analysis compared 590 patients with mCRPC, who were diagnosed and treated in two treatment eras (2004–2007 vs. 2010–2013) at the Dana–Farber Cancer Institute [11]. The authors demonstrated a 41% decreased risk of death in the newer treatment era, with a median OS gain of 6 months. In addition, the cumulative benefit from the newer therapies was more pronounced in longer-term survivors and de novo patients. Although this study provided useful information, all patients had castration-resistant disease, only 216 had de novo mPCa, and they were all managed in a top-level institution.

In another study, Helgstrand and colleagues analyzed the incidence and mortality data of patients with de novo mPCa included in the SEER database and in the Danish Prostate Cancer Registry [13]. In patients diagnosed between 2000 and 2009, the median OS was 22 months in SEER and 30 months in the Danish Registry. The five-year overall mortality was 80.0% in both registries in the period of 2000–2004, remained stable (80.5%) according to SEER in 2005–2008, and decreased to 73.2% according to the Danish Registry in 2005–2009.

Although the monocentric experience of the Dana–Farber Cancer Institute and the Danish data confirmed the potential survival gain offered by newer treatments, the SEER analysis by Helgstrand and colleagues did not show substantial survival changes after 2004.

In the present SEER-based analysis, we investigated whether the introduction of both chemotherapy and ARSi in mCRPC had substantially changed the real-world OS and CSS in the population of patients with de novo mPCa diagnosed in the United States of America in three different time periods (2000–2003—Cohort A, 2004–2010—Cohort B, 2011–2014—Cohort C). Although the patients were allocated to these cohorts regardless of having received a specific treatment, we highlight that docetaxel was approved by the FDA for the treatment of mCRPC in 2004, whereas ARSi was approved from 2011 onwards (Figure 1).

More than 26,000 patients diagnosed between 2000 and 2014 were included in our analysis; of these, 6047 were allocated to Cohort A, 11,815 to Cohort B, and 8572 to Cohort C (Table 1). We found that age had a significant impact on patients' OS and CSS (Tables 2 and 3). In the multivariable model, patients older than 85 showed a double risk of dying compared with patients between 15 and 54 years old, and the hazard ratio for death was also significantly unfavorable in patients aged 75–84. Although this figure might be at least in part attributable to the reduced expected survival, older patients may also be less likely to receive the same treatments as their younger counterparts, especially chemotherapy.

We did not find a significant difference in the OS and CSS between Cohort A and Cohort B (Figure 2). Conversely, we observed a statistically significant improvement in the OS and CSS of patients included in Cohort C, who showed a decreased risk of death of 9%, a decreased risk of cancer-specific death of 8%, and a median OS gain of 4 months compared with Cohort A. The comparison of Cohort C with Cohort B, adjusted for the metastatic stage, also demonstrated an OS improvement of 6% and a CSS improvement of 11%. When compared with the other metastatic stages, we found that patients with M1c disease showed the worst survival, but had a more pronounced OS and CSS improvement in the newer ARSi era compared with M1a or M1b patients (Table 4). Although the reason for this observation remains unknown, the presence of visceral metastases might lead to more aggressive pharmaceutical approaches and more adherence to treatment that could result in increased benefit compared with the other stages.

The median OS gain of chemotherapy and ARSi in randomized trials for mCRPC was 2–4 months in first-line [1,5,6] and 4–5 months in second-line [3,4]. Although our study was not designed to demonstrate the potential benefit of chemotherapy or ARSi, a more robust OS and CSS improvement would have been expected in patients diagnosed in 2011–2014, after the introduction of several agents in clinical practice (Figure 1). A median OS improvement of 4 months in Cohort C compared with Cohort A appears to be quite discouraging. Regardless of cohort analysis, the probability of survival after 3 years from diagnosis was 40.0% in 2000 and 46.8% in 2014 (Figure 3). Similarly, the five-year probability of survival was 24.0% in 2000 and 28.2% in 2012. Several reasons might explain these disappointing results.

First, the degree of benefit seen in clinical trials does not necessarily translate into the real-world setting. Screen failure rates on trials are relatively high and can easily affect the ultimate generalizability of trial results to the real-world population.

Second, our study was based on patients diagnosed with de novo mHSPC who were supposed to receive androgen-deprivation therapy (ADT) as a first-line treatment for metastatic disease, and subsequently docetaxel or ARSi as a first-line treatment for mCRPC. The number of patients who died without receiving a first-line treatment for mCRPC or refused therapies for mCRPC was unknown. The information on the number of lines of treatment, type of treatment, disease burden, number and site of metastases, body mass index, performance status, and comorbidities was not available in the SEER database, and these potential confounders were not included in our analysis. In addition, we acknowledge that some patients could have received chemotherapy or ARSi outside of the defined cohort allocation in the context of clinical trials or some years after mPCa diagnosis.

Third, the medical costs and the health insurance policies might have significantly reduced the extensive use of ARSi and chemotherapy in the general population of patients with de novo mPCa diagnosed and treated in the United States, affecting their survival outcomes. Ramsey and colleagues reported that the cumulative incidence of bankruptcy in the first 5 years after prostate cancer diagnosis is 38% (nearly 50% in metastatic stage), and the risk of mortality is almost twice as high among patients with prostate cancer who file for bankruptcy compared with those who do not [12]. Further studies should investigate whether insurance policies or limited access to healthcare services could contribute to such disappointing survival gains observed in the SEER registry after the introduction of chemotherapy and ARSi.

Fourth, patients with de novo mPCa showed worse time to castration and survival compared with those who relapsed after local therapy, irrespective of treatment received [14,15]. Therefore, the intrinsic aggressiveness of de novo mPCa could have also led to decreased survival gains in this patient population. Although discouraged by international guidelines in recent years, possible premature discontinuation of ARSi and chemotherapy based on PSA progression without clinical or radiographic progression could have also affected the outcome data of patients diagnosed between 2004 and 2014 [16].

Finally, we acknowledge that our study excludes the possible benefit induced by docetaxel or ARSi in mHSPC, given their approval for this setting in the latest years (Figure 1). The earlier use of these agents provided OS gains that exceeded 12 months in randomized trials for mHSPC [8]. Future analyses could also detect additional survival benefits that might be provided by an increased knowledge in the sequencing of agents for mCRPC and by the biomarker-driven selection of patients suitable for specific drugs (i.e., poly (ADP-ribose) polymerase (PARP) inhibitors) [17–19].

4. Patients and Methods

The SEER*Stat software was used to select all patients with de novo mPCa from the SEER Research Data 2000–2017 [20]. Patients were assigned to three cohorts based on the year of diagnosis (2000–2003: Cohort A; 2004–2010: Cohort B; 2011–2014: Cohort C). Patients with prostate cancer were identified using the codes for malignant adenocarcinoma (8140/3) and prostate gland (C61.9). Only patients with a single tumor in medical history were selected. Metastatic patients were identified using a combination of the American Joint Committee on Cancer (AJCC) classification from the 3rd and 6th editions. According to the November 2019 submission of SEER data, the study cut-off for survival data was 31 December 2017. In order to minimize potential bias related to different follow-up among the cohorts, the maximum follow-up was fixed to 5 years, and patients diagnosed from 2015 onwards were excluded. OS was defined as the time from mPCa diagnosis to death from any cause. CSS was defined as the time from mPCa diagnosis to death from prostate cancer. Patient age (SEER standard for survival in prostate cancer: 15–54, 55–64, 65–74, 75–84, 85+), race, year of mPCa diagnosis, metastatic stage, and outcome data were included in the case listing session of SEER*Stat. The variables described were analyzed in univariate analysis using Kaplan–Meier curves and a log-rank test. A p-value ≤ 0.05 was considered statistically significant. Cox proportional hazards models were used to test the effects of covariates on OS and CSS. Only patients who had known values for the variables of interest were included. The chi-square statistic was applied to compare groups. The IBM software Statistical Package for Social Sciences (SPSS) Version 23 and RStudio Version 1.2.5001 were used for data analysis.

5. Conclusions

Our large-scale, retrospective study suggested that the real-world OS and CSS have not drastically changed during the last two decades in patients with de novo mPCa diagnosed in the United States. The median OS of these patients remained poor and did not exceed 2.5 years. Although we acknowledge that several potential confounding factors have not been adjusted in our analysis, our study highlighted that a significant discrepancy might exist between the benefit observed in randomized trials and the real-world data. Several reasons might explain this discrepancy, such as a lack of access to cancer cares, patients' ineligibility or refusal of treatments, insurance issues, or intrinsic aggressiveness of de novo disease. However, given that patients were not allocated according to the receipt of specific treatments, our results should not be used to draw conclusions about the potential efficacy of systemic therapies.

Author Contributions: Conceptualization, C.C.; methodology, D.O., A.R.; formal analysis, C.C., A.R., L.Z.; data curation, L.Z., C.M.; writing—original draft preparation, C.C., D.S.; writing—review and editing, P.B., C.M., E.C., E.Z., D.S.; supervision, F.B., D.O., E.C.; project administration, L.Z. All authors have read and agreed to the published version of the manuscript.

Acknowledgments: C.C. is supported by an ESMO Clinical Research Fellowship (2019–2020). This work has been awarded with a Conquer Cancer Foundation of ASCO Merit Award at 2020 ASCO–GU.

References

1. Tannock, I.F.; de Wit, R.; Berry, W.R.; Horti, J.; Pluzanska, A.; Chi, K.N.; Oudard, S.; Theodore, C.; James, N.D.; Turesson, I.; et al. Docetaxel plus prednisone or mitoxantrone plus prednisone for advanced prostate cancer. *N. Engl. J. Med.* **2004**, *351*, 1502–1512. [CrossRef]
2. De Bono, J.S.; Oudard, S.; Ozguroglu, M.; Hansen, S.; Machiels, J.P.; Kocak, I.; Gravis, G.; Bodrogi, I.; Mackenzie, M.J.; Shen, L.; et al. Prednisone plus cabazitaxel or mitoxantrone for metastatic castration-resistant prostate cancer progressing after docetaxel treatment: A randomised open-label trial. *Lancet* **2010**, *376*, 1147–1154. [CrossRef]

3. De Bono, J.S.; Logothetis, C.J.; Molina, A.; Fizazi, K.; North, S.; Chu, L.; Chi, K.N.; Jones, R.J.; Goodman, O.B., Jr.; Saad, F.; et al. Abiraterone and increased survival in metastatic prostate cancer. *N. Engl. J. Med.* **2011**, *364*, 1995–2005. [CrossRef] [PubMed]
4. Scher, H.I.; Fizazi, K.; Saad, F.; Taplin, M.E.; Sternberg, C.N.; Miller, K.; de Wit, R.; Mulders, P.; Chi, K.N.; Shore, N.D.; et al. Increased survival with enzalutamide in prostate cancer after chemotherapy. *N. Engl. J. Med.* **2012**, *367*, 1187–1197. [CrossRef] [PubMed]
5. Ryan, C.J.; Smith, M.R.; de Bono, J.S.; Molina, A.; Logothetis, C.J.; de Souza, P.; Fizazi, K.; Mainwaring, P.; Piulats, J.M.; Ng, S.; et al. Abiraterone in metastatic prostate cancer without previous chemotherapy. *N. Engl. J. Med.* **2013**, *368*, 138–148. [CrossRef] [PubMed]
6. Beer, T.M.; Armstrong, A.J.; Rathkopf, D.E.; Loriot, Y.; Sternberg, C.N.; Higano, C.S.; Iversen, P.; Bhattacharya, S.; Carles, J.; Chowdhury, S.; et al. Enzalutamide in metastatic prostate cancer before chemotherapy. *N. Engl. J. Med.* **2014**, *371*, 424–433. [CrossRef] [PubMed]
7. Sweeney, C.J.; Chen, Y.H.; Carducci, M.; Liu, G.; Jarrard, D.F.; Eisenberger, M.; Wong, Y.N.; Hahn, N.; Kohli, M.; Cooney, M.M.; et al. Chemohormonal Therapy in Metastatic Hormone-Sensitive Prostate Cancer. *N. Engl. J. Med.* **2015**, *373*, 737–746. [CrossRef] [PubMed]
8. Cattrini, C.; Castro, E.; Lozano, R.; Zanardi, E.; Rubagotti, A.; Boccardo, F.; Olmos, D. Current Treatment Options for Metastatic Hormone-Sensitive Prostate Cancer. *Cancers* **2019**, *11*, 1355. [CrossRef] [PubMed]
9. Mottet, N.; Bellmunt, J.; Briers, E.; Bolla, M.; Bourke, L.; Cornford, P.; De Santis, M.; Henry, A.; Joniau, S.; Lam, T. *Members of the EAU–ESTRO–ESUR–SIOG Prostate Cancer Guidelines Panel. EAU–ESTRO–ESUR–SIOG Guidelines on Prostate Cancer*; Presented at the EAU Annual Congress Amsterdam 2020. 978-94-92671-07-3; EAU Guidelines Office: Arnhem, The Netherlands, 2020.
10. Thompson, A.L.; Sarmah, P.; Beresford, M.J.; Jefferies, E.R. Management of metastatic prostate cancer in the elderly: Identifying fitness for chemotherapy in the post-STAMPEDE world. *Bju Int.* **2017**, *120*, 751–754. [CrossRef] [PubMed]
11. Francini, E.; Gray, K.P.; Shaw, G.K.; Evan, C.P.; Hamid, A.A.; Perry, C.E.; Kantoff, P.W.; Taplin, M.E.; Sweeney, C.J. Impact of new systemic therapies on overall survival of patients with metastatic castration-resistant prostate cancer in a hospital-based registry. *Prostate Cancer Prostatic Dis.* **2019**, *22*, 420–427. [CrossRef] [PubMed]
12. Ramsey, S.D.; Bansal, A.; Fedorenko, C.R.; Blough, D.K.; Overstreet, K.A.; Shankaran, V.; Newcomb, P. Financial Insolvency as a Risk Factor for Early Mortality among Patients with Cancer. *J. Clin. Oncol.* **2016**, *34*, 980–986. [CrossRef] [PubMed]
13. Helgstrand, J.T.; Roder, M.A.; Klemann, N.; Toft, B.G.; Lichtensztajn, D.Y.; Brooks, J.D.; Brasso, K.; Vainer, B.; Iversen, P. Trends in incidence and 5-year mortality in men with newly diagnosed, metastatic prostate cancer-A population-based analysis of 2 national cohorts. *Cancer* **2018**, *124*, 2931–2938. [CrossRef] [PubMed]
14. Francini, E.; Gray, K.P.; Xie, W.; Shaw, G.K.; Valenca, L.; Bernard, B.; Albiges, L.; Harshman, L.C.; Kantoff, P.W.; Taplin, M.E.; et al. Time of metastatic disease presentation and volume of disease are prognostic for metastatic hormone sensitive prostate cancer (mHSPC). *Prostate* **2018**, *78*, 889–895. [CrossRef] [PubMed]
15. Finianos, A.; Gupta, K.; Clark, B.; Simmens, S.J.; Aragon-Ching, J.B. Characterization of Differences Between Prostate Cancer Patients Presenting with De Novo Versus Primary Progressive Metastatic Disease. *Clin. Genitourin. Cancer* **2017**, *16*, 85–89. [CrossRef] [PubMed]
16. Becker, D.J.; Iyengar, A.D.; Punekar, S.R.; Ng, J.; Zaman, A.; Loeb, S.; Becker, K.D.; Makarov, D. Treatment of Metastatic Castration-resistant Prostate Cancer with Abiraterone and Enzalutamide Despite PSA Progression. *Anticancer Res.* **2019**, *39*, 2467–2473. [CrossRef] [PubMed]
17. De Wit, R.; de Bono, J.; Sternberg, C.N.; Fizazi, K.; Tombal, B.; Wulfing, C.; Kramer, G.; Eymard, J.C.; Bamias, A.; Carles, J.; et al. Cabazitaxel versus Abiraterone or Enzalutamide in Metastatic Prostate Cancer. *N. Engl. J. Med.* **2019**, *381*, 2506–2518. [CrossRef] [PubMed]
18. De Bono, J.; Mateo, J.; Fizazi, K.; Saad, F.; Shore, N.; Sandhu, S.; Chi, K.N.; Sartor, O.; Agarwal, N.; Olmos, D.; et al. Olaparib for Metastatic Castration-Resistant Prostate Cancer. *N. Engl. J. Med.* **2020**, *382*, 2091–2102. [CrossRef] [PubMed]

19. Messina, C.; Cattrini, C.; Soldato, D.; Vallome, G.; Caffo, O.; Castro, E.; Olmos, D.; Boccardo, F.; Zanardi, E. BRCA Mutations in Prostate Cancer: Prognostic and Predictive Implications. *J. Oncol.* **2020**, *2020*, 4986365. [CrossRef] [PubMed]

20. Surveillance, Epidemiology, and End Results (SEER) Program (www.seer.cancer.gov) SEER*Stat Database: Incidence-SEER Research Data, 18 Registries, Nov 2019 Sub (2000–2017)-Linked to County Attributes-Time Dependent (1990–2017) Income/Rurality, 1969–2017 Counties; National Cancer Institute, DCCPS, Surveillance Research Program, Released April 2020, Based on the November 2019 Submission. Available online: https://seer.cancer.gov/data/citation.html (accessed on 3 October 2020).

9

Clear Cell Adenocarcinoma of the Urinary Bladder is a Glycogen-Rich Tumor with Poorer Prognosis

Zhengqiu Zhou [1], Connor J. Kinslow [2], Peng Wang [3], Bin Huang [4], Simon K. Cheng [2,5], Israel Deutsch [2,5], Matthew S. Gentry [1,6] and Ramon C. Sun [6,7,*]

1 Department of Molecular and Cellular Biochemistry, University of Kentucky College of Medicine, Lexington, KY 40536, USA; zhengqiu.zhou@uky.edu (Z.Z.); matthew.gentry@uky.edu (M.S.G.)
2 Department of Radiation Oncology, Vagelos College of Physicians and Surgeons, Columbia University Irving Medical Center, New York, NY 10032, USA; cjk2151@cumc.columbia.edu (C.J.K.); sc3225@cumc.columbia.edu (S.K.C.); id2182@cumc.columbia.edu (I.D.)
3 Division of Medical Oncology, Department of Internal Medicine, College of Medicine, University of Kentucky, Lexington, KY 40536, USA; p.wang@uky.edu
4 Department of Biostatistics, College of Public Health, University of Kentucky, Lexington, KY 40536, USA; bhuang@kcr.uky.edu
5 Herbert Irving Comprehensive Cancer Center, Vagelos College of Physicians and Surgeons, Columbia University Irving Medical Center, New York, NY 10032, USA
6 Markey Cancer Center, University of Kentucky, Lexington, KY 40536, USA
7 Department of Neuroscience, University of Kentucky College of Medicine, Lexington, KY 40536, USA
* Correspondence: ramon.sun@uky.edu

Abstract: Clear cell adenocarcinoma (CCA) is a rare variant of urinary bladder carcinoma with a glycogen-rich phenotype and unknown prognosis. Using the National Cancer Institute's surveillance, epidemiology, and end results (SEER) program database, we documented recent trends in incidence, mortality, demographical characteristics, and survival on this rare subtype of urinary bladder cancer. The overall age-adjusted incidence and mortality of CCA was 0.087 (95% confidence interval (CI): 0.069–0.107) and 0.064 (95% CI: 0.049–0.081) respectively per million population. In comparison to non-CCAs, CCAs were more commonly associated with younger age (<60 years old, $p = 0.005$), female ($p < 0.001$), black ethnicity ($p = 0.001$), grade III ($p < 0.001$), and higher AJCC 6th staging ($p < 0.001$). In addition, CCA patients more frequently received complete cystectomy ($p < 0.001$) and beam radiation ($p < 0.001$) than non-CCA patients. Our study showed a poorer prognosis of CCAs compared to all other carcinomas of the urinary bladder ($p < 0.001$), accounted for by higher tumor staging of CCA cases. This study adds to the growing evidence that glycogen-rich cancers may have unique characteristics affecting tumor aggressiveness and patient prognosis. Additional mechanistic studies are needed to assess whether it's the excess glycogen that contributes to the higher stage at diagnosis.

Keywords: glycogen; clear-cell adenocarcinoma; urinary bladder; SEER program database

---

1. Introduction

Glycogen, a multibranched polymer of glucose, serves as our body's main form of carbohydrate storage [1]. In the past decade, glycogen has become well-established that, in addition to its role in maintaining metabolic homeostasis in normal cells, it also has a crucial role in promoting tumor growth, especially under adverse conditions [2]. Under hypoxic conditions, which are commonly encountered by tumors cells, expression of transcription factor HIF1α increases glycogen accumulation [3]. Cancer cells have been shown to mobilize this excess glycogen via a p38α mitogen-activated protein kinase pathway to fuel cellular proliferation and metastasis [4]. Glycogen has also been proposed to maintain the Warburg effect in tumor cells, providing a mechanism for survival during nutrient deprivation [5]. Furthermore, glycogen's inability to metabolize glycogen through small molecule inhibitors was able to induce apoptosis or senescence in tumor cells [6,7]. Altogether, cancer cells utilize glycogen as a way to alter its metabolic programing in order to adapt to the adverse tumor microenvironment and maintain tumor growth.

Aberrant glycogen deposits have been identified in tumors from multiple origins, including cancers of the breast, kidney, uterus, lung, head and neck, bladder, ovary, skin, brain and colorectal tumors [8–12]. They are often identified as "clear cell" due to the transparent and ovoid appearance seen on histological staining. A poorer prognosis has been documented in clear cell carcinomas of the kidney [13], uterus [14], ovaries [15] and breast [16]. However, due to the rarity of some these tumors, the prognostic implications in other types of "clear cell" cancers remain unclear.

Clear cell adenocarcinoma of the urinary bladder (CCA) is a rare histological growth pattern first reported by Dow and Young in 1968 [17]. These tumors contain sheets of uniform ovoid cells with clear cytoplasm containing abundant glycogen [18,19]. Since there are no distinguishing symptoms of CCA, diagnosis is based on histopathological identification of these characteristics. Due to its rarity, information on the characteristics and prognosis of CCA have been limited to case reports, with less than 50 cases reported to date [19–21]. The largest existing literature review was performed by Lu et al., consisting of 38 case reports [21]. The review supported surgical resection as initial treatment for CCA and noted a possible increase in metastasis risk compared to urothelial carcinomas. However, the study determined that the prognosis of CCA was unclear as longer follow up periods were needed to more accurately assess survival characteristics [21]. No incidence and mortality data have been reported yet.

As the first large-scale study to date, we utilized the National Cancer Institute's surveillance, epidemiology, and end results (SEER) program database to conduct a retrospective assessment of incidence, mortality, demographics, and survival for CCA. Based on the previous literature that has shown a link between glycogen rich tumors and tumor aggressiveness [13–16], our study aimed to assess whether similar prognostic outcomes exist for CCAs. Using 91 cases of CCA and 205,106 cases of other urinary bladder cancers (non-CCA) obtained from the SEER Program database, we identified a poorer prognosis attributed to higher staging at time for diagnosis for CCAs. Our study contributes to the growing body of evidence revealing a possible link between glycogen and tumor aggressiveness.

2. Experimental Section

2.1. Data Source

The SEER Program is the National Cancer Institute's authoritative source of information on cancer incidence and survival capturing approximately 34.6% of the US population [22]. It is populated with high quality population-based data from national cancer registries. Vital status is updated annually and routinely undergoes quality-control checks.

2.2. Sample Selection and Coding

Age-adjusted incidence and mortality rates were calculated using the SEER*Stat Software (Version 8.3.6, National Cancer Institute, Bethesda, MD, USA) using all 91 cases of malignant cases of CCA of the urinary bladder and 205, 106 cases of non-CCA from 2004 to 2015 from the SEER Program database [23,24]. Incidence and mortality were age-adjusted by standardizing to the 2000 United States Census population. All other data collection and analysis were conducted as described previously [16,25]. We obtained the November, 2015 submission [26] and November, 2017 submission [27] from the SEER Program database and merged all identified cases of malignant cancers of the bladder identified by International Classification of Diseases-O-3 (ICD-O-3) codes C67.0–C67.9 from January 2004 to December 2015. Carcinomas of the bladder were determined based on the adapted classification scheme for adolescents and young adults. Cases of clear cell adenocarcinoma were identified by ICD-O-3 code 8310.

The following variables were collected and coded: AYA site recode, primary site, ICD-O-3 histology, age at diagnosis, sex, race, grade, American Joint Commission on Cancer (AJCC) 6th Edition Staging, AJCC 6th Edition TNM system, survival months, vital status, bone metastasis at diagnosis, brain metastasis at diagnosis, liver metastasis at diagnosis, lung metastasis at diagnosis, surgery, and radiation. Cases of AJCC 6th stage 0a and 0is were merged and referred to as "stage 0". Ta, Tis were merged and referred to as "Ta/Tis". T1, T1a, T1b, T1 NOS were merged and collectively referred to as "T1". T2, T2a, T2b, T2 NOS were merged and collectively referred to as "T2". T3, T3a, T3b, T3c, T3 NOS were merged and collectively referred to as "T3". T4, T4a, T4b, T4 NOS were merged and collectively referred to as "T4". The surgery codes 10 (local tumor destruction), 20 (local tumor excision), and 30 (partial cystectomy) were merged and collectively referred to as "local procedure/ partial cystectomy". Surgical codes 50 (simple/total/complete cystectomy), 60 (complete cystectomy with reconstruction), and 70 (pelvic exenteration) were combined, and collectively referred to as "complete cystectomy". Surgical codes 80 (cystectomy, NOS) and 90 (surgery, NOS) were combined and collectively referred to as "surgery, NOS". Detailed SEER database surgery codes are available at (https://seer.cancer.gov/manuals/2018/appendixc.html). Cases diagnosed at autopsy or that could have 0 days of follow-up were excluded all analyses except for incidence and mortality calculations.

2.3. *Statistical Analysis*

All statistical analysis was carried out using the IBM SPSS Statistics software package (version 25, International Business Machines Corporation, Armonk, NY, USA). The significance of incidence and mortality trends were calculated using linear regression analysis. Differences in demographic and clinical characteristics between CCA and non-CCA were determined using the Pearson's chi-square test. Median survival times were determined using the Kaplan–Meier method, and the significance was determined using the log-rank test. Multivariable analyses of overall survival were conducted using the Cox proportional hazards ratios (HR) model. Corresponding HR and 95% confidence intervals (CI) were estimated from the model. Two-tailed p-values < 0.05 were considered statistically significant.

3. Results

3.1. *Incidence and Mortality of CCA*

To assess recent trends in the incidence and mortality of CCA, we queried all cases of CCA from 2004 to 2015 in the SEER Program database. Over this period, the age-adjusted the incidence of CCA was 0.087 individuals per 1,000,000 (Supplementary Table S1). Our analysis suggested a downward trend in incidence over this period—a shift from 0.062 per 1,000,000 in 2004 to 0.057 per 1,000,000 individuals in 2015 with an annual decrease rate of 0.003. However, this trend was non-significant ($p = 0.178$, Supplementary Figure S1A). We further assessed incidence separated by gender (Supplementary Table S1). The incidence of CCA among female and males were similar, with a slight female predominance—0.091 and 0.084 per 10,000,000 for females and males respectively from 2004 to 2015 (Supplementary Table S1).

The mortality rate from 2004–2015 was 0.064 individuals per 1,000,000 with an increasing trend of 0.002 per year. This trend was also non-significant ($p = 0.477$, Supplementary Figure S1B, Supplementary Table S1). When separated by gender, male with CCA had higher mortality rate of 0.074 compared to 0.058 in females per 1,000,000 individuals (Table S1).

3.2. *Demographics and Clinical Characteristics*

To compare demographical and clinical characteristics of CCA to non-CCA cancers of the urinary bladder, we utilized cases of malignant carcinomas of the urinary bladder from 2004, when AJCC 6th staging information became available, to 2015, the most recent data available at time of analysis. We obtained 205,197 cases of malignant urinary bladder carcinoma. Of these, 91 cases (0.04%) were identified as CCA. The median follow-up time was 19 months with 45 deaths in these CCA patients.

Amongst 205,106 cases of non-CCA patients, the median follow-up time was 23 months, with 68,951 recorded deaths. The median age at diagnosis of CCA was 70 years old and median age at diagnosis was 72 years old in non-CCA patients.

The demographical and clinical characteristics of the patient population are summarized in Table 1. Our results showed that CCA patients were more likely to be younger age (<60 years of age; $p = 0.005$), female ($p < 0.001$) and black ($p = 0.001$) than non-CCA patients. The larger proportion of female patients is consistent with our incidence analysis. CCA patients also had higher grade ($p < 0.001$), higher AJCC 6th staging ($p < 0.001$) including TNM staging (p values for T, N, M stage were $p < 0.001$, $p < 0.001$ and $p < 0.001$, respectively). The primary site of tumor location was significantly different between CCA and non-CCA patients ($p < 0.001$); CCA patients were more likely to have tumors in the trigone of bladder, bladder neck and urachus, whereas non-CCA tumors appeared mostly in the lateral wall of bladder. As expected with more advanced tumor staging, CCA patients showed higher likelihood of brain ($p < 0.001$) and liver ($p = 0.028$) metastasis. However, very few cases with metastasis were available; only a single case was available for brain metastasis and two cases for liver metastasis. Furthermore, our data showed that non-CCA patients were more likely to receive fewer radical treatments such as local procedure or partial cystectomy, while more CCA patients received complete cystectomies ($p < 0.001$). The majority of non-CCA patients did not receive radiation, while a greater number of CCA patients received beam radiation ($p < 0.001$).

Table 1. Demographical and clinical characteristics comparing clear cell adenocarcinoma to other carcinomas of the urinary bladder.

		Clear Cell Adenocarcinoma (N = 91)		Non-Clear Cell Adenocarcinoma (N = 205,106)		
		Count	**%**	**Count**	**%**	***p*-Value**
Age	0–60	27	29.7	37,649	18.4	0.005
	61+	64	70.3	167,457	81.6	
Sex	Female	54	59.3	49,241	24.0	<0.001
	Male	37	40.7	155,865	76.0	
Race	White	77	84.6	182,492	89.0	0.001
	Black	13	14.3	11,519	5.6	
	Other	1	1.1	8588	4.2	
	Unknown	0	0.0	2507	1.2	
Tumor primary site	Trigone of bladder	9	9.9	12,765	6.2	<0.001
	Dome of bladder	4	4.4	7213	3.5	
	Lateral wall of bladder	6	6.6	41,041	20.0	
	Anterior wall of bladder	5	5.5	4334	2.1	
	Posterior wall of bladder	7	7.7	18,819	9.2	
	Bladder neck	10	11.0	6354	3.1	
	Ureteric orifice	4	4.4	7820	3.8	
	Urachus	1	1.1	310	0.2	
	Overlapping lesion of bladder	13	14.3	21,112	10.3	
	Bladder, NOS	32	35.2	85,338	41.6	
Grade	Grade I	0	0.0	23,684	11.5	<0.001
	Grade II	5	5.5	48,123	23.5	
	Grade III	22	24.2	35,849	17.5	
	Grade IV	25	27.5	59,477	29.0	
	Unknown	39	42.9	37,973	18.5	

Table 1. *Cont.*

		Clear Cell Adenocarcinoma (N = 91)		Non-Clear Cell Adenocarcinoma (N = 205,106)		
		Count	%	Count	%	p-Value
AJCC 6th stage	Stage 0	2	2.2	105,545	51.5	<0.001
	Stage 1	22	24.2	46,332	22.6	
	Stage 2	28	30.8	23,463	11.4	
	Stage 3	9	9.9	8157	4.0	
	Stage 4	17	18.7	14,012	6.8	
	Unknown	13	14.3	7597	3.7	
T stage	Tis/Ta	2	2.2	105,545	51.5	<0.001
	T0	0	0.0	91	0.0	
	T1	26	28.6	49,221	24.0	
	T2	35	38.5	28,776	14.0	
	T3	7	7.7	8046	3.9	
	T4	11	12.1	7713	3.8	
	Unknown	10	11.0	5714	2.8	
N stage	N0	70	76.9	189,973	92.6	<0.001
	N1	2	2.2	3994	1.9	
	N2	6	6.6	3806	1.9	
	N3	1	1.1	166	0.1	
	Unknown	12	13.2	7167	3.5	
M stage	M0	75	82.4	193,071	94.1	<0.001
	M1	11	12.1	7565	3.7	
	Unknown	5	5.5	4470	2.2	
Bone metastasis [a]	No	42	97.7	102,083	97.0	0.697
	Yes	0	0.0	1432	1.4	
	Unknown	1	2.3	1698	1.6	
Brain metastasis [a]	No	41	95.3	103,393	98.3	<0.001
	Yes	1	2.3	122	0.1	
	Unknown	1	2.3	1698	1.6	
Liver metastasis [a]	No	40	93.0	102,600	97.5	0.028
	Yes	2	4.7	926	0.9	
	Unknown	1	2.3	1687	1.6	
Lung metastasis [a]	No	41	95.3	102,153	97.1	0.771
	Yes	1	2.3	1327	1.3	
	Unknown	1	2.3	1733	1.6	
Type of surgical procedure	No surgery	8	8.8	15,265	7.4	<0.001
	Local procedure/partial cystectomy	60	65.9	170,325	83.0	
	Complete cystectomy	22	24.2	18,327	8.9	
	Surgery NOS	0	0.0	504	0.2	
	Unknown if surgery performed	1	1.1	685	0.3	
Type of radiation [b]	None	67	85.9	160,440	94.6	<0.001
	Beam radiation	9	11.5	7485	4.4	
	Other radiation	1	1.3	219	0.1	
	Unknown if radiation received	1	1.3	1389	0.8	

Bolded are statistically significant p-values when comparing between clear cell adenocarcinoma to other carcinomas of the urinary bladder. NA—not applicable. [a] Variable only available for cases diagnosed after 2010. [b] Variable only available for cases diagnosed before 2013.

3.3. *Survival*

The median survival for CCA patients was 34 months with 5- and 10-year survival rates of 41%, 30%, respectively. The median survival for non-CCA patients was 87 months, with corresponding 5- and 10-year survival rates of 61% and 44%, respectively (Figure 1, $p < 0.001$). Using multivariable analysis accounting for age, sex, race, AJCC 6th stage, tumor grade, surgery, and radiation treatment, survival for CCA patients was no longer significantly poorer than non-CCA patients (HR: 0.93; 95% CI: 0.69–1.255; $p = 0.636$, Supplementary Table S2 left half). However, when staging was removed from same multivariable analysis, CCA survival remained significantly shorter than non-CCA patients (HR: 1.435, 95% CI: 1.064–1.936, $p = 0.018$, Supplementary Table S2 right half). Therefore, the histological subtype CCA is not an independent prognostic factor for survival, but instead, it is the more advanced staging in CCA patients accounts for the survival difference between CCA and non-CCA patients.

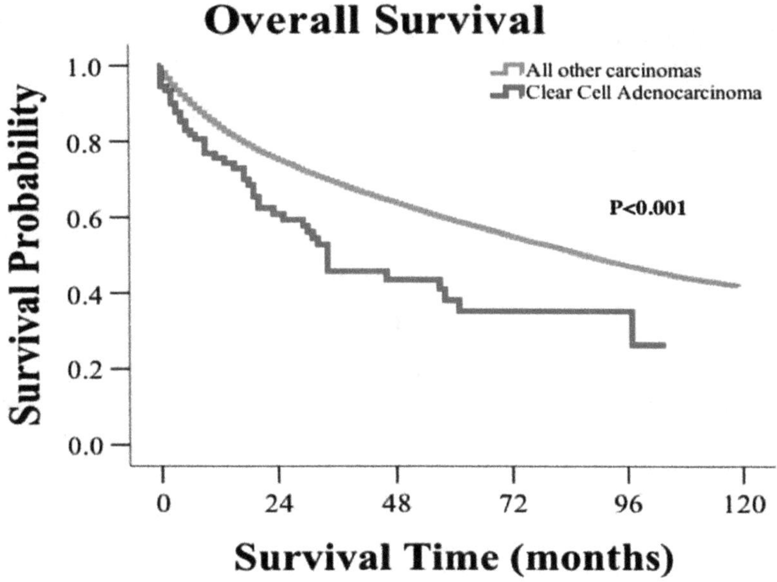

Number at Risk.

Survival months	0	24	48	72	96	120
CCA	205,106	100,972	63,338	35,862	15,121	0
Non-CCA	91	39	19	9	4	0

Figure 1. Kaplan–Meier curve and risk table of clear cell adenocarcinoma in comparison to other carcinomas of the urinary bladder.

To further confirm our finding that the worse prognosis is attributable for the higher staging, we stratified our CCA cases according to AJCC 6th staging and compared survival in patients with non-muscle invasive (AJCC 6th stage 0 and I), muscle-invasive (AJCC 6th stage II and III) and metastatic (AJCC 6th stage IV) pathology. As suspected, when stratified by non-muscle invasive, muscle-invasive, and metastatic cases, the survival durations were no longer significantly different between CCA and non-CCA cases (Table 2, $p = 0.654$, $p = 0.653$, $p = 0.091$ respectively).

Table 2. Survival comparison between clear cell adenocarcinoma and other urinary bladder cancers stratified by stage.

		Median Survival	95% Confidence Interval		
			Lower Bound	Upper Bound	*p*-Value
Non-muscle invasive (Stage 0–1)	Non-CCA	119			0.654
	CCA				
Muscle invasive (Stage 2–3)	Non-CCA	25	24.263	25.737	0.653
	CCA	32	16.308	47.692	
Metastatic (Stage 4)	Non-CCA	9	8.736	9.264	0.091
	CCA	18	13.315	22.685	

Moreover, when surgical procedure was assessed in each subgroup of patients stratified by staging, a significant difference in the survival of muscle-invasive CCA patients was observed. Patients receiving total cystectomy showed significantly greater survival probability than those receiving local procedures or partial cystectomy ($p = 0.028$, Figure 2A). However, for metastatic cases, no survival difference was observed based on surgical treatment received ($p = 0.269$, Figure 2B). Survival comparisons for non-muscle invasive cases were unable to be conducted due to the large number of censored events, i.e., patients that did not die during the follow-up period.

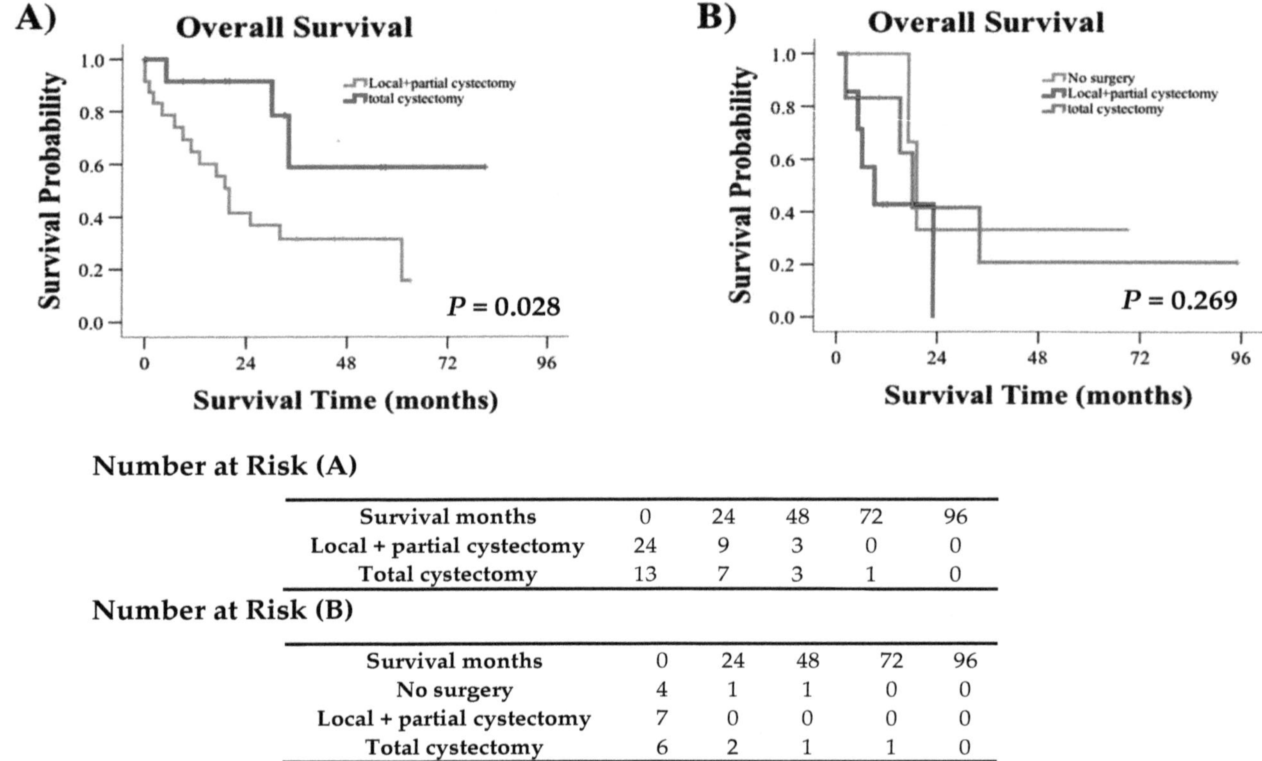

Number at Risk (A)

Survival months	0	24	48	72	96
Local + partial cystectomy	24	9	3	0	0
Total cystectomy	13	7	3	1	0

Number at Risk (B)

Survival months	0	24	48	72	96
No surgery	4	1	1	0	0
Local + partial cystectomy	7	0	0	0	0
Total cystectomy	6	2	1	1	0

Figure 2. Kaplan–Meier curves and risk tables demonstrating survival for (**A**) muscle invasive cases of CCA defined by AJCC 6th stage II and III and (**B**) metastatic CCA cases defined by AJCC 6th stage IV.

4. Discussion

Using the SEER program database, we documented incidence, mortality, demographics, and survival on a rare subtype of urinary bladder cancer. We identified that CCAs were more commonly associated with younger age, higher grade, female gender, black ethnicity, and have a higher risk of brain and liver metastasis. Although it was not present in any of the cases reported in the SEER program database, bone metastasis in CCAs has been reported in several previously published case reports [28,29]. The most common location of CCA identified from our study was from trigone and bladder neck. This finding is consistent with previous reviews that also documented these as common tumor locations [21,28]. More importantly, our study showed a poorer prognosis of CCAs compared to all other carcinomas of the urinary bladder attributable to the higher tumor staging of the CCA cases. The poorer prognosis was irrespective of age, sex, race, grade, surgery and radiation treatment. In muscle invasive cases of CCA, type of surgical treatment was a significant factor in determining survival—There was improved survival when treated with complete cystectomies, which is consistent with standard of care for carcinomas of the urinary bladder [30].

The capability for glycogen to enhance tumor survival in adverse conditions may result in a faster invasion of CCA, hence, higher staging at diagnosis. Glycogen stores provide an excess glucose supply that can be utilized in the hypoxic conditions of tumor microenvironment [7]. The glycogen breakdown also generates nucleotides critical for cell proliferation such as NAPDH, an essential reducing agent, through the pentose phosphate pathway [7]. Furthermore, the glycogen shunt has been proposed to sustain the Warburg effect, a phenomenon that causes cells to use glucose in glycolysis instead of oxidative phosphorylation even in presence of plentiful oxygen in cells [31]. During periods of decreased glucose availability, the glycogen shunt sustains the production of glycolytic intermediates and ATP through the Warburg effect, hence maintaining tumor growth in nutrient deprived conditions [5].

Recently, the glycogen debranching enzyme amylo-α-1, 6-glucosidase, 4-α-glucanotransferase (AGL) was shown to have tumor suppressor functions in a model of urothelial bladder cancer [32]. Loss of AGL increased tumor growth in vitro and in xenografted tumors accompanied by an increase in abnormal glycogen structures (limit dextrin) and decrease in normal glycogen. The study also showed an increase in aerobic glycolysis and increased lactate, consistent with a shift towards the Warburg effect. Similar to our results, patients with reduced AGL expression was also associated with a decrease in overall survival, but was no longer predictive of survival when examined in a multivariate model that included age, sex, stage, and grade [32]. The similarities of our findings in CCA suggest that the manipulation of glycogen accumulations in urothelial bladder tumors may induce characteristics that mimic CCA.

While most urinary bladder cancers are male predominant [33], it was an interesting finding that CCA seemed to have a female predominance. The higher proportion of female patients supports a possible mullerian origin of CCA which has been previously proposed due to its association with endometriosis and histological resemblance to clear cell cancers of female genital tract [19,34]. Moreover, it is well known that females with urinary bladder cancers are generally diagnosed with more advanced disease and have poorer prognosis than males [33,35]. However, our findings suggested that it was CCA males instead who had higher mortality than females. Collectively, the gender disparity between CCA and other urinary bladder cancers suggest that CCA is an entity with differing characteristics to other urinary bladder cancers. More mechanistic and clinical studies are needed to improve our understanding of how gender and its associated factors relate to CCA pathology and prognosis.

At this time, no tailored therapy exists for CCA. Patients typically undergo some form of surgical resection such as transurethral resection, total cystectomy, partial cystectomy or radical surgery accompanied by chemotherapy and/or radiation [30]. Our study suggests that those with muscle invasive disease had survival benefit from total cystectomy rather than partial cystectomy, although prospective studies are needed to confirm these findings. Further understanding of cancer glycogen metabolism may help us with new avenues of tailored disease treatment. No information with regards to chemotherapy treatment was included in this manuscript due to a lack of reliable data in the SEER program database at this time.

5. Conclusions

As the first large-scale study to date, we assessed the incidence, mortality, demographical/clinical characteristics, and survival of CCA, a rare, glycogen-rich variant of urinary bladder cancer. We found a poorer prognosis of CCAs compared to all other carcinomas of the urinary bladder that was attributable to the higher staging of these tumors. However, the limitations of the study include the retrospective study design, small number of cases of interest (i.e., CCA) in comparison to control cases (i.e., non-CCA), and reliability of the SEER program database. Additional prospective clinical studies are needed to confirm these findings. Mechanistic studies that assess signaling pathways linking glycogen and rate of tumor growth would be beneficial for improving the understanding of the link between glycogen and poorer patient prognosis, and help to identify novel, targeted therapies for these glycogen-rich cancers.

Author Contributions: Z.Z. conducted the data analysis and drafted the manuscript. C.J.K. assisted with data analysis. P.W., S.K.C. and I.D. assisted in providing clinical insights for the manuscript. B.H. provided guidance on statistical analyses. M.S.G. and R.C.S. conceptualized the manuscript. All authors have read and agreed to the published version of the manuscript.

Acknowledgments: Special thanks to Gentry lab and Vander Kooi lab for the numerous discussions and continuous support.

References and Notes

1. Young, L.E.A.; Brizzee, C.O.; Macedo, J.K.A.; Murphy, R.D.; Contreras, C.J.; DePaoli-Roach, A.A.; Roach, P.J.; Gentry, M.S.; Sun, R.C. Accurate and sensitive quantitation of glucose and glucose phosphates derived from storage carbohydrates by mass spectrometry. *Carbohydr. Polym.* **2019**, *230*, 115651. [CrossRef]
2. Schulze, A.; Harris, A.L. How cancer metabolism is tuned for proliferation and vulnerable to disruption. *Nature* **2012**, *491*, 364–373. [CrossRef] [PubMed]
3. Pelletier, J.; Bellot, G.; Gounon, P.; Lacas-Gervais, S.; Pouyssegur, J.; Mazure, N.M. Glycogen Synthesis is Induced in Hypoxia by the Hypoxia-Inducible Factor and Promotes Cancer Cell Survival. *Front. Oncol.* **2012**, *2*, 18. [CrossRef] [PubMed]
4. Curtis, M.; Kenny, H.A.; Ashcroft, B.; Mukherjee, A.; Johnson, A.; Zhang, Y.; Helou, Y.; Batlle, R.; Liu, X.; Gutierrez, N.; et al. Fibroblasts Mobilize Tumor Cell Glycogen to Promote Proliferation and Metastasis. *Cell Metab* **2019**, *29*, 141–155. [CrossRef] [PubMed]
5. Shulman, R.G.; Rothman, D.L. The Glycogen Shunt Maintains Glycolytic Homeostasis and the Warburg Effect in Cancer. *Trends Cancer* **2017**, *3*, 761–767. [CrossRef]
6. Lee, W.N.; Guo, P.; Lim, S.; Bassilian, S.; Lee, S.T.; Boren, J.; Cascante, M.; Go, V.L.; Boros, L.G. Metabolic sensitivity of pancreatic tumour cell apoptosis to glycogen phosphorylase inhibitor treatment. *Br. J. Cancer* **2004**, *91*, 2094–2100. [CrossRef] [PubMed]
7. Favaro, E.; Bensaad, K.; Chong, M.G.; Tennant, D.A.; Ferguson, D.J.; Snell, C.; Steers, G.; Turley, H.; Li, J.L.; Gunther, U.L.; et al. Glucose utilization via glycogen phosphorylase sustains proliferation and prevents premature senescence in cancer cells. *Cell Metab.* **2012**, *16*, 751–764. [CrossRef]
8. Rousset, M.; Zweibaum, A.; Fogh, J. Presence of Glycogen and Growth-related Variations in 58 Cultured Human Tumor Cell Lines of Various Tissue Origins. *Cancer Res.* **1981**, *41*, 1165–1170.
9. Rousset, M.; Chevalier, G.; Rousset, J.-P.; Dussaulx, E.; Zweibaum, A. Presence and Cell Growth-related Variations of Glycogen in Human Colorectal Adenocarcinoma Cell Lines in Culture. *Cancer Res.* **1979**, *39*, 531–534.
10. Staedel, C.; Beck, J.-P. Resurgence of glycogen synthesis and storage capacity in cultured hepatoma cells. *Cell Differ.* **1978**, *7*, 61–71. [CrossRef]
11. Altemus, M.A.; Yates, J.A.; Wu, Z.; Bao, L.; Merajver, S.D. Glycogen accumulation in aggressive breast cancers under hypoxia [abstract]. *Mol. Cell. Biol.* **2018**, *78* (Suppl. 13), 1446.
12. Sun, R.C.; Fan, T.W.M.; Deng, P.; Higashi, R.M.; Lane, A.N.; Le, A.-T.; Scott, T.L.; Sun, Q.; Warmoes, M.O.; Yang, Y. Noninvasive liquid diet delivery of stable isotopes into mouse models for deep metabolic network tracing. *Nat. Commun.* **2017**, *8*, 1646. [CrossRef] [PubMed]
13. Cheville, J.C.; Lohse, C.M.; Zincke, H.; Weaver, A.L.; Blute, M.L. Comparisons of outcome and prognostic features among histologic subtypes of renal cell carcinoma. *Am. J. Surg. Pathol.* **2003**, *27*, 612–624. [CrossRef] [PubMed]
14. Gadducci, A.; Cosio, S.; Spirito, N.; Cionini, L. Clear cell carcinoma of the endometrium: A biological and clinical enigma. *Anticancer Res.* **2010**, *30*, 1327–1334. [PubMed]
15. Sugiyama, T.; Kamura, T.; Kigawa, J.; Terakawa, N.; Kikuchi, Y.; Kita, T.; Suzuki, M.; Sato, I.; Taguchi, K. Clinical characteristics of clear cell carcinoma of the ovary: A distinct histologic type with poor prognosis and resistance to platinum-based chemotherapy. *Cancer* **2000**, *88*, 2584–2589. [CrossRef]
16. Zhou, Z.; Kinslow, C.J.; Hibshoosh, H.; Guo, H.; Cheng, S.K.; He, C.; Gentry, M.S.; Sun, R.C. Clinical Features, Survival and Prognostic Factors of Glycogen-Rich Clear Cell Carcinoma (GRCC) of the Breast in the U.S. Population. *J. Clin. Med.* **2019**, *8*, 246. [CrossRef]
17. Dow, J.A.; Young, J.D., Jr. Mesonephric adenocarcinoma of the bladder. *J. Urol.* **1968**, *100*, 466–469. [CrossRef]
18. Young, R.H.; Scully, R.E. Clear cell adenocarcinoma of the bladder and urethra. A report of three cases and review of the literature. *Am. J. Surg. Pathol.* **1985**, *9*, 816–826. [CrossRef]
19. Adeniran, A.J.; Tamboli, P. Clear cell adenocarcinoma of the urinary bladder: A short review. *Arch. Pathol. Lab. Med.* **2009**, *133*, 987–991.
20. Venyo, A.K. Primary Clear Cell Carcinoma of the Urinary Bladder. *Int. Sch. Res. Not.* **2014**, *2014*, 593826. [CrossRef]
21. Lu, J.; Xu, Z.; Jiang, F.; Wang, Y.; Hou, Y.; Wang, C.; Chen, Q. Primary clear cell adenocarcinoma of the bladder with recurrence: A case report and literature review. *World J. Surg. Oncol.* **2012**, *10*, 33. [CrossRef] [PubMed]

22. National Cancer Institute Surveillance. Epidemiology and End Result Program. Overview of the SEER Program. Available online: https://seer.cancer.gov/about/overview.html (accessed on 19 June 2016).
23. National Cancer Institute. DCCPS, Surveillance Research Program. Surveillance, Epidemiology, and End Results (SEER) Program (www.seer.cancer.gov). SEER*Stat Database: Incidence—SEER 18 Regs Research Data + Hurricane Katrina Impacted Louisiana Cases, Nov 2017 Sub (2000–2015) <Katrina/Rita Population Adjustment>—Linked To County Attributes—Total U.S., 1969–2016 Counties, released April 2018, based on the November 2017 Submission.
24. National Cancer Institute. DCCPS, Surveillance Research Program. Surveillance, Epidemiology, and End Results (SEER) Program (www.seer.cancer.gov) SEER*Stat Database: Incidence-Based Mortality—SEER 18 Regs (Excl Louisiana) Research Data, Nov 2017 Sub (2000–2015) <Katrina/Rita Population Adjustment>—Linked To County Attributes—Total U.S., 1969–2016 Counties, Released April 2018, based on the November 2017 Submission.
25. Kinslow, C.J.; Bruce, S.S.; Rae, A.I.; Sheth, S.A.; McKhann, G.M.; Sisti, M.B.; Bruce, J.N.; Sonabend, A.M.; Wang, T.J.C. Solitary-fibrous tumor/hemangiopericytoma of the central nervous system: A population-based study. *J. Neurooncol.* **2018**, *138*, 173–182. [CrossRef] [PubMed]
26. National Cancer Institute. DCCPS, Surveillance Research Program. Surveillance, Epidemiology, and End Results (SEER) Program (www.seer.cancer.gov) SEER*Stat Database: Incidence—SEER 18 Regs Research Data + Hurricane Katrina Impacted Louisiana Cases, Nov 2015 Sub (1973–2013 Varying)—Linked To County Attributes—Total U.S., 1969–2014 Counties, released April 2016, based on the November 2015 Submission.
27. National Cancer Institute. DCCPS, Surveillance Research Program. Surveillance, Epidemiology, and End Results (SEER) Program (www.seer.cancer.gov) SEER*Stat Database: Incidence—SEER 18 Regs Research Data + Hurricane Katrina Impacted Louisiana Cases, Nov 2017 Sub (1973–2015 Varying)—Linked To County Attributes—Total U.S., 1969–2016 Counties, released April 2018, based on the November 2017 Submission.
28. Matsuoka, Y.; Machida, T.; Oka, K.; Ishizaka, K. Clear cell adenocarcinoma of the urinary bladder inducing acute renal failure. *Int. J. Urol.* **2002**, *9*, 467–469. [CrossRef] [PubMed]
29. Honda, N.; Yamada, Y.; Nanaura, H.; Fukatsu, H.; Nonomura, H.; Hatano, Y. Mesonephric adenocarcinoma of the urinary bladder: A case report. *Hinyokika Kiyo* **2000**, *46*, 27–31. [PubMed]
30. National Comprehensive Cancer Network. NCCN Clinical Practice Guidelines in Oncology (NCCN Guidelines). Bladder Cancer. Version 1.2019. Available online: https://www.partnershipagainstcancer.ca/db-sage/sage20181257/# (accessed on 19 June 2018).
31. Warburg, O. On the origin of cancer cells. *Science* **1956**, *123*, 309–314. [CrossRef]
32. Guin, S.; Pollard, C.; Ru, Y.; Ritterson Lew, C.; Duex, J.E.; Dancik, G.; Owens, C.; Spencer, A.; Knight, S.; Holemon, H.; et al. Role in tumor growth of a glycogen debranching enzyme lost in glycogen storage disease. *J. Natl. Cancer Inst.* **2014**, *106*. [CrossRef]
33. Dobruch, J.; Daneshmand, S.; Fisch, M.; Lotan, Y.; Noon, A.P.; Resnick, M.J.; Shariat, S.F.; Zlotta, A.R.; Boorjian, S.A. Gender and Bladder Cancer: A Collaborative Review of Etiology, Biology, and Outcomes. *Eur. Urol.* **2016**, *69*, 300–310. [CrossRef]
34. Drew, P.A.; Murphy, W.M.; Civantos, F.; Speights, V.O. The histogenesis of clear cell adenocarcinoma of the lower urinary tract. Case series and review of the literature. *Hum. Pathol.* **1996**, *27*, 248–252. [CrossRef]

10

Unusual Faces of Bladder Cancer

Claudia Manini [1] and José I. López [2,*]

[1] Department of Pathology, San Giovanni Bosco Hospital, 10154 Turin, Italy; claudiamaninicm@gmail.com
[2] Department of Pathology, Biocruces-Bizkaia Health Research Institute, Cruces University Hospital, Barakaldo, 48903 Bizkaia, Spain
* Correspondence: jilpath@gmail.com

Simple Summary: The spectrum of architectural and cytological findings in UC is wide, although transitional cell carcinoma, either papillary or flat, low- or high-grade, constitutes the majority of cases in routine practice. Some of these changes are just mere morphological variations, but others must be recognized since they have importance for the patient. The goal of this review is to compile this histological variability giving to the general pathologist a general idea of this morphological spectrum in a few pages. The review also updates the literature focusing specifically on the morphological and immunohistochemical clues useful for the diagnosis and some selected molecular studies with prognostic and/or diagnostic implications.

Abstract: The overwhelming majority of bladder cancers are transitional cell carcinomas. Albeit mostly monotonous, carcinomas in the bladder may occasionally display a broad spectrum of histological features that should be recognized by pathologists because some of them represent a diagnostic problem and/or lead prognostic implications. Sometimes these features are focal in the context of conventional transitional cell carcinomas, but some others are generalized across the tumor making its recognition a challenge. For practical purposes, the review distributes the morphologic spectrum of changes in architecture and cytology. Thus, nested and large nested, micropapillary, myxoid stroma, small tubules and adenoma nephrogenic-like, microcystic, verrucous, and diffuse lymphoepithelioma-like, on one hand, and plasmacytoid, signet ring, basaloid-squamous, yolk-sac, trophoblastic, rhabdoid, lipid/lipoblastic, giant, clear, eosinophilic (oncocytoid), and sarcomatoid, on the other, are revisited. Key histological and immunohistochemical features useful in the differential diagnosis are mentioned. In selected cases, molecular data associated with the diagnosis, prognosis, and/or treatment are also included.

Keywords: bladder cancer; diagnosis; differential diagnosis; prognosis; histopathology; immunohistochemistry

---

1. Introduction

Bladder cancer is a frequent neoplasm [1] in which tobacco use, pollution, and other varied agents have been directly implicated in its genesis and development [2]. Most of them are composed of transitional cells of low/intermediate grade, papillary architecture, and invasion limited to the lamina propria and submucosa. However, a smaller but significant number of cases do display dismal features like high-grade, non-papillary growth patterns, and muscularis propria invasion, with these patients pursuing an aggressive clinical course.

Aside from transitional cell carcinoma (TCC), other histological subtypes, like conventional squamous cell carcinoma, adenocarcinoma, and neuroendocrine carcinoma, are quite frequently seen in clinical practice, alone or in combination, particularly in the context of high-grade cases. These cases are not the subject of this review.

Although TCC is a histologically monotonous neoplasm composed in the vast majority of cases by easily recognizable transitional cells, a small subset of cases displays a broad spectrum of architectural and/or cytological characteristics that should be recognized since some of them carry diagnostic difficulties and/or prognostic implications [3] (Table 1). This recognition is increasingly important now that very promising advances linking morphological variants with genomic signatures are being identified [4].

Table 1. Unusual features in bladder cancer with prognostic profiles.

Architectural Changes	Prognostic Profiles
	Worse prognosis - Nested - Large nested - Micropapillary
	Not worse prognosis - Myxoid stromal change - Small tubules - Nephrogenic adenoma-like - Microcystic - Verrucous - Diffuse lymphoepithelioma-like
Cytological changes	
	Worse prognosis - Plasmacytoid - Signet-ring - Basaloid-squamous - Yolk-sac -Trophoblastic - Rhabdoid - Giant pleomorphic - Clear - Sarcomatoid
	Not worse prognosis - Lipid/lipoblast - Giant osteoclast-like - Eosinophilic (oncocytoid)

Clinical practice allows the pathologist to face unusual histological subtypes of urothelial carcinomas (UC), and conventional TCC displaying focal/extensive morphologic variations of uncertain significance. This narrative collects 25 years of personal experience of the authors in the routine diagnosis of bladder cancer.

2. Architectural Changes

2.1. *Nested and Large Nested Architecture*

Talbert and Young reported in 1989 three cases of a deceptively benign bladder carcinoma characterized by small packed cellular aggregates closely resembling von Brunn nests and nephrogenic adenoma [5]. Isolated cases of this histological subtype of bladder cancer had previously appeared in the literature, always being referred to as of von Brunn nest origin [6]. Now, nested UC is well recognized and fully characterized by histological, immunohistochemical, and molecular perspectives [7,8]. Under the microscope, nested UC appears as a non-papillary neoplastic growth of bland cells with scarce atypia arranged in small nests (Figure 1a) showing an evident infiltrating growth pattern at different levels of the bladder wall. Typically, the tumor does not induce a stromal reaction nor is accompanied by inflammatory infiltrates. Problems to recognize nested UC may arise in small superficial biopsies if crushing artifacts are present or if the infiltrative nature is not seen.

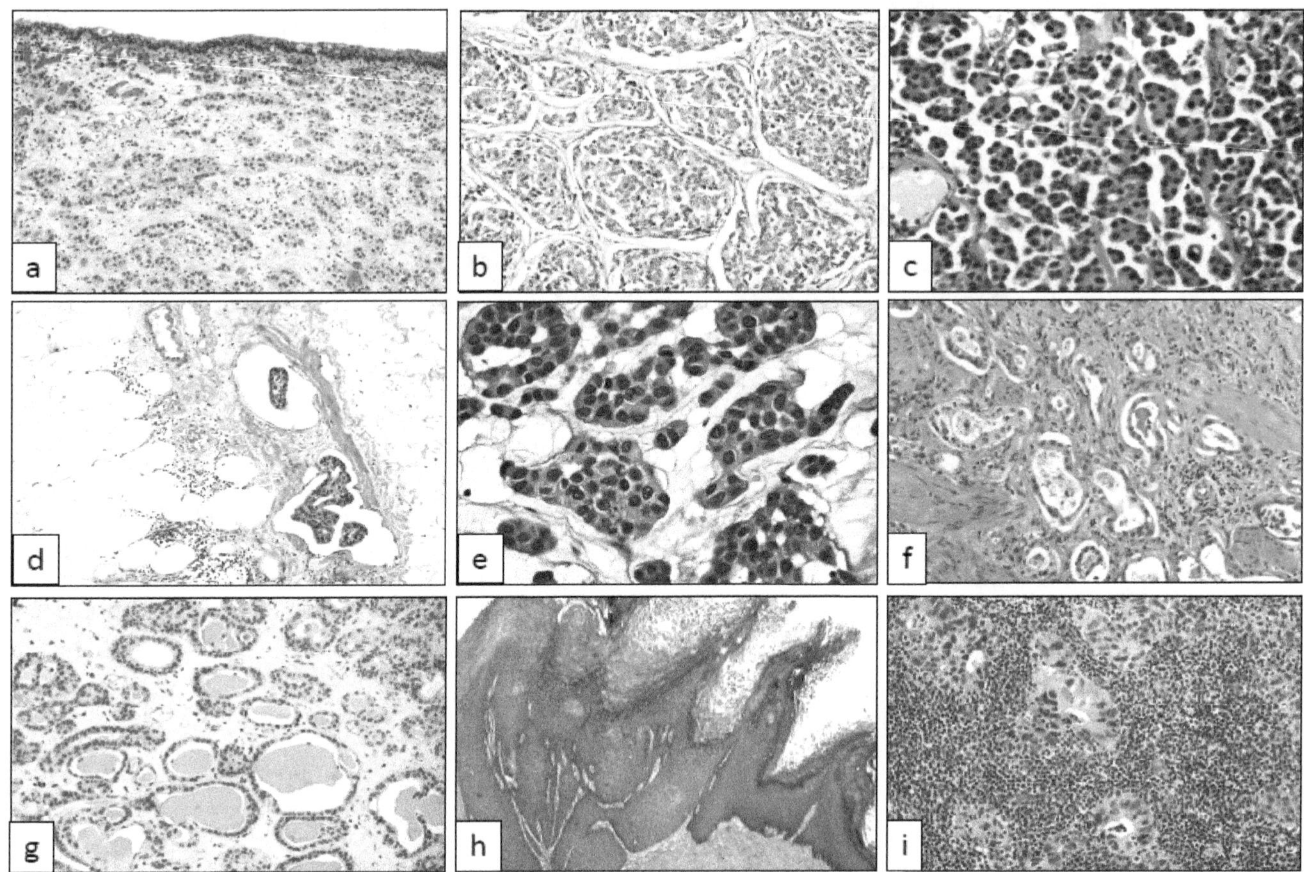

Figure 1. Architectural changes in bladder cancer (with original magnifications included). (**a**) Nested pattern (×100), (**b**) large nested pattern (×100), (**c**) micropapillary pattern (×250), (**d**) vascular invasion in the micropapillary pattern (×100), (**e**) myxoid basophilic stroma (×400), (**f**) small tubules (×100), (**g**) microcystic pattern (×100), (**h**) verrucous pattern (×40), and (**i**) lymphoepithelioma-like pattern (×250).

Cox and Epstein described in 2011 the large nested variant of UC reporting the characteristic histology of a tumor resembling large von Brunn nests with inverted growth in 23 patients [9]. Some isolated cases of this UC variant have been reported since then, and only two more series of cases have been published so far [10,11]. The large nested UC shares with the nested UC the same morphologic characteristics and clinical aggressiveness but the nests are larger (Figure 1b), with a growth pattern mimicking conventional inverted UC. These similarities have been advised to merge them into the same group in the last WHO classification of UC [12]. Interestingly, large nested UC displays a luminal phenotype, positive with FOXA1, GATA3, and CK 20 [12]. *FGFR3* and *TERT* genes are frequently mutated in this UC subtype [12].

2.2. Micropapillary Architecture

UC may sometimes display a micropapillary architecture. Delicate, thin, and fragile papillae without stromal axis are the hallmark of this morphological variant of UC (Figure 1c). To note, the invasive component of micropapillary UC shows nests with cells detached from the basal membrane, a typical artifact in this tumor that mimics lymphatic invasion and is associated with biological aggressiveness [13]. The vascular invasion is a very frequent histological finding (Figure 1d). Aside from rare pure examples, the majority of cases are mixed with a conventional transitional cell carcinoma, usually high grade. Like the rest of micropapillary carcinomas across the body [14], this histological subtype of UC has a dismal prognosis, even worse than conventional high-grade UC at the same stage [15], and typically presents with advanced stages at diagnosis. Although exceptional, micropapillary carcinomas from other sites may metastasize to the urinary bladder [16], making the correct diagnosis more difficult.

The first description of this variant of UC was made in 1994 by Amin et al. [17], where they stressed the histological similarities of this bladder tumor with the classic papillary serous carcinoma of the ovary. After that, many series have been published all along the urinary tract, including the renal pelvis and ureter [18,19].

Abundant immunohistochemical and molecular analyses have been performed in micropapillary UC [20–22] all confirming its aggressive potential. Although initially thought to be a variant of adenocarcinoma by some authors [23], Yang et al. have very recently reported that the micropapillary UC is not a variant of adenocarcinoma [22].

2.3. *Myxoid Stromal Change*

UC may display focal myxoid changes in the stroma (Figure 1e) mimicking the colloid adenocarcinomas seen in other sites. This change has been previously reported [24,25] and when observed in transurethral resection specimens, may lead to an erroneous interpretation of colonic adenocarcinoma invading the bladder wall. Solid cell nests immersed in a basophilic edematous stroma are the hallmark of this histological change, which is usually focal but can be generalized in some isolated cases. Again, immunohistochemistry is of much help in cases in which the transitional phenotype of the tumor is not evident on hematoxylin-eosin slides. GATA3 positivity, co-expression of CK7 and CK20, and CDX-2 negativity should resolve the diagnostic dilemma in doubtful cases [24]. Attention must be paid, however, to the occasional CK7 positivity of some colorectal adenocarcinomas, a finding that is a sign of dismal prognosis [26].

2.4. *Small Tubules and Nephrogenic Adenoma-Like Architecture*

Very occasionally, UC is composed of low-grade cells arranged in small tubules resembling *cystitis glandularis* or nephrogenic adenoma (Figure 1f) [27]. The bland cytologic features of this histologic subtype contrast with its frank infiltrative nature, even reaching the muscularis propria in some cases. Since nephrogenic adenoma may display also a concerning pseudo-infiltrative growth [28], an immunohistochemical study with PAX-8, CK7, p63, and napsin A [29] may be useful to make the differential diagnosis in problematic cases. The clinical significance of this histologic change is not established so far.

2.5. *Microcystic Architecture*

The microcystic histology has been rarely reported in the literature at UC. Aside from a handful of single case reports, the largest series published to date analyzes 20 cases [30]. The limited examples reported up to now show a bland histologic appearance, with round to oval cysts which often contain eosinophilic intraluminal secretion covered by low columnar or flattened urothelial cells (Figure 1g). Despite its deceptive bland histology, microcystic UC displays the same aggressiveness of conventional UC at the same stage. The main differential diagnosis is nephrogenic adenoma and adenocarcinoma of the bladder. In this sense, a basic immunohistochemical panel including p63 positivity and CK7/20 co-expression coupled with napsin A and PAX-8 negativities will resolve the eventual diagnostic troubles.

2.6. *Verrucous Architecture*

Genuine verrucous carcinoma is a rare tumor subtype in the urinary tract [31], however, conventional well-differentiated squamous cell carcinoma with "verrucous" architectural features is a much more common event. Since the difference between them has prognostic implications their correct identification by the pathologist matters. Verrucous carcinoma may recur but never metastasize. Some cases are related to HPV infection, others to schistosomiasis, but there are also cases unrelated to any known specific etiology [32].

The diagnosis of a verrucous carcinoma in the urinary tract, as elsewhere, is subjected to very strict histological criteria. Only low-grade keratinizing squamous cell carcinomas with superficial verrucous architecture should be considered (Figure 1h). Verrucous carcinomas may display a pushing border of growth into the lamina propria, but a true invasion is lacking. Noteworthy, any high-grade area across the tumor or frank stromal infiltration makes the diagnosis of verrucous carcinoma unsuitable.

2.7. Diffuse Architecture with Lymphoepithelioma-Like Changes

Lymphoepithelioma is the classical histological term referring to an undifferentiated carcinoma first described in the nasopharyngeal region of Asian patients [33]. Some of them are related to Epstein-Barr virus infection. Since then, analog histology has been described in many carcinomas widely distributed in the body. Aside from multiple case reports, several series of this tumor subtype in the bladder [33–36] and the upper urinary tract [37] have been published in the literature. Remarkably, the theoretical relationship of lymphoepithelioma-like UC with Epstein–Barr virus infection is no longer sustainable in cases arising in the urinary tract after the results obtained with FISH analyses in the largest series [35–37].

The tumor shows a diffuse growth of ill-defined islands of poorly-differentiated cells with badly defined cytoplasmic borders, large nuclei, and patent nucleoli. The stroma is heavily infiltrated by lymphocytes occasionally showing lymphoepithelial lesion (Figure 1i). By immunohistochemistry, GATA3, cytokeratins 34βE12, AE1-AE3, and CK7, p53 and p63 are positive in a variable number of cases, whereas TTF-1, CD30, and CK20 are negative [36,37]. The prognosis does not differ from conventional UC at the same stage.

3. Cytological Changes

3.1. Plasmacytoid Cells

Plasmacytoid UC is an aggressive tumor. This cytologic variant of UC can present as pure tumors or mixed with conventional UC and/or with other non-conventional UC. For example, mixed micropapillary and plasmacytoid UC cases have been occasionally reported [38]. Histological similarities with multiple myeloma were noticed since the first report by Sahin et al. in 1991 [39]. Since this original description, several large series have been published so far all of them confirming its dismal prognosis [40].

In its typical presentation, the tumor appears as flat, non-papillary, highly cellular masses growing diffusely in the urinary tract wall with infiltrative edges and frequent vascular invasion images. Neoplastic cells are non-cohesively arranged and show lateralized cytoplasm, nuclear atypia, and high mitotic count (Figure 2a). In doubtful cases, or patients with a previous history of plasma cell dyscrasia, immunohistochemistry is of help revealing its epithelial, non-plasmacytic, nature. Briefly, GATA-3 and CK7 are positive and CD 38 is negative. Positive immunostaining with CD 138 may be observed in this neoplasm, but this finding does not preclude the diagnosis of plasmacytoid UC [41].

HER2 overexpression has been observed by FISH in plasmacytoid UC [42]. Contrary to what happens in most UC, plasmacytoid variants do not seem to harbor *TP53* gene mutations in a sequencing analysis [41]. On the other hand, *TERT* gene promoter mutations have been detected [43]. A study using whole-exome sequencing has detected somatic alterations in the *CDH1* gene of 84% of plasmacytoid UC, a finding of clinical aggressiveness that seems to be specific to this tumor variant [44].

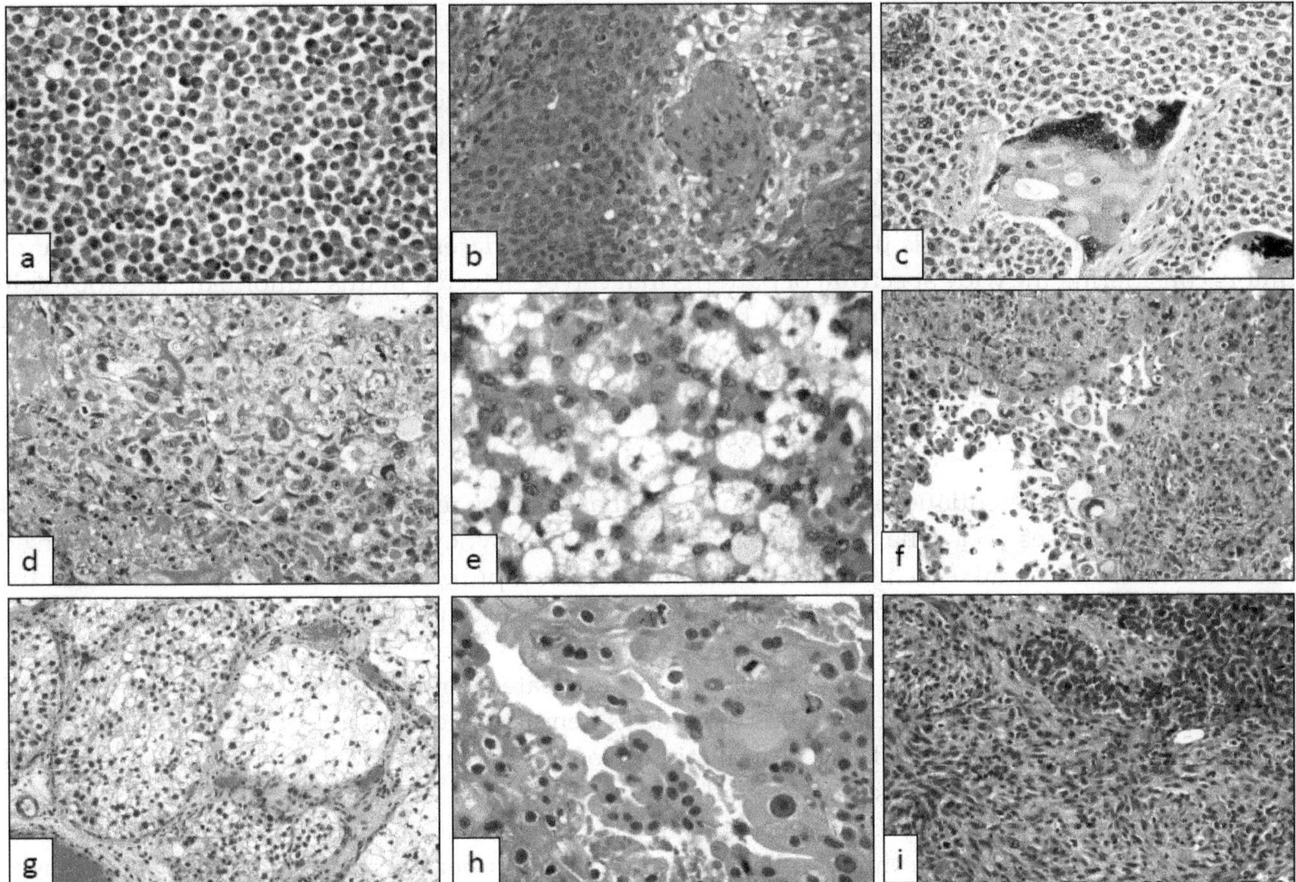

Figure 2. Cytological changes in bladder cancer. (**a**) Plasmacytoid cells (×250), (**b**) basaloid and squamous cells (×250), (**c**) syncytiotrophoblastic cells (×250), (**d**) trophoblastic cells (×250), (**e**) lipoblastic-like cells (×400), (**f**) pleomorphic giant cells (×250), (**g**) clear cells (×100), (**h**) eosinophilic (oncocytoid) cells (×400), and (**i**) sarcomatoid cells (×250).

3.2. Signet-Ring Cells

Since signet-ring cell features are very rare in UC, and their identification in transurethral resection specimens can raise the possibility of a metastatic seed from a neoplasm originating in the digestive tract. A careful search of the classical urothelial features (nests of transitional cells, papillae, in situ carcinoma in the surface epithelium, etc.) in the biopsy, if present, may be of help in the differential diagnosis. Otherwise, the clinical context of the patient and a basic immunohistochemical panel, for example, CK7/20, GATA-3, CDX-2, and p63, should resolve the dilemma. The analysis of the national Surveillance, Epidemiology, and End Results (SEER) database of 318 such cases confirms the worse prognosis of this histologic variant compared with conventional UC [45].

3.3. Basaloid-Squamous Cells

Basaloid-squamous cell carcinomas are aggressive neoplasms mainly located in the head and neck [46] and anal [47] regions. The tumor is extraordinarily uncommon in the urinary tract, with only a handful of single cases published to date [48–51]. Everywhere, most basaloid squamous cell carcinomas are associated with HPV infection [51].

Histologically, the tumor is deeply infiltrative and shows a typical biphasic pattern (Figure 2b). Basaloid atypical cells with high mitotic rate and scarce cytoplasm are arranged in lobes and nests showing peripheral palisading and stromal reaction. Basaloid nests are centered by squamous islands with evident keratinization. p16 is intensely positive in tumor cells.

3.4. Yolk Sac Cells

A very limited number of UC with yolk sac tumor differentiation has been reported in the literature [52–55]. The yolk sac differentiation represents an example of a somatic differentiation present in non-gonadal neoplasms [56]. A varied spectrum of patterns have been identified in these tumors: microcystic, vitelline, glandular enteric-like, hepatoid, solid, sarcomatoid, etc. An enteroblastic differentiation seems to be the most frequent histology in somatically derived yolk sac tumors [56].

Immunohistochemistry is useful to identify yolk sac differentiation in UC and other somatic tumors considering the wide spectrum of patterns that can be detected in this tumor. Alpha-fetoprotein and SALL4 are consistently positive. CK7, however, is negative. Markers of intestinal differentiation, like CDX2, are usually positive in enteroblastic areas and Her Par-1 in hepatoid ones. A polysomic abnormality in 12p has been detected in one recently published case [55].

3.5. Trophoblastic Cells

Trophoblastic differentiation is a rare event in UC that has been recently reviewed by Przybycin et al. in a series of 16 cases [57]. The spectrum includes isolated syncytiotrophoblast cells interspersed in a conventional UC, mixed choriocarcinoma and UC, and pure choriocarcinoma. Same as in the yolk sac differentiation, trophoblastic changes are examples of somatically derived differentiations in non-gonadal tumors.

Syncytiotrophoblasts are detected as isolated multinucleated giant cells immersed in high-grade UC (Figure 2c). Choriocarcinoma differentiation appears as hemorrhagic areas at low-power magnification. A closer view of these areas reveals the typical mixture of trophoblastic and syncytiotrophoblastic cells immersed in a necro-hemorrhagic background (Figure 2d).

By immunohistochemistry, β-hCG is expressed in trophoblastic and syncytiotrophoblastic cells, as well as in the malignant urothelial cells in a significant number of cases. Interestingly, increased levels of seric β-hCG in patients with UC is an independent prognostic factor [58]. GATA3 positivity has been detected in more than 70% of trophoblastic tumors in a large series [59] and appears as a useful marker to be included in the diagnostic panel. SALL4 is focally positive in less than 50% of the cases [57] and is negative in the larger syncytiotrophoblastic cells [60]. HSD3B1, a novel marker specific to trophoblastic differentiation [61], has been detected in 100% of the cases [57].

3.6. Rhabdoid Cells

Rhabdoid tumors have been documented in many different topographies across the body [62], always linked to biological aggressiveness and bad prognosis. Its histogenesis is still unclear. A handful of rhabdoid tumors of the bladder have been published, particularly in children and young adults [63–65]. There are, however, isolated cases reported in adulthood [66–68].

Aside from genuine rhabdoid tumors, a focal *rhabdoid* phenotype can be observed sometimes in UC [68], where large and ovoid cells with large atypical nuclei and lateralized eosinophilic cytoplasm may appear growing without any specific pattern usually in high-grade neoplasms. A possible rhabdomyoblastic dedifferentiation in the context of a sarcomatoid UC should be ruled out, at least theoretically, in these cases.

By immunohistochemistry, rhabdoid cells are positive for CK7, CK20, vimentin, E-cadherin, and β-catenin, p63, and INI-1 [68].

3.7. Lipid/Lipoblast-Like Cells

These two terms refer to a rare variant of UC composed of lipidic appearing tumor cells intermingled with transitional cells in variable proportions. It was first recognized by Mostofi et al. in 1999 [69]. Since then only single case reports and two short series [70,71] have been published. The longest series so far analyzes 27 cases collected from different international institutions [71]. Lipidic-appearing cells may resemble either adipocytes or adipoblasts (Figure 2e) and usually take part in a high-grade UC, not otherwise specified. Immunohistochemistry confirms the epithelial nature in all cases, including the co-expression of CK7 and CK20 [70,71].

3.8. Giant Cells

Giant cells are rarely observed in UC and only single case reports and a few short series have been published so far [72–74]. Two morphological variants have been described: osteoclast-like and giant pleomorphic cells, both of them associated with high-grade neoplasms. For practical purposes, these cells must be distinguished from trophoblastic and syncytiotrophoblastic cells appearing in some UC (see above). The presence of these giant cells in UC may be focal in the context of a high-grade UC or diffuse across the tumor, making difficult the correct diagnosis. A dedifferentiated sarcomatoid UC (see below) diagnosis can be considered in some of these cases.

Pleomorphic giant cell carcinoma have been described in many sites of the body and is a tumor subtype with dismal prognosis everywhere. Giant cell tumor areas in UC show a diffuse growth of cells with extreme pleomorphism and high mitotic count (Figure 2f). Cytoplasmic vacuolization and emperipolesis can be detected. Unusually, these tumors are at advanced stages at diagnosis, with deep infiltration in the bladder wall and frequent lymphatic dissemination [72]. Fifty percent of the patients reported in the series of Samaratunga et al. died of disease within the first year of follow-up [73]. By immunohistochemistry, the co-expression of CK7/20 and GATA3 positivity are retained in these tumors.

Osteoclast-like giant cells can be rarely observed in tumors originating in many sites of the body. In the bladder, they appear very occasionally in the context of high-grade UC. Contrary to the observed in pleomorphic giant cells, osteoclastic-like giant cells devoid of atypia and mitosis and show a reactive, non-neoplastic appearance. Whether these cells are truly neoplastic or reactive in the context of the tumor is a classical controversy that has been recently elucidated [74]. In this study, osteoclast-like giant cells are negative for GATA3, thrombomodulin, uroplakin II, and cytokeratin AE1/AE3, thus confirming their non-epithelial differentiation [74].

3.9. Clear Cells

Only single cases and a short series of 10 cases [75] of clear cell UC have been published so far. An advanced stage at diagnosis and an aggressive clinical course is the rule in these patients. Clear cell change, however, is regularly mentioned in several papers reviewing the varied morphology of UC in the bladder and upper urinary tract [76–80].

Clear cell change in UC reflects intracytoplasmic glycogen accumulation that in some cases is extreme this way resembling the typical clear cells observed in clear cell renal cell carcinoma. Usually, clear cell nests are intermingled in the tumor with conventional transitional cells (Figure 2g), which makes its correct identification easier. However, if the clear cell change is generalized or if transurethral resection specimens do not contain pieces of evidence of the urothelial origin of the tumor, the possibility of metastasis in the bladder of a clear cell renal cell carcinoma should be always taken into account [81].

3.10. Eosinophilic (Oncocytoid) Cells

An eosinophilic change can be observed in some UC resembling the cells of renal oncocytomas [82]. These cases show large granular and deeply eosinophilic elements with focal apocrinoid features (Figure 2h). Frequent nuclear pleomorphism is also seen, but true atypia is lacking. Mitoses are scarce, or absent, giving an overall impression of a low-grade tumor. Immunohistochemistry is that of the conventional UC, and neuroendocrine markers are negative. Anyway, further descriptions are needed to delineate better this histologic feature. At least for practical purposes, this histologic feature should be distinguished from oncocytic carcinoid tumors of the urinary bladder [83], an extraordinarily rare entity in the urinary bladder.

3.11. Sarcomatoid Cells

Sarcomatoid dedifferentiation is a relatively common finding in high-grade UC. Recent studies have approached the correlation between morphology and genomics in sarcomatoid bladder cancer through analyzing the epithelial to mesenchymal transition process concluding that UC developing sarcomatoid transformation are carcinomas of basal-type [84]. Practically all possible differentiations have been reported in the literature, from undifferentiated spindle cell (Figure 2i) to osteosarcoma. The epithelial component may be scarce or even not identified in some cases, so the diagnosis of primary sarcoma in the urinary bladder should be made with caution in transurethral resection specimens.

An excellent review of this topic based on a MEDLINE database study has been recently published [85].

4. Conclusions

This narrative collects the varied spectrum of morphological features that can be found in UC. These changes have been organized in architectural and cytological for didactic purposes, but mixtures of them are eventually found in real practice. The goal of this overview is to offer in a few pages the essentials for recognizing them giving diagnostic clues based on morphological and immunohistochemical keys.

Author Contributions: C.M. and J.I.L. have designed, reviewed, written, and approved the final version of the manuscript. Both authors have read and agreed to the published version of the manuscript.

References

1. Siegel, R.L.; Miller, K.D.; Jemal, A. Cancer statistics, 2020. *CA Cancer J. Clin.* **2020**, *70*, 7–30. [CrossRef] [PubMed]
2. Teoh, J.Y.; Huang, J.; Ko, W.Y.; Lok, V.; Choi, P.; Ng, C.F.; Sengupta, S.; Mostafid, H.; Kamat, A.M.; Black, P.C.; et al. Global trends of bladder cancer incidence and mortality, and their associations with tobacco use and gross domestic products per capita. *Eur. Urol.* **2020**. [CrossRef]
3. Lobo, N.; Shariat, S.F.; Guo, C.C.; Fernandez, M.I.; Kassouf, W.; Choudhury, A.; Gao, J.; Williams, S.B.; Galsky, M.D.; Taylor III, J.A.; et al. What is the significance of variant histology in urothelial carcinoma? *Eur. Urol. Focus.* **2020**, *6*, 653–663. [CrossRef]
4. Al-Ahmadie, H.; Netto, G.J. Updates on the genomics of bladder cancer and novel molecular taxonomy. *Adv. Anat. Pathol.* **2020**, *27*, 36–43. [CrossRef]
5. Talbert, M.L.; Young, R.H. Carcinomas of the urinary bladder with deceptively benign-appearing foci. A report of three cases. *Am. J. Surg. Pathol.* **1989**, *13*, 374–381. [CrossRef] [PubMed]
6. Stern, J.B. Unusual benign bladder tumor of von Brunn nest origin. *Urology* **1979**, *14*, 288–289. [CrossRef]
7. Lin, O.; Cardillo, M.; Dalbagni, G.; Linkov, I.; Hutchinson, B.; Reuter, V.E. Nested variant of urothelial carcinoma: A clinicopathologic and immunohistochemical study of 12 cases. *Mod. Pathol.* **2003**, *16*, 1289–1298. [CrossRef] [PubMed]
8. Levy, D.R.; Cheng, L. The expanding molecular and mutational landscape of nested variant of urothelial carcinoma. *Histopathology* **2020**, *76*, 638–639. [CrossRef] [PubMed]
9. Cox, R.; Epstein, J.I. Large nested variant of urothelial carcinoma: 23 cases mimicking von Brunn nests and inverted growth pattern of noninvasive papillary urothelial carcinoma. *Am. J. Surg. Pathol.* **2011**, *35*, 1337–1342. [CrossRef] [PubMed]
10. Compérat, E.; McKenney, J.K.; Hartmann, A.; Hes, O.; Bertz, S.; Varinot, J.; Brimo, F. Large nested variant of urothelial carcinoma: A clinicopathological study of 36 cases. *Histopathology* **2017**, *71*, 703–710. [CrossRef]
11. Hacihasanoglu, E.; Behzatoglu, K. Large nested urothelial carcinoma: A clinicopathological study of 22 cases on transurethral resection materials. *Ann. Diagn. Pathol.* **2019**, *42*, 7–11. [CrossRef] [PubMed]
12. Weyerer, V.; Eckstein, M.; Compérat, E.; Juette, H.; Gaisa, N.T.; Allory, Y.; Stöhr, R.; Wullich, B.; Rouprêt, M.; Hartmann, A.; et al. Pure large nested variant of urothelial carcinoma (LNUC) is the prototype of an *FGFR3* mutated aggressive urothelial carcinoma with luminal-papillary phenotype. *Cancers* **2020**, *12*, 763. [CrossRef] [PubMed]

13. Shah, T.S.; Kaag, M.; Raman, J.D.; Chan, W.; Tran, T.; Kunchala, S.; Shuman, L.; DeGraff, D.J.; Chen, G.; Warrick, J.I. Clinical significance of prominent retraction clefts in invasive urothelial carcinoma. *Hum. Pathol.* **2017**, *61*, 90–96. [CrossRef] [PubMed]
14. Nassar, H. Carcinomas with micropapillary morphology. Clinical significance and current concepts. *Adv. Anat. Pathol.* **2004**, *11*, 297–303. [CrossRef] [PubMed]
15. Jin, D.; Jin, K.; Qiu, S.; Zhou, X.; Yuan, Q.; Yang, L.; Wei, Q. Prognostic values of the clinicopathological characteristics and survival outcomes in micropapillary urothelial carcinoma of the bladder: A SEER database analysis. *Cancer Med.* **2020**, *9*, 4897–4906. [CrossRef] [PubMed]
16. Ramalingam, P.; Middleton, L.P.; Tamboli, P.; Troncoso, P.; Silva, E.G.; Ayala, A.G. Invasive micropapillary carcinoma of the breast metastatic to the urinary bladder and endometrium: Diagnostic pitfalls and review of the literature of tumors with micropapillary features. *Ann. Diagn. Pathol.* **2003**, *7*, 112–119. [CrossRef]
17. Amin, M.B.; Ro, J.Y.; El-Sharkawy, T.; Lee, K.M.; Troncoso, P.; Silva, E.G.; Ordóñez, N.G.; Ayala, A.G. Micropapillary variant of transitional cell carcinoma of the urinary bladder. Histologic pattern resembling ovarian papillary serous carcinoma. *Am. J. Surg. Pathol.* **1994**, *18*, 1224–1232. [CrossRef]
18. Holmäng, S.; Thomsen, J.; Johansson, S.L. Micropapillary carcinoma of the renal pelvis and ureter. *J. Urol.* **2006**, *175*, 463–466. [CrossRef]
19. Perez-Montiel, D.; Hes, O.; Michal, M.; Suster, S. Micropapillary urothelial carcinoma of the upper urinary tract: Clinicopathologic study of five cases. *Am. J. Clin. Pathol.* **2006**, *126*, 86–92. [CrossRef]
20. Guo, C.C.; Dadhania, V.; Zhang, L.; Majewski, T.; Bondaruk, J.; Sykulski, M.; Wronowska, W.; Gambin, A.; Wang, Y.; Zhang, S.; et al. Gene Expression Profile of the Clinically Aggressive Micropapillary Variant of Bladder Cancer. *Eur. Urol.* **2016**, *70*, 211–220. [CrossRef]
21. Zinnall, U.; Weyerer, V.; Compérat, E.; Camparo, P.; Gaisa, N.T.; Knuechel-Clarke, R.; Perren, A.; Lugli, A.; Toma, M.; Baretton, G.; et al. Micropapillary urothelial carcinoma: Evaluation of HER2 status and immunohistochemical characterization of the molecular subtype. *Hum. Pathol.* **2018**, *80*, 55–64. [CrossRef] [PubMed]
22. Yang, Y.; Kaimakliotis, H.Z.; Williamson, S.R.; Koch, M.O.; Huang, K.; Barboza, M.P.; Zhang, S.; Wang, M.; Idrees, M.T.; Grignon, D.J.; et al. Micropapillary urothelial carcinoma of urinary bladder displays immunophenotypic features of luminal and p53-like subtypes and is not a variant of adenocarcinoma. *Urol. Oncol.* **2020**, *38*, 449–458. [CrossRef] [PubMed]
23. Johansson, S.L.; Borghede, G.; Holmäng, S. Micropapillary bladder carcinoma: A clinicopathological study of 20 cases. *J. Urol.* **1999**, *161*, 1798–1802. [CrossRef]
24. Tavora, F.; Epstein, J.I. Urothelial carcinoma with abundant myxoid stroma. *Hum. Pathol.* **2009**, *40*, 1391–1398. [CrossRef] [PubMed]
25. Gilg, M.M.; Wimmer, B.; Ott, A.; Langner, C. Urothelial carcinoma with abundant myxoid stroma. Evidence for mucinous production by cancer cells. *Virchows Arch.* **2012**, *461*, 99–101. [CrossRef] [PubMed]
26. Fei, F.; Li, C.; Cao, Y.; Liu, K.; Du, J.; Gu, Y.; Wang, X.; Li, Y.; Zhang, S. CK7 expression associates with the location, differentiation, lymph node metastasis, and the Dukes' stage of primary colorectal cancers. *J. Cancer* **2019**, *10*, 2510–2519. [CrossRef]
27. Young, R.H.; Oliva, E. Transitional cell carcinomas of the urinary bladder that may be underdiagnosed. A report of four invasive cases exemplifying the homology between neoplastic and non-neoplastic transitional cell lesions. *Am. J. Surg. Pathol.* **1996**, *20*, 1448–1454. [CrossRef] [PubMed]
28. Santi, R.; Angulo, J.C.; Nesi, G.; de Petris, G.; Kuroda, N.; Hes, O.; López, J.I. Common and uncommon features of nephrogenic adenoma revisited. *Pathol. Res. Pract.* **2019**, *215*, 152561. [CrossRef]
29. Sharifai, N.; Abro, B.; Chen, J.F.; Zhao, M.; He, H.; Cao, D. Napsin A is a highly sensitive marker for nephrogenic adenoma: An immunohistochemical study with a specificity test in genitourinary tumors. *Hum. Pathol.* **2020**, *102*, 23–32. [CrossRef] [PubMed]
30. Lopez-Beltrán, A.; Montironi, R.; Cheng, L. Microcystic urothelial carcinoma: Morphology, immunohistochemistry and clinical behaviour. *Histopathology* **2014**, *64*, 872–879. [CrossRef]
31. Park, S.; Reuter, V.E.; Hansel, D.E. Non-urothelial carcinomas of the bladder. *Histopathology* **2019**, *74*, 97–111. [CrossRef] [PubMed]

32. Flores, M.R.; Ruiz, M.R.; Florian, R.E.; De Leon, W.; Jose, L.S. Pan-urothelial verrucous carcinoma unrelated to schistosomiasis. *BMJ Case Rep.* **2009**, *2009*, bcr08.2008.0787. [CrossRef] [PubMed]
33. Holmäng, S.; Borghede, G.; Johansson, S.L. Bladder carcinoma with lymphoepithelioma-like differentiation: A report of 9 cases. *J. Urol.* **1998**, *159*, 779–782. [CrossRef]
34. López-Beltrán, A.; Luque, R.J.; Vicioso, L.; Anglada, F.; Requena, M.J.; Quintero, A.; Montironi, R. Lymphoepithelioma-like carcinoma of the urinary bladder: A clinicopathologic study of 13 cases. *Virchows Arch.* **2001**, *438*, 552–557. [CrossRef] [PubMed]
35. Tamas, E.F.; Nielsen, M.E.; Schoenberg, M.P.; Epstein, J.I. Lymphoepithelioma-like carcinoma of the urinary tract: A clinicopathological study of 30 pure and mixed cases. *Mod. Pathol.* **2007**, *20*, 828–834. [CrossRef] [PubMed]
36. Williamson, S.R.; Zhang, S.; Lopez-Beltran, A.; Shah, R.B.; Montironi, R.; Tan, P.H.; Wang, M.; Baldridge, L.A.; MacLennan, G.T.; Cheng, L. Lymphoepithelioma-like carcinoma of the urinary bladder: Clinicopathologic, immunohistochemical and molecular features. *Am. J. Surg. Pathol.* **2011**, *35*, 474–483. [CrossRef] [PubMed]
37. López-Beltrán, A.; Paner, G.; Blanca, A.; Montironi, R.; Tsuzuki, T.; Nagashima, Y.; Chuang, S.S.; Win, K.T.; Madruga, L.; Raspollini, M.R.; et al. Lymphoepithelioma-like carcinoma of the upper urinary tract. *Virchows Arch.* **2017**, *470*, 703–709. [CrossRef]
38. Park, S.; Cho, M.S.; Kim, K.H. A case report of urothelial carcinoma with combined micropapillary and plasmacytoid morphology in the urinary bladder. *Diagn. Cytopathol.* **2016**, *44*, 124–127. [CrossRef]
39. Sahin, A.A.; Myhre, M.; Ro, J.Y.; Sneige, N.; Dekmezian, R.H.; Ayala, A.G. Plasmacytoid transitional cell carcinoma. Report of a case with initial presentation mimicking multiple myeloma. *Acta Cytol.* **1991**, *35*, 277–280.
40. Kim, D.K.; Kim, J.W.; Ro, J.Y.; Lee, H.S.; Park, J.Y.; Ahn, H.K.; Lee, J.Y.; Cho, K.S. Plasmacytoid variant of urothelial carcinoma of the bladder: A systematic review and meta-analysis of clinicopathological features and survival outcomes. *J. Urol.* **2020**, *204*, 215–223. [CrossRef]
41. Raspollini, M.R.; Sardi, I.; Giunti, L.; Di Lollo, S.; Baroni, G.; Stomaci, N.; Menghetti, I.; Franchi, A. Plasmacytoid urothelial carcinoma of the urinary bladder: Clinicopathologic, immunohistochemical, ultrastructural, and molecular analysis of a case series. *Hum. Pathol.* **2011**, *42*, 1149–1158. [CrossRef] [PubMed]
42. Kim, B.; Kim, G.; Song, B.; Lee, C.; Park, J.H.; Moon, K.C. HER2 protein overexpression and gene amplification in plasmacytoid urothelial carcinoma of the urinary bladder. *Dis. Markers.* **2016**, *2016*, 8463731. [CrossRef] [PubMed]
43. Palsgrove, D.N.; Taheri, D.; Springer, S.U.; Cowan, M.; Guner, G.; Mendoza Rodriguez, M.A.; Rodriguez Pena, M.D.C.; Wang, Y.; Kinde, I.; Cunha, I.; et al. Targeted sequencing of plasmacytoid urothelial carcinoma reveals frequent TERT promoter mutations. *Hum. Pathol.* **2019**, *85*, 1–9. [CrossRef] [PubMed]
44. Al-Ahmadie, H.A.; Iyer, G.; Lee, B.H.; Scott, S.N.; Mehra, R.; Bagrodia, A.; Jordan, E.J.; Gao, S.P.; Ramirez, R.; Cha, E.K.; et al. Frequent somatic *CDH1* loss-of-function mutations in plasmacytoid-variant bladder cancer. *Nat. Genet.* **2016**, *48*, 356–358. [CrossRef] [PubMed]
45. Jin, D.; Qiu, S.; Jin, K.; Zhou, X.; Cao, Q.; Yang, L.; Wei, Q. Signet-Ring Cell Carcinoma as an Independent Prognostic Factor for Patients with Urinary Bladder Cancer: A Population-Based Study. *Front. Oncol.* **2020**, *10*, 653. [CrossRef] [PubMed]
46. Ereño, C.; Gaafar, A.; Garmendia, M.; Etxezarraga, C.; Bilbao, F.J.; Lopez, J.I. Basaloid squamous cell carcinoma of the head and neck. A clinicopathological and follow-up study of 40 cases and review of the literature. *Head Neck Pathol.* **2008**, *2*, 83–91. [CrossRef]
47. Graham, R.P.; Arnold, C.A.; Naini, B.V.; Lam-Himlin, D.M. Basaloid squamous cell carcinoma of the anus revisited. *Am. J. Surg. Pathol.* **2016**, *40*, 354–360. [CrossRef]
48. Vakar-Lopez, F.; Abrams, J. Basaloid squamous cell carcinoma occurring in the urinary bladder. *Arch. Pathol. Lab. Med.* **2000**, *124*, 455–459.
49. Hagemann, I.S.; Lu, J.; Lewis, J.S., Jr. Basaloid squamous cell carcinoma arising in [corrected] the renal pelvis. *Int. J. Surg. Pathol.* **2008**, *16*, 199–201. [CrossRef]
50. Neves, T.R.; Soares, M.J.; Monteiro, P.G.; Lima, M.S.; Monteiro, H.G. Basaloid squamous cell carcinoma in the urinary bladder with small cell carcinoma. *J. Clin. Oncol.* **2011**, *29*, e440–e442. [CrossRef]

51. Ginori, A.; Barone, A.; Santopietro, R.; Barbanti, G.; Cecconi, F.; Tripodi, S.A. Human papillomavirus-related basaloid squamous cell carcinoma of the bladder associated with genital tract human papillomavirus infection. *Int. J. Urol.* **2015**, *22*, 222–225. [CrossRef] [PubMed]
52. Samaratunga, H.; Samaratunga, D.; Dunglison, N.; Perry-Keene, J.; Nicklin, J.; Delahunt, B. Alpha-fetoprotein-producing carcinoma of the renal pelvis exhibiting hepatoid and urothelial differentiation. *Anticancer Res.* **2012**, *32*, 4987–4991. [PubMed]
53. Ravishankar, S.; Malpica, A.; Ramalingam, P.; Euscher, E.D. Yolk sac tumor in extragonadal pelvic sites: Still a diagnostic challenge. *Am. J. Surg. Pathol.* **2017**, *41*, 1–11. [CrossRef] [PubMed]
54. Melms, J.C.; Thummalapalli, R.; Shaw, K.; Ye, H.; Tsai, L.; Bhatt, R.S.; Izar, B. Alpha-fetoprotein (AFP) as a tumor marker in a patient with urothelial cancer with exceptional response to anti-PD-L1 therapy and an escape lesion mimic. *J. Immunother. Cancer* **2018**, *6*, 89. [CrossRef] [PubMed]
55. Espejo-Herrera, N.; Condom-Mundó, E. Yolk sac tumor differentiation in urothelial carcinoma of the urinary bladder: A case report and differential diagnosis. *Diagn. Pathol.* **2020**, *15*, 68. [CrossRef] [PubMed]
56. McNamee, T.; Damato, S.; McCluggage, W.G. Yolk sac tumours of the female genital tract in older adults derive commonly from somatic epithelial neoplasms: Somatically derived yolk sac tumours. *Histopathology* **2016**, *69*, 739–751. [CrossRef] [PubMed]
57. Przybycin, C.G.; McKenney, J.K.; Nguyen, J.K.; Shah, R.B.; Umar, S.A.; Harik, L.; Shih, I.M.; Cox, R.M. Urothelial carcinomas with trophoblastic differentiation, including choriocarcinoma. Clinicopathologic series of 16 cases. *Am. J. Surg. Pathol.* **2020**, *44*, 1322–1330.
58. Douglas, J.; Sharp, A.; Chau, C.; Head, J.; Drake, T.; Wheater, M.; Geldart, T.; Mead, G.; Crabb, S.J. Serum total hCGβ level is an independent prognostic factor in transitional cell carcinoma of the urothelial tract. *Br. J. Cancer* **2014**, *110*, 1759–1766. [CrossRef]
59. Banet, N.; Gown, A.M.; Shih, I.M.; Li, Q.K.; Roden, R.B.S.; Nucci, M.R.; Cheng, L.; Przybycin, C.G.; Nasseri-Nik, N.; Wu, L.S.F.; et al. GATA-3 expression in trophoblastic tissues. An immunohistochemical study of 445 cases, including diagnostic utility. *Am. J. Surg. Pathol.* **2015**, *39*, 101–108. [CrossRef]
60. Miettinen, M.; Wang, Z.; McCue, P.A.; Sarlomo-Rikala, M.; Rys, J.; Biernat, W.; Lasota, J.; See, Y.S. SALL4 expression in germ cell and non-germ cell tumors. A systematic immunohistochemical study of 3215 cases. *Am. J. Surg. Pathol.* **2014**, *38*, 410–420. [CrossRef]
61. Mao, T.L.; Kurman, R.J.; Jeng, Y.M.; Husng, W.; Shih, I.M. HSD3B1 as a novel trophoblast-associated marker that assists in the differential diagnosis of trophoblastic tumors and tumorlike lesions. *Am. J. Surg. Pathol.* **2008**, *32*, 236–242. [CrossRef] [PubMed]
62. Wick, M.R.; Ritter, J.H.; Dehner, L.P. Malignant rhabdoid tumors: A clinicopathologic review and conceptual discussion. *Sem. Diagn. Pathol.* **1995**, *12*, 233–248.
63. Warren, K.S.; Oxley, J.; Koupparis, A. Pure malignant rhabdoid tumor of the bladder. *Can. Urol. Assoc. J.* **2014**, *8*, e260–e262. [CrossRef] [PubMed]
64. Sterling, M.E.; Long, C.J.; Bosse, K.R.; Bagatell, R.; Shukla, A.R. A rapid progression of disease after surgical excision of a malignant rhabdoid tumor of the bladder. *Urology* **2015**, *85*, 664–666. [CrossRef] [PubMed]
65. Assadi, A.; Alzubaidi, A.; Lesmana, H.; Brennan, R.C.; Ortiz-Hernandez, V.; Gleason, J.M. Pure bladder malingnant rhabdoid tumor successfully treated with partial cystectomy, radiation, and chemotherapy: A case report and review of the literature. *J. Pediatr. Hematol. Oncol.* **2020**. [CrossRef] [PubMed]
66. Parwani, A.V.; Herawi, M.; Volmar, K.; Tsai, S.H.; Epstein, J.I. Urothelial carcinoma with rhabdoid features: Report of 6 cases. *Hum. Pathol.* **2006**, *37*, 168–172. [CrossRef]
67. Fukumura, Y.; Fujii, H.; Mitani, K.; Sakamoto, Y.; Matsumoto, T.; Suda, K.; Yao, T. Urothelial carcinoma of the renal pelvis with rhabdoid features. *Pathol. Int.* **2009**, *59*, 322–325. [CrossRef]
68. Tajima, S. Rhabdoid variant of urotelial carcinoma of the urinary bladder: A case report with emphasis on immunohistochemical analysis regarding the formation of rhabdoid morphology. *Int. J. Clin. Exp. Pathol.* **2015**, *8*, 9638–9642.
69. Mostofi, F.K.; Davis, C.J.; Sesterhenn, I.A. *World Health Organization International Histological Classification of Tumours: Histological Typing of Urinary Bladder Tumours*, 2nd ed.; Springer: Berlin/Heidelberg, Germany, 1999.
70. Leroy, X.; Gonzalez, S.; Zini, L.; Aubert, S. Lipoid-cell variant of urothelial carcinoma: A clinicopathologic and immunohistochemical study of five cases. *Am. J. Surg. Pathol.* **2007**, *31*, 770–773. [CrossRef]

71. López-Beltrán, A.; Amin, M.B.; Oliveira, P.S.; Montironi, R.; Algaba, F.; McKenney, J.K.; de Torres, I.; Mazerolles, C.; Wang, M.; Cheng, L. Urothelial carcinoma of the bladder. Lipid cell variant: Clinicopathologic findings and LOH analysis. *Am. J. Surg. Pathol.* **2010**, *34*, 371–376. [CrossRef]
72. López-Beltrán, A.; Blanca, A.; Montironi, R.; Cheng, L.; Regueiro, J.C. Pleomorphic giant cell carcinoma of the urinary bladder. *Hum. Pathol.* **2009**, *40*, 1461–1466. [CrossRef] [PubMed]
73. Samatunga, H.; Delahunt, B.; Egevad, L.; Adamson, M.; Hussey, D.; Malone, G.; Hoyle, K.; Nathan, T.; Kerle, D.; Ferguson, P.; et al. Pleomorphic giant cells carcinoma of the urinary bladder: An extreme form of tumour de-differentiation. *Histopathology* **2016**, *68*, 533–540. [CrossRef] [PubMed]
74. Priore, S.F.; Schwartz, L.E.; Epstein, J.I. An expanded immunohistochemical profile of osteoclast-rich undifferentiated carcinoma of the urinary tract. *Mod. Pathol.* **2018**, *31*, 984–988. [CrossRef] [PubMed]
75. Mai, K.T.; Baterman, J.; Djordjevic, B.; Flood, T.A.; Belanger, E.C. Clear cell urothelial carcinoma: A study of 10 cases and meta-analysis of the entity. Evidence of mesonephric differentiation. *Int. J. Surg. Pathol.* **2017**, *25*, 18–25. [CrossRef]
76. Pérez-Montiel, D.; Wakely, P.E.; Hes, O.; Michal, M.; Suster, S. High-grade urothelial carcinoma of the renal pelvis: Clinicopathologic study of 108 cases with emphasis on unusual morphologic variants. *Mod. Pathol.* **2006**, *19*, 494–503. [CrossRef]
77. Amin, M.B. Histological variants of urothelial carcinoma: Diagnostic, therapeutic and prognostic implications. *Mod. Pathol.* **2009**, *24*, 6–15. [CrossRef]
78. Hayashi, H.; Mann, S.; Kao, C.S.; Grignon, D.; Idrees, M. Variant morphology in upper urinary tract urothelial carcinoma: A 14-year case series of biopsy and resection specimens. *Hum. Pathol.* **2017**, *65*, 209–216. [CrossRef]
79. López-Beltrán, A.; Henriques, V.; Montironi, R.; Cimadamore, A.; Raspollini, M.R.; Cheng, L. Variants and new entities of bladder cancer. *Histopathology* **2019**, *74*, 77–96. [CrossRef]
80. Rolim, I.; Henriques, V.; Rolim, N.; Blanca, A.; Marques, R.C.; Volavsek, M.; Carvalho, I.; Montironi, R.; Cimadamore, A.; Raspollini, M.R.; et al. Clinicopathologic analysis of upper urinary tract carcinoma with variant histology. *Virchows Arch.* **2020**, *477*, 111–120. [CrossRef]
81. Sim, S.J.; Ro, J.Y.; Ordonez, N.G.; Park, Y.W.; Kee, K.H.; Ayala, A.G. Metastatic renal cell carcinoma to the bladder: A clinicopathologic and immunohistochemical study. *Mod. Pathol.* **1999**, *12*, 351–355.
82. Tajima, S. Urothelial carcinoma with oncocytic features: An extremely rare case presenting a diagnostic challenge in urine cytology. *Int. J. Clin. Exp. Pathol.* **2015**, *8*, 8591–8597. [PubMed]
83. McCabe, J.E.; Das, S.; Dowling, P.; Hamid, B.N.; Pettersson, B.A. Oncocytic carcinoid tumour of the bladder. *J. Clin. Pathol.* **2005**, *58*, 446–447. [PubMed]
84. Genitsch, V.; Kollár, A.; Vandekerkhove, G.; Blarer, J.; Furrer, M.; Annala, M.; Herberts, C.; Pycha, A.; de Jong, J.J.; Liu, Y.; et al. Morphologic and genomic characterization of urothelial to sarcomatoid transition in muscle-invasive bladder cancer. *Urol. Oncol.* **2019**, *37*, 826–836. [CrossRef] [PubMed]
85. Malla, M.; Wang, J.F.; Trepeta, R.; Feng, A.; Wang, J. Sarcomatoid carcinoma of the urinary bladder. *Clin. Genitourin. Cancer* **2016**, *14*, 366–372. [CrossRef]

11

The Role of Daily Adaptive Stereotactic MR-Guided Radiotherapy for Renal Cell Cancer

Shyama U. Tetar [1,†], Omar Bohoudi [1,†], Suresh Senan [1], Miguel A. Palacios [1], Swie S. Oei [1], Antoinet M. van der Wel [1], Berend J. Slotman [1], R. Jeroen A. van Moorselaar [2], Frank J. Lagerwaard [1] and Anna M. E. Bruynzeel [1,*]

1 Department of Radiation Oncology, Amsterdam University Medical Centers, 1081 HZ Amsterdam, The Netherlands; su.tetar@amsterdamumc.nl (S.U.T.); o.bohoudi@amsterdamumc.nl (O.B.); s.senan@amsterdamumc.nl (S.S.); m.palacios@amsterdamumc.nl (M.A.P.); ss.oei@amsterdamumc.nl (S.S.O.); a.vanderwel1@amsterdamumc.nl (A.M.v.d.W.); bj.slotman@amsterdamumc.nl (B.J.S.); fj.lagerwaard@amsterdamumc.nl (F.J.L.)

2 Department of Urology, Amsterdam University Medical Centers, 1081 HV Amsterdam, The Netherlands; rja.vanmoorselaar@amsterdamumc.nl

* Correspondence: ame.bruynzeel@amsterdamumc.nl

† These authors joined first authors.

Simple Summary: Standard treatment for localized renal cell carcinoma (RCC) is surgery. Stereotactic radiotherapy given in a few high dose fractions is a promising treatment for this indication and could be an alternative option for patients unsuitable for surgery. Stereotactic MR-guided radiotherapy (MRgRT) is clinically implemented as a new technique for precise treatment delivery of abdominal tumors, like RCC. In this study, we evaluated the clinical impact of stereotactic MRgRT given in five fractions of 8 Gy and routine plan re-optimization for 36 patients with large primary RCCs. Our evaluation showed good oncological results with minimal side-effects. Even in this group with large tumors, daily plan re-optimization was only needed in a minority of patients who can be identified upfront. This is a favorable result since online MRgRT plan adaptation is a time-consuming procedure. In these patients, MRgRT delivery will be faster, and these patients could be candidates for even less fractions per treatment.

Abstract: Novel magnetic-resonance-guided radiotherapy (MRgRT) permits real-time soft-tissue visualization, respiratory-gated delivery with minimal safety margins, and time-consuming daily plan re-optimisation. We report on early clinical outcomes of MRgRT and routine plan re-optimization for large primary renal cell cancer (RCC). Thirty-six patients were treated with MRgRT in 40 Gy/5 fractions. Prior to each fraction, re-contouring of tumor and normal organs on a pretreatment MR-scan allowed daily plan re-optimization. Treatment-induced toxicity and radiological responses were scored, which was followed by an offline analysis to evaluate the need for such daily re-optimization in 180 fractions. Mean age and tumor diameter were 78.1 years and 5.6 cm, respectively. All patients completed MRgRT with an average fraction duration of 45 min. Local control (LC) and overall survival rates at one year were 95.2% and 91.2%. No grade ≥3 toxicity was reported. Plans without re-optimization met institutional radiotherapy constraints in 83.9% of 180 fractions. Thus, daily plan re-optimization was required for only a minority of patients, who can be identified upfront by a higher volume of normal organs receiving 25 Gy in baseline plans. In conclusion, stereotactic MRgRT for large primary RCC showed low toxicity and high LC, while daily plan re-optimization was required only in a minority of patients.

Keywords: MR-guided; radiotherapy; MRgRT; stereotactic ablative radiotherapy; stereotactic ablative radiation therapy (SABR); renal cell cancer; RCC; online adaptive

1. Introduction

A radical or partial nephrectomy is the preferred standard curative treatment for localized renal cell carcinoma (RCC) [1–4]. Ablative local treatment, such as radiofrequency ablation (RFA), cryoablation (CA), or microwave ablation (MWA), is an alternative in elderly patients who present with a high surgical risk due to several comorbidities [3]. Radiotherapy does not have a prominent role in current international and national guidelines in treating primary RCC [1–4]. In recent years, stereotactic ablative radiation therapy (SABR) has been evaluated in several smaller retrospective and prospective studies [5–14], usually in RCC patients unsuitable for surgery. Outcomes of a multi-institutional pool from nine institutions, utilizing either single or multi-fractionated treatment in 223 patients, have been reported by the International Radiosurgery Oncology Consortium for Kidney (IROCK) [15]. SABR for RCC was found to be well tolerated, achieved local control (LC) rates exceeding 95% at four years of follow-up and grade ≥3 toxicity rates of 1.3%, and had an average decrease in glomerular filtration rate of 5.5 mL per minute. The majority of the tumors in this pooled analysis was ≤4 cm and clinical data for larger tumors is limited. A retrospective analysis of a subgroup of 95 patients with tumors >4 cm was recently published [16], but with the exception of these data, clinical outcomes on cT1b-T2 RCC SABR are scarce. Due to the inherent limitations to a pooled analyses, the Trans-Tasman Radiation Oncology Group (TROG) and the Australian and New Zealand Urogenital and Prostate Cancer Trials Group (ANZUP) have initiated a prospective, multi-institutional phase II study in 70 patients with biopsy-confirmed medical inoperable RCC patients [17]. Full accrual has recently been completed, and the data of this trial are eagerly awaited.

Technical challenges in renal SABR include the management of intra-fractional motion, and potential solutions using an internal target volume-approach, fiducial-assisted robotic SABR or abdominal compression [18] have been described. Magnetic-resonance (MR)-guided radiotherapy (MRgRT) has been considered a promising option because of its improved visualization of kidney tumors in relation to critical adjacent organs such as a small bowel, duodenum, and stomach and the opportunity of real-time tumor tracking and automated gated delivery [18,19]. MRgRT also facilitates daily plan re-optimization as a means to reduce organs at risk (OAR) doses when abdominal organs are near the primary tumor. Furthermore, MRgRT is an outpatient treatment for which no invasive procedures or anesthesia is required. However, to the best of our knowledge, clinical data on MR-guided SABR for localized RCC have not been reported.

Stereotactic MRgRT with routine daily plan adaptation was clinically implemented at our center in 2016 for a variety of clinical indications. The aim of the current paper is to describe our technique, early clinical outcomes, and the role of daily plan adaptation in MRgRT for patients with primary large RCC.

2. Materials and Methods

Data from all patients treated with MRgRT on the MRIdian-system (ViewRay Inc., Mountain View, CA, USA) at the Amsterdam University Medical Centers are collected within a prospective institutional review board approved database. Between May 2016 and February 2020, a total of 51 patients were treated for a primary RCC (n = 36), local recurrences (n = 5), renal metastases from other primary tumors (n = 3), or a diagnosis of urothelial carcinoma (n = 7). This analysis is restricted to the remaining 36 patients who were treated for primary RCC.

All patients underwent stereotactic adaptive MRgRT delivered to a dose of 40 Gy in five fractions in a two-week period. Implanted fiducials were not required, and the adaptive workflow was similar to that which had been described previously for pancreatic tumors [20]. Briefly, for simulation, both a MR-scan (0.35T True-FISP, TR/TE: 3.37 ms/1.45 ms, FA: 60°, 17-s with 1.6 mm × 1.6 mm × 3.0 mm resolution) and computed tomography (CT)-scan (slice thickness of 2 mm) are acquired during a shallow-inspiration breath-hold. Geometric accuracy of the MRIdian system is < 0.1 cm in a sphere of 10 cm radius around the isocenter, and <0.15 cm in a sphere of 17.5 cm radius. Every patient was brought as close to the isocenter as possible for each fraction, and the maximum distance from the tumor or any other critical structure to the isocenter was always below 10 cm. Geometric accuracy was assessed with two different dedicated phantoms for spatial integrity measurements. Contouring of the primary tumor (also called gross tumor volume; GTV) and OAR is performed on breath-hold MR-images with the aid of diagnostic imaging, generally contrast-enhanced CT scans. The PTV (planning target volume) is derived from the GTV plus an isotropic 3-mm margin. A co-planar baseline plan consisting of between 30 and 42 intensity modulated radiotherapy (IMRT)-segments is generated, using the MRIdian treatment planning software. Dose calculation was executed with a VMC and EGSnrc code-based Monte-Carlo algorithm (statistical uncertainty of 1% and a grid size of 0.3 cm × 0.3 cm × 0.3 cm) using the deformed electron density map from the simulation CT scan. Institutional target coverage and OAR constraints are summarized in Table 1.

Table 1. Dose prescription for institutional target coverage and normal tissue constraints. The constraints represent the cut-off doses for radiotherapy planning with the aim of dose sparing in the surrounding organs (contralateral kidney, liver, duodenum, bowel, and stomach) while, at the same time, aiming to achieve a high dose in the tumor with the margin, which is represented as the planning target volume. Organs at risk are only re-contoured within 2 cm of the tumor and, for an adaptive setting, only the dose in these structures are optimized.

Structure	Dose to Volume			
Planning Target Volume	≥50	% at	38	Gy
	≤1	cc at	50	Gy
Kidney Contralateral	≤25	% at	12	Gy
Liver	≤50	% at	12	Gy
Duodenum, Bowel, Stomach in 2 cm	≤0.1	cc at	36	Gy
	≤1	cc at	33	Gy

We perform routine plan re-optimization using the daily pre-SABR breath-hold MR-imaging acquired in the treatment position. After rigid registration on the GTV, OAR contours are propagated to the repeat MR using deformable image registration. The ViewRay deformable image registration algorithm uses an intensity-based algorithm, which minimizes a cost function that measures the similarity between the images including a regularization term in order to obtain smoother deformation fields and prevent sharp discontinuities. The GTV and OAR contours are checked and adjusted where needed within a 2-cm distance of the PTV by the attending radiation oncologist. Next, the baseline IMRT plan is recalculated on the new anatomy ("predicted plan"), and subsequently re-optimized using the target and OAR optimization objectives of the baseline plan ("re-optimized plan"). Plan re-optimization prioritizes avoiding high doses to OARs, even when this is at the cost of decreased PTV coverage. Both the predicted and re-optimized plans are reviewed, and the re-optimized plan is selected for the actual delivery.

MRgRT delivery is performed using respiratory gating during subsequent breath-hold periods in shallow inspiration. The tracking structure for gating is either the primary tumor, or the kidney itself on a single sagittal plane (Figure 1), depending on the visibility on this sagittal plane. Gating is augmented by visual and/or auditory feedback provided to patients during treatment [21]. Visual feedback is performed with the aid of an in-room MR compatible monitor on which both the tracking structure (GTV or kidney) and the gating boundary (3 mm), generally corresponding to the PTV, is projected in real-time. The 2D MR images during treatment were acquired with a True FISP sequence with the MRIdian (0.35 T) at a frequency of four frames-per-second (TR: 2.1 ms, TE: 0.91 ms, FA: 60°).

FOV was 0.35 cm × 0.35 cm and the slice thickness was 0.7 cm. Due to the low magnetic field and low FA, "real-time" MR images of the patient were performed without interruption during the beam-on time. A previous analysis showed a treatment duty cycle efficiency between 67% and 87% for upper abdominal tumors [22].

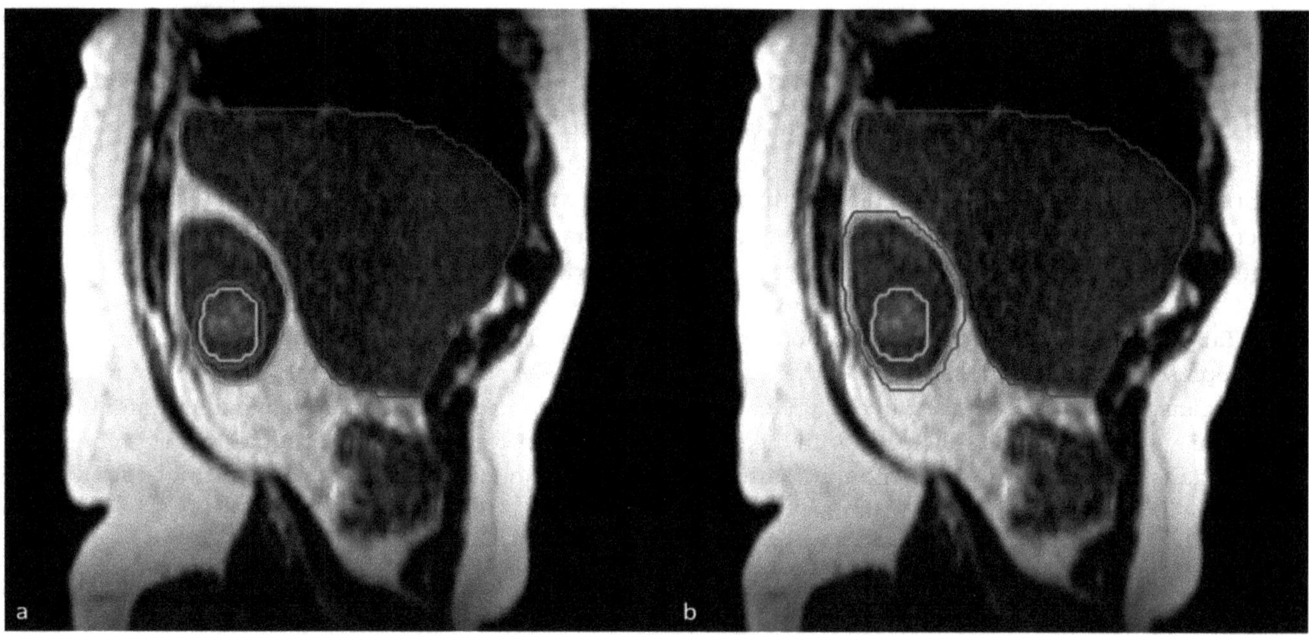

Figure 1. Sagittal plane for tumor tracking: either (**a**) tracking on gross tumor volume (green) or (**b**) tracking on the whole kidney (orange). A boundary of 3 mm (red) for gated delivery.

Baseline patient and tumor characteristics and follow-up data including LC, renal function, and toxicity were collected. Acute and late toxicity was scored using the Common Terminology Criteria for Adverse Events (CTCAE) version 4.0. Follow-up imaging was assessed by a CT-scan or ultrasound, and the tumor response was classified according to RECIST 1.1. criteria.

An offline analysis was performed to evaluate the need for daily plan re-optimization in MRgRT for RCC in a total of 180 fractions. For this purpose, predicted and re-optimized plans were analyzed for adherence with planning target objectives and OAR constraints, i.e., a V_{38Gy} of the GTV ≥ 90%, and $V_{33Gy} \leq 1$ cc for stomach, duodenum, and bowel. Re-optimization was defined as "needed" when the predicted plan violated the above-mentioned GTV and/or OAR constraints, which was subsequently corrected by re-optimization. In contrast, plan re-optimization was defined as "redundant" when predicted plans already complied with the planning objectives. In addition, the value of plan re-optimization was analyzed on a patient level by studying the number of fractions per patient that were considered suboptimal.

Statistical Analysis

Descriptive statistics were used for baseline patient and tumor characteristics. The change in renal function (eGFR) from baseline versus post-treatment at the latest available time point in follow-up was evaluated using the paired sampled *t*-test. Local, regional, distant disease control and overall survival (OS) were estimated using the Kaplan-Meier method. OS was calculated as the time between the first fraction of MRgRT and the date of the last follow-up. LC was calculated as the time between the first fraction of MRgRT and the date of last imaging. Statistical analysis used for plan comparisons was performed using the Wilcoxon Signed-Rank test. A *p*-value of < 0.05 was considered to be statistically significant. Decision tree analysis (CHAID, Chi-square automatic interaction detection) was used to explore predictive pretreatment characteristics and most significant cut-off values to identify patients for whom daily re-optimization was needed. Baseline volumetric, geometric, and dosimetric parameters, i.e., GTV size (cc), laterality (left, right), location (interpolar, upper or lower pole), V_{33Gy}, V_{30Gy}, V_{25Gy}, and V_{20Gy} for each OAR structure separately or combined in one structure were used as input variables. The qualitative re-optimization benefit variable ("redundant" or "needed") was selected as the target variable for decision tree analysis. The significance level for node splitting was set at $p < 0.05$. Stopping parameters to prevent over-fitting were applied by setting the minimum number of records in a leaf to be at least 10% of the data set. The Statistical Package for the Social Sciences (SPSS) version 26 (IBM® SPSS Statistics, Armonk, NY, USA) was used to perform all statistical analyses.

3. Results

3.1. Clinical Outcomes

All 36 patients were referred for SABR after discussion in a multidisciplinary tumor board, and reasons for referral included a high surgical risk due to comorbidity ($n = 9$), which is unsuitable for other ablative therapies due to tumor size ($n = 10$) or location ($n = 5$), patient preference ($n = 5$), co-existing second malignancy ($n = 3$), use of anti-coagulants ($n = 2$), and chronic stage ≥IV kidney disease ($n = 2$). Baseline patient characteristics are summarized in Table 2. The mean age of this cohort was 78.1 years with a preponderance of men (66.7%). The mean tumor diameter was 5.6 cm (range 2.4–9.3 cm) with 86.1% of tumors measuring ≥4 cm in the largest dimension of which 23 patients have a cT1b tumor and 8 patients have a cT2a tumor. Five patients (13.9%) had metastasized renal cell carcinoma (RCC) at the time of diagnosis. Pathologic confirmation of RCC before treatment was achieved in approximately half of patients (55.6%) of which the majority was diagnosed with Fuhrman grade 2 ($n = 14$). Other patients with histology included Fuhrman grade 1 ($n = 1$), Fuhrman grade 3 ($n = 1$), a RCC with sarcomatoid features ($n = 1$), and a chromophobe tumor ($n = 1$). In two patients, no grading was available because pathologic confirmation was obtained from systemic metastases. All patients were able to complete adaptive MRgRT with an average time per fraction of 45 min. An overview of the average duration of the different components of adaptive MRgRT for RCC is shown in Figure 2. Three patients completed treatment while tracking on the kidney instead of the tumor.

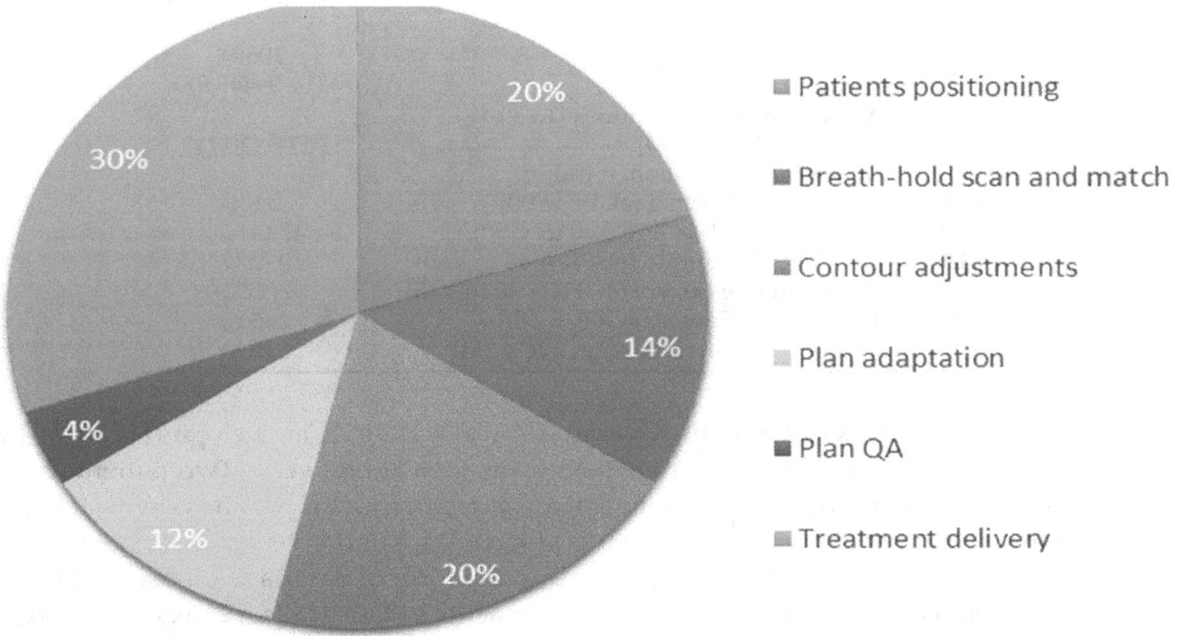

Figure 2. Pie-chart of the average duration of the different components of breath-hold gated adaptive MR-guided radiotherapy with an average time per fraction of 45 min.

Table 2. Baseline patient characteristics ($n = 36$). Abbreviations: RCC = renal cell carcinoma, GTV = gross tumor volume, PTV = planning target volume, CKD = chronic kidney disease.

	Mean Age (Range), Years	**78.1 (58–95)**
	Sex, *n* (%)	
	Male	24 (66.7)
	Female	12 (33.3)
	WHO performance status, *n* (%)	
	0	3 (7.9)
	1	21 (58.3)
	2	12 (33.3)
	Charlson comorbidity, *n* (%)	
	Mean (SD)	6.4 (2.5)
	2–3	3 (8.3)
	4–6	18 (50)
	7–9	10 (27.8)
	10–13	5 (13.9)
	Histology RCC, *n* (%)	
	Yes	20 (55.6)
	No	16 (44.4)
	Tumor Laterality, *n* (%)	
	Left	13 (36.1)
	Right	23 (63.9)
	Tumor location, *n* (%)	
	Interpolar	13 (36.1)
	Lower pole	13 (36.1)
	Upper pole	10 (27.8)
	Tumor size largest dimension, cm	
	Mean (SD)	5.6 (1.6)
	Median (range)	5.5 (2.4–9.3)
	T-stage, *n* (%)	
	cT1a	5 (13.9)
	cT1b	23 (63.9)
	cT2a	8 (22.2)
	GTV, cc	
	Mean (range)	79.7 (7.7–350.4)
	PTV, cc	
	Mean (range)	108.6 (14.3–445.9)
	Renal function (eGFR), ml/min/1.73 m^2	
	Mean (SD)	55.8 (20.1)
	CKD classification, *n* (%)	
I	Normal (eGFR ≥ 90)	0 (0)
II	Mild (eGFR ≥ 60 to < 90)	15 (41.7)
IIIa	Mild-Moderate (eGFR ≥ 45 to <60)	10 (27.8)
IIIb	Moderate-Severe (eGFR ≥ 30 to <45)	8 (22.2)
IV	Severe (eGFR < 30)	2 (5.6)
V	Kidney failure (eGFR < 15)	1 (2.8)

The median follow-up was 16.4 months. Overall survival was 91.2% at one year (Figure 3), LC was 95.2% (Figure 3), and freedom from any progression was 91% at one year. Two patients had local recurrences. One patient had progressive distant disease at recurrence for which systemic therapy was delivered, and the second patient with an isolated local recurrence underwent radiofrequency ablation as salvage. Treatment-related acute toxicity grade ≥ 2 in the form of nausea was observed in a single patient, which responded to oral ondansetron. No other acute or late grade ≥2 toxicity was reported. The mean eGFR at baseline was 55.3 (SD ±19.0) mL/min/1.73 m^2. With a mean interval of 16 months and mean eGFR post-MRgRT was 49.3 (SD ± 19.1) mL/min/1.73 m^2, which indicates a decrease of 6.0 mL/min/1.73 m^2. No patient in this cohort required dialysis during follow-up.

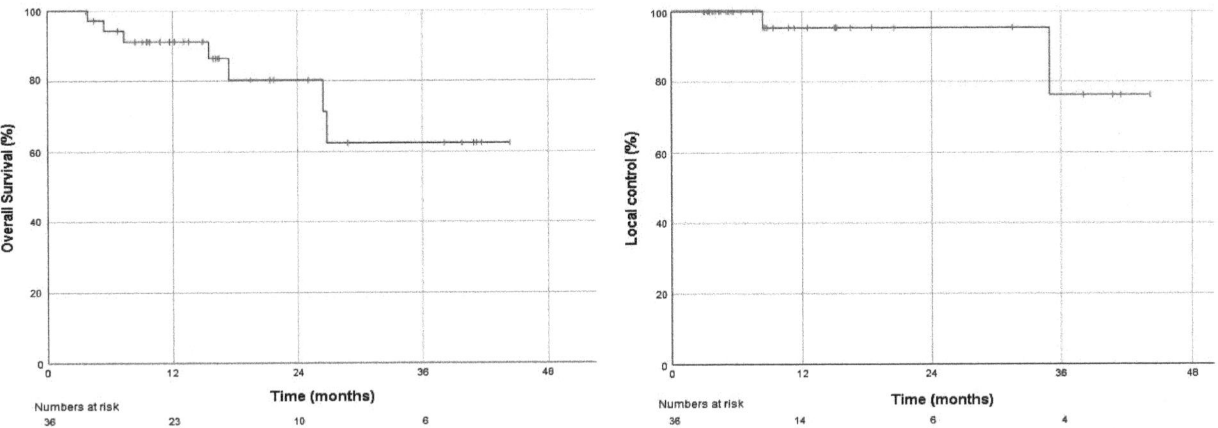

Figure 3. Kaplan-Meier plots for overall survival (left) and local control (right).

3.2. The Need for Daily Plan Re-Optimization

In 151 out of 180 fractions (83.9%), the predicted plans (without re-optimization) met all institutional target and OAR constraints. In these fractions, predicted and re-optimized plans were of similar quality with a mean GTV V_{38Gy} of 98.8% and 99.1%, respectively, and mean V_{33Gy} of 0 cc for both stomach, duodenum, and bowel. In the other 29 fractions, predicted plans were suboptimal with insufficient GTV coverage in two out of 180 fractions (1.1%) exceeding OAR constraints in 25 fractions (13.9%), and both insufficient GTV coverage and exceeded OAR constraints in another two fractions (1.1%). There was no significant difference in suboptimal predicted plans for left-sided or right-sided RCC ($p = 0.56$). For these suboptimal plans, on-couch re-optimization corrected the GTV V_{38Gy} from a mean of 88.7% (predicted) to 97.4% (re-optimized). Similarly, re-optimization corrected OAR $V_{33Gy} \leq 1$ cc violations from on average V_{33Gy} of 4.1 (predicted plans) to 0.3 cc (re-optimized plans). Analysis on a patient basis showed that the 29 insufficient predicted fractions were distributed among 11 patients (11/36, 30.6%). However, three or more suboptimal fractions were seen in only five patients (13.9%).

Decision tree analysis identified the baseline OAR V_{25Gy} (combined structure of stomach, bowel, and duodenum) as the most significant predictor variable for daily adaptive planning needs with 0.5 cc as an optimal cut-off value ($p < 0.001$). In all cases with a baseline OAR V_{25Gy} of ≤ 0.5 cc, plan adaptation was redundant as the predicted plans already complied with institutional constraints. In patients with baseline OAR V_{25Gy} of more than 0.5 cc, plan re-optimization was needed in 32.2% of fractions in order to fulfill the preset target coverage and OAR constraints (Table 3). The correct classification rate of the decision tree was 86.1% with a sensitivity of 100% and a specificity of 67.7%. The difference between re-optimized and predicted dose parameters for target (GTV $V_{95\%}$) and OAR (V_{33Gy}) stratified for split group 1 and 2 (Table 3) is shown in Figure 4.

Table 3. Results in the Chi-square automatic interaction detection (CHAID) tree table.

	Redundant *n* (%)	Needed *n* (%)	Total *n* (%)	Predictive Variable	Split Values	Chi-Square	df	*p*-Value
Parent node: all cases	151 (83.9)	29 (16.1)	180 (100)					
Split group 1	90 (100)	0 (0)	90 (100)	OAR V_{25Gy}	≤0.5 cc	34.6	1	<0.001
Split group 2	61 (67.8)	25 (32.2)	90 (100)	OAR V_{25Gy}	>0.5 cc	34.6	1	<0.001

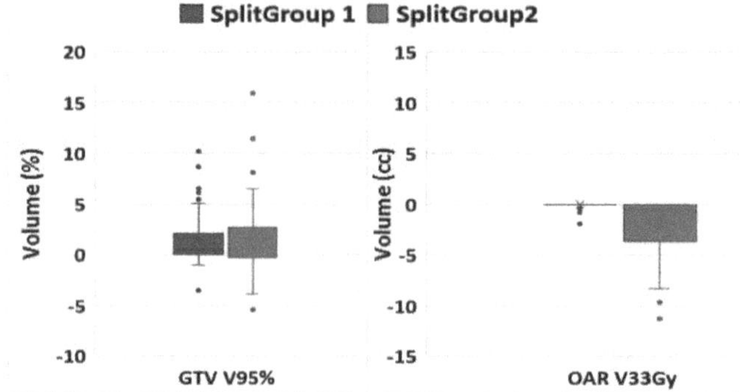

Figure 4. Difference of DVH parameters. Boxplots showing the relative volume difference in GTV $V_{95\%}$ (%) and absolute difference in OAR V_{33Gy} (cc) of the re-optimized compared to the predicted plans stratified for Split group 1 (re-optimization not needed) and 2 (re-optimization needed). Abbreviations: DVH = dose volume histogram, GTV = gross target volume, OAR = organs at risk.

4. Discussion

To the best of our knowledge, this is the first series of patients treated for primary RCC using MRgRT with routine daily plan re-optimization. We applied a commonly used fractionation scheme of 40 Gy in five fractions [18,23,24] in an overall treatment time of two weeks. Only a single patient reported nausea as acute toxicity, and no grade ≥ 2 late toxicity was observed. Despite the inclusion of large tumors, mostly T1b and T2, which had a mean tumor diameter of 5.6 cm and were generally unsuitable for other local therapies, we observed an LC rate of 95.2%. Our local response scoring has been according to the RECIST 1.1 criteria, and 83.3% had stable disease. In addition, 11.1% had partial remission, while 5.6% showed local progression. Fast tumor size regression is uncommon after SABR as previously reported by Sun and colleagues [11]. This preponderance of stable disease is in accordance with their paper. Both LC and OS are reported to be poorer for larger primary RCC than for the smaller lesions [25,26]. Despite this observation, our LC rate is within the high range of what was reported in recent systematic reviews, meta-analyses, and pooled analyses of SABR for primary RCC [15,24,27].

MRgRT with daily plan re-optimization was feasible with an average fraction duration of 45 min, even in poorer condition patients with multiple co-existing diseases. Despite this prolonged treatment duration, all patients were able to complete treatment, which indicates good tolerability. Our fractionation scheme of 40 Gy in five fractions is commonly used and seems safe without severe toxicity. With a mean interval of well over one year, the mean decline in eGFR in our study was only 6.0 (SD ± 9.8) mL/min/1.73 m^2. This value corresponds well with the mean decline in eGFR of 5.5 (SD ± 13.3) mL/min/1.73 m^2 that was described in previous SABR studies [15,28]. This limited decline in renal function in our patients with relatively large RCC may well be the result of this gated approach with small mobility boundaries, instead of using internal target volumes incorporating full tumor motion.

MRgRT also offers the advantage of using plan re-optimization for each delivered fraction at the cost of additional time. Our offline analysis showed that daily plan re-optimization was required in only 16% of fractions in which the predicted plan failed to meet the predetermined high-dose OAR constraints or target coverage objectives. Decision tree analysis showed that patients for whom daily plan re-optimization is not required can be identified upfront on the basis of a V_{25Gy} of the combined OAR of less than 0.5 cc in the baseline plan. It is, however, unlikely that an isolated single fraction violating high OAR dose or target constraints will be clinically relevant, and three out of five insufficient predicted plans were seen in only 14% of patients. Performing MRgRT without plan re-optimization indicates that the re-contouring, plan adaptation, and plan quality assurance phases can be omitted, which would enable respiratory-gated MRgRT fractions to be completed in 30 min. Furthermore, when plan adaptation is redundant, this indicates that the presence of the radiation oncologist at the MR Linac is not necessary. As a result of our analysis, we are currently introducing the found V_{25Gy} selection criterion in clinical practice.

The main limitation of our study is the relative short and unstructured patient follow-up. The limited number of RCC patients reflects the limited role of SABR in current international treatment guidelines, as only patients unsuitable for or refusing other local treatments are referred for curative radiation therapy. Another limitation includes the absence of pathology in half of our patients. Incomplete pathology confirmation is partly inherent to our patient population with generally frail elderly patients, which is unsuitable for other treatment modalities. Moreover, in a number of patients, a diagnostic biopsy was considered contra-indicated because of anticoagulant use or the anatomical location of the tumor. All patients had been discussed in a multidisciplinary tumor board with access to all available diagnostic imaging. Contrast enhanced multi-phasic CT has a high sensitivity and specificity for characterization and detection of RCC [3,29] and this specific imaging was available for all patients without pathological confirmation.

Prior to the MRgRT era, the need for radiologists to implant fiducial markers has also been an obstacle for referral for SABR. Our data show that MRgRT can be a valid alternative in patients unsuitable for the more commonly used local treatments, because of patient vitality or tumor size. The only contra-indication for MRgRT is having MR-incompatible devices. The main advantage of MRgRT is that it is an outpatient, non-invasive treatment for which not even the placement of fiducial markers is necessary. Whether MRgRT can also be considered as an alternative to partial nephrectomy or cryotherapy needs to be addressed in a prospective randomized study, which should also evaluate quality of life and cost-effectiveness. With regard to the favorable outcome in the data on SABR literature as well as the current analysis on MRgRT, a more prominent role of SABR in the treatment guidelines for RCC appears warranted.

5. Conclusions

In conclusion, hypo-fractionated MRgRT for large RCC resulted in high LC and very low toxicity rates. Gated treatment without the need for anesthesia or fiducials appeared well tolerated. Even in this group with large RCCs, daily plan re-optimization was not needed for the majority of patients, who can be identified upfront by a combined OAR V_{25Gy} of ≤ 0.5 cc in the baseline plans. This is a favorable result since online MRgRT plan adaptation is a time-consuming procedure. In this group of patients, MRgRT delivery will be faster, and these patients could be candidates for further hypofractionation [30].

Author Contributions: Conceptualization, S.U.T., O.B., F.J.L., and A.M.E.B.; Methodology, O.B. and F.J.L.; Software, O.B. and F.J.L.; Formal analysis, S.U.T., O.B., and F.J.L.; Investigation, S.U.T and O.B.; Resources, S.U.T., S.S.O., A.M.v.d.W., and A.M.E.B.; Data curation, S.U.T., O.B., and F.J.L.; Writing—original draft preparation, S.U.T., O.B., F.J.L., and A.M.E.B.; Writing—review and editing, S.S., M.A.P., S.S.O., A.M.v.d.W., R.J.A.v.M., and B.J.S.; Visualization, S.U.T. and O.B.; Supervision, F.J.L. and A.M.E.B.; Project administration, S.U.T., O.B., F.J.L., and A.M.E.B. All authors have read and agreed to the published version of the manuscript.

References

1. Escudier, B.; Porta, C.; Schmidinger, M.; Rioux-Leclercq, N.; Bex, A.; Khoo, V.; Grünwald, V.; Gillessen, S.; Horwich, A.; ESMO Guidelines Committee. Renal cell carcinoma: ESMO Clinical Practice Guidelines for diagnosis, treatment and follow-up. *Ann. Oncol.* **2019**, *30*, 706–720. [CrossRef] [PubMed]
2. Campbell, S.; Uzzo, R.G.; Allaf, M.E.; Bass, E.B.; Cadeddu, J.A.; Chang, A.; Clark, P.E.; Davis, B.J.; Derweesh, I.H.; Giambarresi, L.; et al. Renal Mass and Localized Renal Cancer: AUA Guideline. *J. Urol.* **2017**, *198*, 520–529. [CrossRef] [PubMed]
3. Ljungberg, B.; Albiges, L.; Bensalah, K.; Bex, A.; Giles, R.H.; Hora, M.; Kuczyk, M.A.; Lam, T.; Marconi, L.; Merseburger, A.S.; et al. *European Association of Urology Guidelines on Renal Cell Carcinoma*; EAU Annual Congress: Amsterdam, The Netherlands, 2020; ISBN 978-94-92671-07-3.

4. Motzer, R.J.; Jonasch, E.; Agarwal, N.; Bhayani, S.; Bro, W.P.; Chang, S.S.; Choueiri, T.K.; Costello, B.A.; Derweesh, I.H.; Fishman, M.; et al. Kidney Cancer, Version 2.2017, NCCN Clinical Practice Guidelines in Oncology. *J. Natl. Compr. Canc. Netw.* **2017**, *15*, 804–834. [CrossRef] [PubMed]
5. Peddada, A.V.; Anderson, D.; Blasi, O.C.; McCollough, K.; Jennings, S.B.; Monroe, A.T. Nephron-Sparing Robotic Radiosurgical Therapy for Primary Renal Cell Carcinoma: Single-Institution Experience and Review of the Literature. *Adv. Radiat. Oncol.* **2019**, *5*, 204–211. [CrossRef] [PubMed]
6. Siva, S.; Pham, D.; Kron, T.; Bressel, M.; Lam, J.; Tan, T.H.; Chesson, B.; Shaw, M.; Chander, S.; Gill, S.; et al. Stereotactic ablative body radiotherapy for inoperable primary kidney cancer: A prospective clinical trial. *BJU Int.* **2017**, *120*, 623–630. [CrossRef]
7. Staehler, M.; Bader, M.; Schlenker, B.; Casuscelli, J.; Karl, A.; Roosen, A.; Stief, C.G.; Bex, A.; Wowra, B.; Muacevic, A. Single fraction radiosurgery for the treatment of renal tumors. *J. Urol.* **2015**, *193*, 771–775. [CrossRef]
8. Ponsky, L.; Lo, S.S.; Zhang, Y.; Schluchter, M.; Liu, Y.; Patel, R.; Abouassaly, R.; Welford, S.; Gulani, V.; Haaga, J.R.; et al. Phase I dose-escalation study of stereotactic body radiotherapy (SBRT) for poor surgical candidates with localized renal cell carcinoma. *Radiother. Oncol.* **2015**, *117*, 183–187. [CrossRef]
9. Pham, D.; Thompson, A.; Kron, T.; Foroudi, F.; Kolsky, M.S.; Devereux, T.; Lim, A.; Siva, S. Stereotactic ablative body radiation therapy for primary kidney cancer: A 3-dimensional conformal technique associated with low rates of early toxicity. *Int. J. Radiat. Oncol. Biol. Phys.* **2014**, *90*, 1061–1068. [CrossRef]
10. Kaidar-Person, O.; Price, A.; Schreiber, E.; Zagar, T.M.; Chen, R.C. Stereotactic Body Radiotherapy for Large Primary Renal Cell Carcinoma. *Clin. Genitourin. Cancer* **2017**, *15*, e851–e854. [CrossRef]
11. Sun, M.R.; Brook, A.; Powell, M.F.; Kaliannan, K.; Wagner, A.A.; Kaplan, I.D.; Pedrosa, I. Effect of Stereotactic Body Radiotherapy on the Growth Kinetics and Enhancement Pattern of Primary Renal Tumors. *AJR Am. J. Roentgenol.* **2016**, *206*, 544–553. [CrossRef]
12. Chang, J.H.; Cheung, P.; Erler, D.; Sonier, M.; Korol, R.; Chu, W. Stereotactic Ablative Body Radiotherapy for Primary Renal Cell Carcinoma in Non-surgical Candidates: Initial Clinical Experience. *Clin. Oncol.* **2016**, *28*, e109–e114. [CrossRef] [PubMed]
13. Beitler, J.J.; Makara, D.; Silverman, P.; Lederman, G. Definitive, high-dose-perfraction, conformal, stereotactic external radiation for renal cell carcinoma. *Am. J. Clin. Oncol.* **2004**, *27*, 646–648. [CrossRef] [PubMed]
14. McBride, S.M.; Wagner, A.A.; Kaplan, I.D. A phase 1 dose-escalation study of robotic radiosurgery in inoperable primary renal cell carcinoma. *Int. J. Radiat. Oncol. Biol. Phys.* **2013**, *87*, S84. [CrossRef]
15. Siva, S.; Louie, A.V.; Warner, A.; Muacevic, A.; Gandhidasan, S.; Ponsky, L.; Ellis, R.; Kaplan, I.; Mahadevan, A.; Chu, w.; et al. Pooled analysis of stereotactic ablative radiotherapy for primary renal cell carcinoma: A report from the international radiosurgery oncology consortium for kidney (IROCK). *Cancer* **2018**, *124*, 934–942. [CrossRef] [PubMed]
16. Siva, S.; Correa, R.J.; Warner, A.; Staehler, M.; Ellis, R.J.; Ponsky, L.; Kaplan, I.D.; Mahadevan, A.; Chu, W.; Gandhidasan, S.; et al. Stereotactic Ablative Radiotherapy for ≥T1b Primary Renal Cell Carcinoma: A Report from the International Radiosurgery Oncology Consortium for Kidney (IROCK). *Int. J. Radiat. Oncol. Biol. Phys.* **2020**, in press journal pre-proof. [CrossRef] [PubMed]
17. Siva, S.; Chesson, B.; Bressel, M.; Pryor, D.; Higgs, B.; Reynolds, H.M.; Hardcastle, N.; Montgomery, R.; Vanneste, B.G.; Khoo, V.; et al. TROG 15.03 Phase II Clinical Trial of Focal Ablative STereotactic Radiosurgery for Cancers of the Kidney—FASTRACK II. *BMC Cancer* **2018**, *18*, 1030. [CrossRef] [PubMed]
18. Rühle, A.; Andratschke, N.; Siva, S.; Guckenberger, M. Is there a role for stereotactic radiotherapy in the treatment of renal cell carcinoma? *Clin. Transl. Radiat. Oncol.* **2019**, *18*, 104–112. [CrossRef]
19. Corradini, S.; Alongi, F.; Andratschke, N.; Belka, C.; Boldrini, L.; Cellini, F.; Debus, J.; Guckenberger, M.; Hoerner-Rieber, J.; Lagerwaard, F.J.; et al. MR-guidance in clinical reality: Current treatment challenges and future perspectives. *Radiat. Oncol.* **2019**, *14*, 92. [CrossRef]
20. Bohoudi, O.; Bruynzeel, A.; Senan, S.; Cuijpers, J.; Slotman, B.; Lagerwaard, F.; Palacios, M. Fast and robust online adaptive planning in stereotactic MR-guided adaptive radiation therapy (SMART) for pancreatic cancer. *Radiother. Oncol.* **2017**, *125*, 439–444. [CrossRef]
21. Tetar, S.; Bruynzeel, A.; Bakker, R.; Jeulink, M.; Slotman, B.; Oei, S.; Haasbeek, C.; De Jong, K.; Senan, S.; Lagerwaard, F.J. Patient-reported Outcome Measurements on the Tolerance of Magnetic Resonance Imaging-guided Radiation Therapy. *Cureus* **2018**, *10*, e2236. [CrossRef]

22. Koste, J.R.V.S.D.; Palacios, M.A.; Bruynzeel, A.M.; Slotman, B.; Senan, S.; Lagerwaard, F.J. MR-guided Gated Stereotactic Radiation Therapy Delivery for Lung, Adrenal, and Pancreatic Tumors: A Geometric Analysis. *Int. J. Radiat. Oncol. Biol. Phys.* **2018**, *102*, 858–866. [CrossRef] [PubMed]
23. Francolini, G.; Detti, B.; Ingrosso, G.; Desideri, I.; Becherini, C.; Carta, G.A.; Pezzulla, D.; Caramia, G.; Dominici, L.; Maragna, V.; et al. Stereotactic Body Radiation Therapy (SBRT) on Renal Cell Carcinoma, an Overview of Technical Aspects, Biological Rationale and Current Literature. *Crit. Rev. Oncol. Hematol.* **2018**, *131*, 24–29. [CrossRef]
24. Siva, S.; Pham, D.; Gill, S.; Corcoran, N.M.; Foroudi, F. A systematic review of stereotactic radiotherapy ablation for primary renal cell carcinoma. *BJU Int.* **2012**, *110*, E737–E743. [CrossRef] [PubMed]
25. Siva, S.; Staehler, M.; Correa, R.; Warner, A.; Ellis, R.; Gandhidasan, S.; Ponsky, L.; Kaplan, I.; Mahadevan, A.; Chu, W.; et al. Stereotactic Body Radiotherapy for Large Primary Renal Cell Carcinoma: A Report from the International Radiosurgery Oncology Consortium for Kidney (IROCK). *Int. J. Radiat. Oncol. Biol. Phys.* **2019**, *105*, E257–E258. [CrossRef]
26. Wegner, R.E.; Abel, S.; Vemana, G.; Mao, S.; Fuhrer, R. Utilization of Stereotactic Ablative Body Radiation Therapy for Intact Renal Cell Carcinoma: Trends in Treatment and Predictors of Outcome. *Adv. Radiat. Oncol.* **2019**, *5*, 85–91. [CrossRef] [PubMed]
27. Correa, R.J.; Louie, A.V.; Zaorsky, N.G.; Lehrer, E.J.; Ellis, R.; Ponsky, L.; Kaplan, I.; Mahadevan, A.; Chu, W.; Swaminath, A.; et al. The Emerging Role of Stereotactic Ablative Radiotherapy for Primary Renal Cell Carcinoma: A Systematic Review and Meta-Analysis. *Eur. Urol. Focus* **2019**, *5*, 958–969. [CrossRef]
28. Siva, S.; Jackson, P.; Kron, T.; Bressel, M.; Lau, E.; Hofman, M.; Shaw, M.; Chander, S.; Pham, D.; Lawrentshuk, N.; et al. Impact of stereotactic radiotherapy on kidney function in primary renal cell carcinoma: Establishing a dose-response relationship. *Radiother. Oncol.* **2016**, *118*, 540–546. [CrossRef]
29. Musaddaq, B.; Musaddaq, T.; Gupta, A.; Ilyas, S.; Von Stempel, C. Renal Cell Carcinoma: The Evolving Role of Imaging in the 21st Century. *Semin. Ultrasound CT MR* **2020**, *41*, 344–350. [CrossRef]
30. Grant, S.R.; Lei, X.; Hess, K.R.; Smith, G.L.; Matin, S.F.; Wood, C.G.; Nguyen, Q.; Frank, S.J.; Anscher, M.S.; Smith, B.D.; et al. Stereotactic Body Radiation Therapy for the Definitive Treatment of Early Stage Kidney Cancer: A Survival Comparison with Surgery, Tumor Ablation, and Observation. *Adv. Radiat. Oncol.* **2020**, *5*, 495–502. [CrossRef]

12

Recovery from Anesthesia after Robotic-Assisted Radical Cystectomy: Two Different Reversals of Neuromuscular Blockade

Claudia Claroni [1,*], Marco Covotta [1], Giulia Torregiani [1], Maria Elena Marcelli [1], Gabriele Tuderti [2], Giuseppe Simone [2], Alessandra Scotto di Uccio [3], Antonio Zinilli [4] and Ester Forastiere [1]

1 Department of Anaesthesiology, IRCCS Regina Elena National Cancer Institute, 00144 Rome, Italy; marco.covotta@gmail.com (M.C.); giulia.torregiani@gmail.com (G.T.); mariaelena.marcelli@gmail.com (M.E.M.); ester.forastiere@ifo.gov.it (E.F.)

2 Department of Urology, IRCCS Regina Elena National Cancer Institute, 00144 Rome, Italy; gabriele.tuderti@gmail.com (G.T.); puldet@gmail.com (G.S.)

3 School of Medicine, University Hospital Center "Tor Vergata", 00133 Rome, Italy; allascotto@gmail.com

4 IRCrES, Research Institute on Sustainable Economic Growth of the National Research Council of Italy, 00185 Rome, Italy; antonio.zinilli@ircres.cnr.it

* Correspondence: claroni@icloud.com

Abstract: During robot-assisted radical cystectomy (RARC), specific surgical conditions (a steep Trendelenburg position, prolonged pneumoperitoneum, effective myoresolution until the final stages of surgery) can seriously impair the outcomes. The aim of the study was to evaluate the incidence of postoperative nausea and vomiting (PONV) and ileus and the quality of cognitive function at the awakening in two groups of patients undergoing different reversals. In this randomized trial, patients that were American Society of Anesthesiologists physical status (ASA) ≤III candidates for RARC for bladder cancer were randomized into two groups: In the sugammadex (S) group, patients received 2 mg/kg of sugammadex as reversal of neuromuscolar blockade; in the neostigmine (N) group, antagonization was obtained with neostigmine 0.04 mg/kg + atropine 0.02 mg/kg. PONV was evaluated at 30 min, 6 and 24 h after anesthesia. Postoperative cognitive functions and time to resumption of intestinal transit were also investigated. A total of 109 patients were analyzed (54 in the S group and 55 in the N group). The incidence of early PONV was lower in the S group but not statistically significant (S group 25.9% vs. N group 29%; $p = 0.711$). The Mini-Mental State test mean value was higher in the S group vs. the N group (1 h after surgery: 29.3 (29; 30) vs. 27.6 (27; 30), $p = 0.007$; 4 h after surgery: 29.5 (30; 30) vs. 28.4 (28; 30), $p = 0.05$). We did not observe a significant decrease of the PONV after sugammadex administration versus neostigmine use. The Mini-Mental State test mean value was greater in the S group.

Keywords: anesthesia recovery periods; bladder cancer; cognitive impairment; gamma-cyclodextrins; neuromuscular blockade; robotic radical cystectomy

---

1. Introduction

The diffusion of robot-assisted laparoscopic techniques has made it possible to perform surgical procedures with greater precision, and has reduced the need for transfusions, postoperative complications and hospitalization time [1]. In particular, robot-assisted radical cystectomy (RARC) has rapidly spread as the gold standard in the treatment of urothelial tumors, becoming a credible alternative to open cystectomy which is burdened by a high rate of complications [2].

Due to the particular surgical conditions and because of its recent application, there still are many anesthetic implications that must be examined thoroughly—patients have to satisfy specific clinical requirements, identified through careful anesthesiologic assessments [3].

During RARC, the anesthesiologist must be prepared to manage any hemodynamic, cerebrovascular and respiratory changes resulting from the surgical conditions that the robotic procedure requires, such as the prolonged use of pneumoperitoneum, the steep Trendelenburg position in which the patient is placed, and the lengthening of surgical times [4]. In addition, an effective myoresolution until the final stages of surgery is necessary to establish ideal surgical conditions [5] and the factors that can impair the quality and time of awakening [6]. To overcome this effect, a reversal of neuromuscular blockade (NMB) is routinely used in our clinical practice.

Currently, the effectiveness of the rocuronium/sugammadex combination for the reversal of the NMB has been widely demonstrated in terms of time and quality of neuromuscular and respiratory functions [7,8].

Neostigmine has been associated with an increased incidence of postoperative nausea and vomiting (PONV), although there is no definitive agreement on the need to avoid its use to reduce the incidence of PONV [9]. On the other hand, neostigmine has an important muscarinic effect on gastrointestinal (GI) receptors, and, by increasing the availability of acetylcholine, increases the GI motility.

In our study, we investigated if the use of a different kind of NMB reversal can influence the early postoperative period after a prolonged major surgery, such as RARC, affected by alterations on mechanical ventilation, cerebral perfusion, and vascular resistances [10]. Our aim is particularly focused on PONV and ileus, with attention to the recent collective effort to build an enhanced recovery after surgery (ERAS) path applicable specifically in the interventions of RARC [11].

The hypothesis is that the continuous infusion of rocuronium followed by sugammadex administration as NMB reversal in patients undergoing robotic radical cystectomy can improve the quality of awakening in terms of postoperative outcomes and cognitive function, compared to use of neostigmine as reversal.

The primary end point was to compare the incidence of PONV. Secondary end points were postoperative cognitive functions and time to resumption of intestinal transit (ROI).

2. Experimental Section

A mono-center prospective, two-arm parallel, randomized trial was conducted at the IRCCS Regina Elena National Cancer Institute. The study was approved by the Central Ethics Committee Lazio1, in May 2017, with Protocol n. CE/2288/17, and registered with ClinicalTrial.gov identifier NCT03144453. The clinical investigation was conducted according to the principles expressed in the Declaration of Helsinki.

2.1. Patients and Procedures

American Society of Anesthesiologists physical status (ASA) ≤III patients, candidates of RARC for bladder cancer, were enrolled after having given written informed consent. The exclusion criteria were age <18 years, inability to provide informed consent, BMI >30, and a history of cerebrovascular diseases.

Patients were randomly divided into two treatment groups by an operator who is not directly involved in the study using a specific dedicated software, developed in-house by a GW Basic (Microsoft Corporation, USA) programmer, which generates an assignment code verified immediately before arrival in the operating room. Surgeons were blinded to the intervention and blinded observers recorded the outcome.

In both groups, all patients were premedicated with midazolam 0.02 mg/kg and received dexamethasone 8 mg for anti-emesis. General anesthesia was induced with fentanyl 3–5 g/kg, propofol 2 mg/kg and a bolus of rocuronium 0.7 mg/kg was administered. After tracheal intubation, anesthesia was maintained with a mixture of sevoflurane/oxygen/air, adjusted to provide an end-tidal sevoflurane of 1.5–2 vol.%, remifentanil was adapted according to a target-controlled infusion (TCI) range of 2–4 ng/mL. Curarization started with rocuronium 5 g/kg/min and was set to maintain the post-tetanic count between 1 and 2. At the end of surgery, after skin closure, neuromuscular function was allowed to recover spontaneously and, at reappearance of the second twitch (T2), patients received a NMB reversal.

In the sugammadex group (S group), at T2 reappearance, patients received 2 mg/kg of sugammadex.

In the neostigmine group (N group), at T2 reappearance, antagonization was obtained with the standard NMB reversal agent: neostigmine 0.04 mg/kg and atropine 0.02 mg/kg to block the peripheral muscarinic side-effects of neostigmine.

All patients were extubated when the train-of-four (TOF) ratio was 0.9 or higher.

Nasogastric tube was removed after surgery, before the awakening.

In both groups, fluid therapy regimen was mainly restrictive, with a basal infusion of crystalloid variable from 2 to 4 mL/kg/h. Mean arterial blood pressure (MAP) was regulated by titrating remifentanil and fluid administration in order to maintain target values between 65 and 95 mmHg.

The standard monitoring for all patients consisted of continuous ECG, heart rate (HR) and MAP measurements, pulse oximetry (SpO2), inspired and expired gas, and capnometry. Neuromuscular function was measured using a TOF-Watch acceleromyograph (Organon ltd, Dublin, Ireland). After induction of general anesthesia, but before administering any NMB agent, the calibration of the acceleromyograph was performed according to the manufacturer's guidelines. The ulnar nerve received neuromuscular stimulation via two electrodes applied to the skin of the distal underarm, to the left and to the right of the ulnar nerve.

The surgical procedure was performed routinely following the standards of the Department of Urology at our hospital [12].

After surgery, patients requiring rescue anti-emetic therapy received ondansetron 4 mg, which was followed by metoclopramide 20 mg, if necessary.

All patients received intravenous morphine patient-controlled analgesia using the CADD®-Solis device (Smith Medical, Kent, UK) postoperatively. Patient-controlled analgesia was set on the demand mode without a loading dose. The dose of morphine was set at 0.02 mg/kg with a time-lock interval of 15 min.

All patients received morphine 0.07 mg/kg and 1000 mg acetaminophen at the time of surgical wound closure, followed by 1000 mg intravenous acetaminophen every 6 h for up to 5 days.

2.2. *Measurements*

Baseline data were collected, which included risk of PONV by Apfel score, neoadjuvant chemotherapy, and anxiety and depression by the Hospital Anxiety and Depression Scale.

During anesthesia, main parameters (MAP, HR, SpO2 and etCO2) and time to recovery from NMB reversal were recorded. Duration of surgery, amount of opioid consumption, comorbidities, and total amount of intensive care unit admission were also observed.

In the postoperative period, PONV (intended as number of episodes of nausea, vomiting or bloating) was evaluated after 30 min in post-anesthesia care unit (PACU), 6 and 24 h after anesthesia.

The assessment of consciousness at awakening and postoperative cognitive function was carried out by The Observer's Assessment of Alertness/Sedation Scale (OASS) at 15 min, 30 min, and 1 h after anesthesia, and through the Mini Mental State test (MMSt) at 1 and 4 h after anesthesia.

Early postoperative pulmonary failure (including bronchospasm, postoperative PaO2 <60 mmHg, a PaO2:FIO2 ratio ≥ 300 mmHg, or arterial oxyhemoglobin saturation measured with pulse oximetry $<90\%$ and requiring oxygen therapy) was noted after 24 h after anesthesia.

Time to resumption of intestinal transit, defined as time to return of peristalsis and time to first passage of flatus, antiemetics, and morphine consumption were recorded. Nurses detected peristalsis and gastrointestinal symptoms every 2 h and patients were asked to warn staff of the perception of bowel activity.

2.3. *Statistical Analysis*

The primary outcome was the cumulative incidence of PONV in the first 6 postoperative hours. Based on data from our department after this type of surgery using single-drug PONV prophylaxis and reversal of neuromuscular block with neostigmine, and according with previous study [13,14], we estimated that experience PONV would be 30% in neostigmine group and 8% in the sugammadex group. Based on power = 80% and $a = 0.05$, a sample size of 98 patients at least ($n = 49$ per group) was required.

For scores continuous, we used a two-sample Kolmogorov–Smirnov test, while for the ordinal categorical variable we used the Mann–Whitney U-test. *P*-values ≤ 0.05 were regarded as statistically significant. Data were analyzed using SPSS software (IBM, New York, United States).

3. Results

In the period between May 2017 and December 2018, a total of 109 patients were randomized: 54 patients to the S group and 55 to the N group.

The flowchart of the patients who participated in the study is demonstrated in Figure 1. The demographics and clinical characteristics were balanced for both treatment arms and are presented in Table 1. Intraoperative and perioperative data recorded are shown in Table 2.

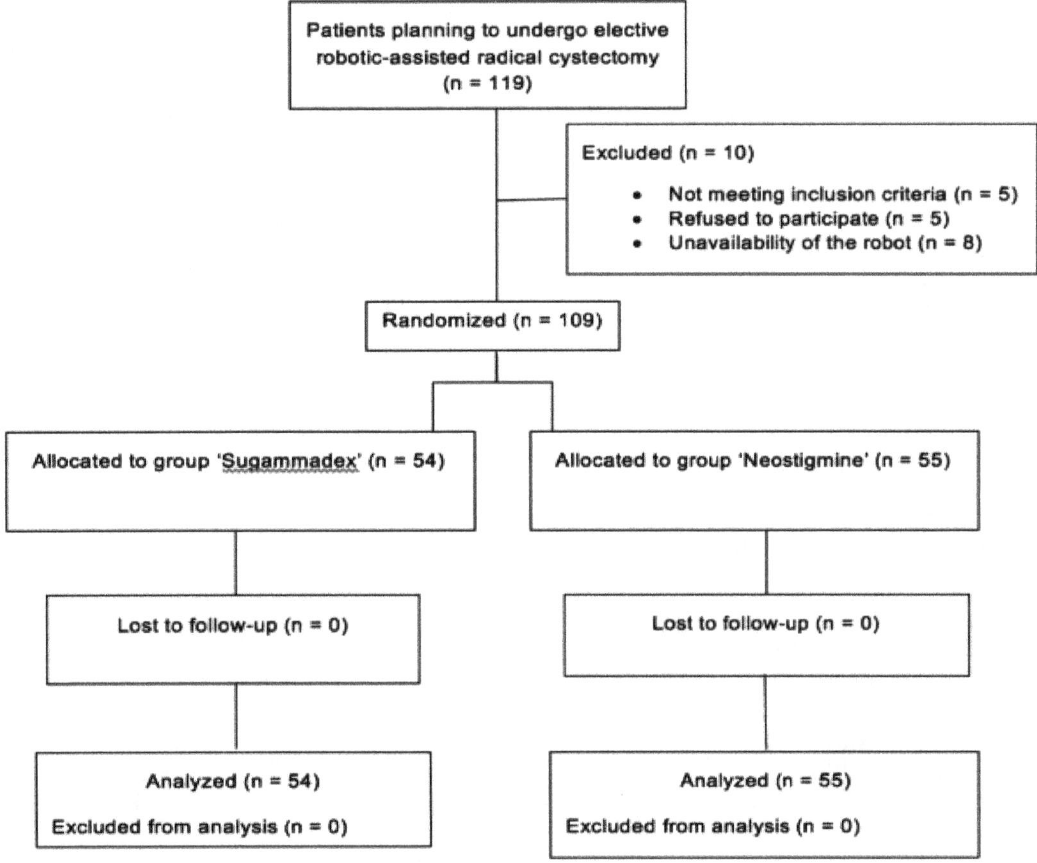

Figure 1. Patient disposition.

Time to recovery from TOF 2 to TOF ratio >0.9 was significantly lower in the S group. The incidence of early PONV was lower in the S group but not statistically significant ($p = 0.711$). The values were similar between the two groups for the incidence of late PONV.

The mean MMSt value was significantly higher in the S group compared with the N group at 1 h after anesthesia [mean and 25–75th percentile, 29.3 (29; 30) vs. 27.6 (27; 30); $p = 0.007$] and at 4 h after anesthesia [29.5 (30; 30) vs. 28.4 (28; 30); $p = 0.048$]. Thus, S group obtained better MMSt values during all measurements of time. The mean OASS value was significantly higher in the S group compared with the N group 1 h after the end of anesthesia (median and 25–75th percentile, 5 (5; 5) vs. 5 (4; 5); $p = 0.02$), but no differences were observed in the first measurement, 30 min after the end of anesthesia (Table 3).

Table 1. Demographic and clinical characteristics.

	S Group (n = 54)	N Group (n = 55)
Age (years), mean (SD)	62.8 (8.9)	60.2 (9.4)
BMI (kg/m^2), mean (SD)	26.3 (3.5)	26.2 (4)
Gender (n), male/female	42/12	40/14
ASA status (n): I/II/III	5/40/9	9/41/5
Apfel risk score (n): I/II/III/IV	20/30/4/0	19/32/4/0
Comorbidities, n (%)		
Hypertension	18 (33.3)	11 (20)
Dysthyroidism	3 (5.5)	4 (7.2)
Previous MI	5 (9.2)	2 (3.6)
Diabetes	6 (11.1)	3 (5.4)
COPD	3 (5.5)	2 (3.6)
Neoadiuvant chemotherapy, n (%)	14 (25.9)	11 (20)
Tumor stage (pT), n (%)		
Tis	8 (14.8)	7 (12.7)
Ta	3 (5.5)	3 (5.4)
T1	7 (13)	8 (14.8)
T2	13 (24)	14 (25.4)
T3	17 (31.4)	16 (29)
T4	6 (11.1)	7 (12.7)
HADS > 8, n (%)	25 (46.2)	27 (49)

BMI: body mass index; ASA: American Society of Anesthesiologists; COPD: chronic obstructive pulmonary disease; HADS: Hospital Anxiety and Depression Scale.

Table 2. Intraoperative and perioperative variables.

	S Group (n = 54)	N Group (n = 55)	p-Value
$EtCO_2$ (mmHg)	28.9 (3)	28.6 (3.4)	0.603
SpO_2 (%)	98.6 (1.3)	98.5 (1.5)	0.821
HR (bpm)	68.3 (15.1)	68.9 (13.9)	0.622
MAP (mmHg)	87 (15.3)	88.2 (15.5)	0.854
Estimated blood loss (mL)	209 (31)	218 (37)	0.200
Surgery time (min)	340.7(80)	326.7 (81.9)	0.437
Anesthesia time (min)	378 (83)	361 (81)	0.526
Recovery time from TOF 2 to TOF Ratio > 0.9 (min)	3.2 (1)	8 (2.8)	<0.001 *
Early PONV 0–6 h, n (%)			
Cumulative incidence	14 (25.9)	16 (29)	0.711
Nausea	10 (18.5)	9 (16.3)	0.767
Vomiting	4 (7.4)	5 (9)	0.750
Late PONV 6–24 h, n (%)			
Cumulative incidence	10 (18.5)	11 (20)	0.845
Nausea	7 (13)	8 (14.5)	0.810
Vomiting	3 (5.5)	3 (5.4)	0.982
Antiemetics consumption (mg)			
Ondansetron	2.6 (3)	3.8 (4.4)	0.105
Metoclopramide	3.7 (4.9)	4.7 (5.7)	0.358
Morphine consumption (mg)			
0–6 h	3 (2.4)	3.7 (2.6)	0.154
0–24 h	6.2 (3)	5.5 (2.8)	0.177
Early postoperative pulmonary failure, n (%)	3 (5.5)	4 (7.2)	0.715
Time to resumption of intestinal transit, days (IQR)	3 (3–5)	3 (3–5)	0.761
Length of stay, days (IQR)	8 (7.5–12.25)	8 (6–12)	0.682

* p-value < 0.05; $EtCO_2$: end tidal CO_2; SpO_2: pulse oximetry; HR: heart rate; MAP: mean arterial pressure; TOF: train-of-four; PONV: postoperative nausea and vomiting; IQR: interquartile range.

Table 3. Consciousness at awakening and postoperative cognitive function.

	S Group (n = 54)	N Group (n = 55)	p-Value
		OASS ¢	
15 min	3 (3; 4)	3 (3; 4)	0.16
30 min	5 (4; 5)	4 (3; 5)	0.06
60 min	5 (5; 5)	5 (4; 5)	0.023 *
		MMSt ♯	
Preop	29.3 (30; 30)	29.2 (29; 30)	0.78
1 h	29.3 (29; 30)	27.6 (27; 30)	0.007 *
4 h	29.5 (30; 30)	28.4 (28; 30)	0.048 *

♯ Data expressed as mean (IQR); ¢ Data expressed as median (IQR); p-value: two-sample Kolmogorov–Smirnov Test; * p-value < 0.05; OASS: Observer's Assessment of Alertness/Sedation Scale; MMSt: Mini Mental State test: IQR: interquartile range.

In Figure 2, we can observe that the trend in both MMSt and OASS is different between the two groups. The MMSt trend remained steadily higher since the awakening, while the values of OASS in S group were significantly increased after the first postoperative hour. The incidence of postoperative pulmonary failure was similar in each group. There were no significant differences between the groups for time to resumption of intestinal transit. Postoperative ondansetron and metoclopramide were similar in each group, as well as analgesic consumption.

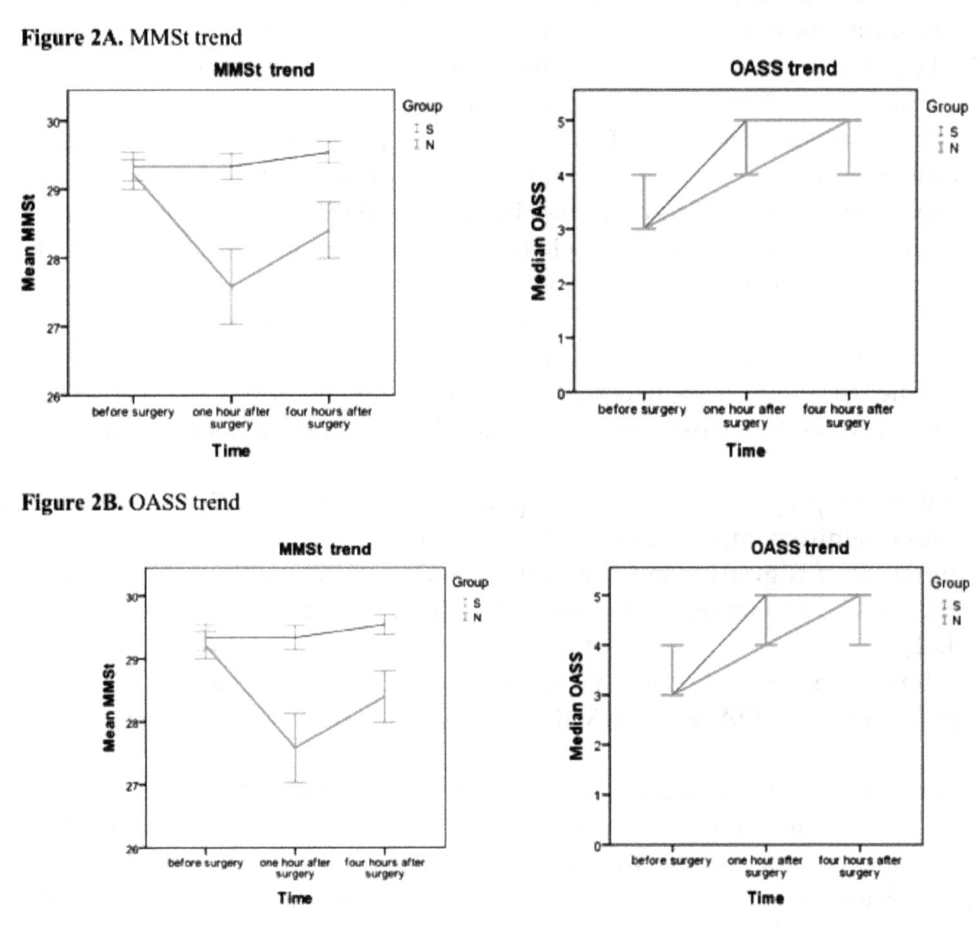

Figure 2. (**A**) MMSt and (**B**) OASS trend (error bars: 95% CI). Blue line: S group. Green line: N group.

4. Discussion

In our study, we attempted to evaluate the quality of recovery from anesthesia in two groups of patients who underwent robotic-assisted laparoscopic cystectomy. Prolonged myoresolution was carried out with continuous infusion of rocuronium: In one group, NMB reversal was obtained with sugammadex and in the other group, the association neostigmine/atropine was used.

Our results show that the incidence of PONV was greater in the N group, although non-statistically significant. Even time to resumption of intestinal transit was overlapping in the two groups.

In the past, studies concerning the reduction of PONV following the use of sugammadex have had conflicting results. Inhibiting cholinesterase action causes neostigmine increases concentration of acetylcholine, the principal excitatory neurotransmitter in the GI tract. Acetylcholine acts by increasing gastric secretions and esophageal pressure and increases the risk of symptoms such as nausea and vomiting, but also allows an increase in GI motility [15]. The prevention of PONV and the rapid restoration of intestinal function are fundamental topics in the development of ERAS protocols, which have shown efficacy in reducing complications and improving outcomes in many surgeries [16]. Nowadays, there are no definitive protocols specific to robotic surgery, and protocols applied in colorectal surgery are often used for cystectomy [10].

Our results agree with those of Peach et al. [17], which, in a large clinical trial of 304 women, did not find a lower incidence of PONV with the use of sugammadex compared with neostigmine. In contrast, Yağan et al. [13] found that the use of sugammadex had lower incidences of PONV in the first postoperative hour and less anti-emetic use at 24 h. In addition, in the study by Koyuncu et al. [18], sugammadex reduces PONV compared with neostigmine and atropine, but only slightly and transiently. While in the Yağan study [13], the population had undergone various types of surgery (more than half underwent head and neck surgery) and in the Koyuncu study [18] patient were candidates for extremity surgery, in the Peach study [17] patients underwent laparoscopic surgery, which, as in robotic cystectomy, involves a certain degree of postoperative ileus, a physiological arrest of GI transit in response to surgical stress and intestinal manipulation. Neostigmine can increase motility only if acetylcholine release and smooth muscle function are relatively preserved, while postoperative ileus induces the activation of presynaptic noradrenergic receptors and impairs the functionality of the enteric nervous system and the sympathetic nerves [19,20]. This could have determined the absence of the expected effects on intestinal and gastric motility.

Moreover, in the study by Yağan, neostigmine doses were higher than those used in our study [13], and the correlation between the neostigmine dose and PONV is now considered a key factor to control the symptoms [9].

Two scales were employed as awakening quality indicators: MMSt and OASS. The MMSt was considered to assess cognitive impairment because it is a rapid and simple to perform test that provides accurate measurements of cognitive status both in subjects with normal functions and in subjects with cognitive alterations [21], and its use to assess subtle changes in cognitive function after anesthesia is often reported [22].

Our results have unexpectedly shown a significant increase of the average value of MMSt in the considered time frames. The OASS mean value also significantly increased in the S group until 1 h after surgery.

The reversal action of sugammadex is based on the structure of cyclodextrins, consisting of a lipophilic central cavity able to encapsulate the steroid rings of the rocuronium molecule, forming an inactive complex that is no longer able to interact with the neuromuscular junction [23]. Based on its structural characteristics, the fact that the sugammadex molecule or the sugammadex/rocuronium complex could interact in any way with the anesthetic drugs or with the cholinergic system was excluded [24]. The apparent rapid awakening at a cognitive level, that some other authors and we have detected [25,26], could be explained in the light of the so-called Afferentation Theory [27], for which general activation of muscle receptors can induce a massive cerebral stimulation of the monoaminergic wakefulness centers. It is also known as the Spindle Theory [23], since it has been postulated that tension and stretch receptors in muscle spindles may be the terminations that transmit static and dynamic variations to the encephalon, acting on various cortical and mesencephalic areas. However, some studies have not been able to demonstrate changes in the depth of anesthesia after sugammadex administration [28], thus the results of studies regarding sugammadex's impact on recovery from general anesthesia remain conflicting and insufficient [29].

In the past, many studies demonstrated an existing relationship between the structure of cyclodextrins and neuroprotection: statins and cyclodextrins, influence the transmission of neural signals, interfering with the production of inflammatory molecules [30]. Ultimately, one could speculate that sugammadex gives an additional effect by interacting with the lipid molecules of the neuronal membrane, reducing exocytosis. This protective effect could be more readily detectable in a surgery, such as robotic cystectomy, which requires more than 2 h in steep Trendelenburg and alterations of cerebrovascular circulation due to prolonged pneumoperitoneum [10]. In the future, it could be interesting to analyze if the use of sugammadex can be optimized, employing it in elderly populations or in surgeries that require high abdominal pressure or extreme conditions.

A limit of our study mainly regards the same limitations related to the neurophysiological tests administered in the postoperative period. These tests may be subject to the learning effect bias and to the variability in the sessions following the preoperative one, considered baseline, and from one session to another. We tried to minimize this variability by administering the test in the same environment, with no external distractions, and patients who needed extra doses of opioids for pain were excluded.

5. Conclusions

In conclusion, our results were not able to demonstrate a significant decrease of the PONV or a more rapid ROI after sugammadex administration versus neostigmine use. We observed a significant increase in MMSt values, suggesting improved quality of awakening with the use of sugammadex in patients undergoing robotic radical cystectomy. Regarding OASS observations in both groups, we obtained higher values in the group receiving sugammadex. Further studies on elderly populations and different types of surgery will be needed in the future, especially with the aim to provide a comprehensive ERAS pathway for cystectomy based on the available evidence.

Author Contributions: Conceptualization, C.C. and E.F.; methodology, C.C.; formal analysis, C.C.; investigation, C.C., M.C. and G.T. (Giulia Torregiani); data curation, M.E.M., A.S.d.U., A.Z., G.T. (Gabriele Tuderti) and G.S.; writing—original draft preparation, C.C.; writing—review and editing, C.C., M.C. and G.T. (Giulia Torregiani); supervision, E.F.

References

1. Leow, J.J.; Chang, S.L.; Meyer, C.P.; Wang, Y.; Hanske, J.; Sammon, J.D.; Cole, A.P.; Preston, M.A.; Dasgupta, P.; Menon, M.; et al. Robot-assisted Versus Open Radical Prostatectomy: A Contemporary Analysis of an All-payer Discharge Database. *Eur. Urol.* **2016**, *70*, 837–845. [CrossRef]
2. Trentman, T.L.; Fassett, S.L.; McGirr, D.; Anderson, B.; Chang, Y.H.H.; Nateras, R.N.; Castle, E.P.; Rosenfeld, D.M. Comparison of anesthetic management and outcomes of robot-assisted versus open radical cystectomy. *J. Robot. Surg.* **2013**, *7*, 273–279. [CrossRef]
3. Oksar, M.; Akbulut, Z.; Ocal, H.; Balbay, M.D.; Kanbak, O. Anesthetic considerations for robotic cystectomy: A prospective study. *Braz. J. Anesthesiol.* **2014**, *64*, 109–115. [CrossRef]
4. Cockcroft, J.O.; Berry, C.B.; McGrath, J.S.; Daugherty, M.O. Anesthesia for Major Urologic Surgery. *Anesthesiol. Clin.* **2015**, *33*, 165–172. [CrossRef]
5. Martini, C.H.; Boon, M.; Bevers, R.F.; Aarts, L.P.; Dahan, A. Evaluation of Surgical Conditions During Laparoscopic Surgery in Patients with Moderate vs. Deep Neuromuscular Block. *Surv. Anesthesiol.* **2014**, *58*, 222–223. [CrossRef]
6. Boon, M.; Martini, C.H.; Aarts, L.P.; Bevers, R.F.; Dahan, A. Effect of variations in depth of neuromuscular blockade on rating of surgical conditions by surgeon and anesthesiologist in patients undergoing laparoscopic renal or prostatic surgery (BLISS trial): Study protocol for a randomized controlled trial. *Trials* **2013**, *14*, 63. [CrossRef]

7. Geldner, G.; Niskanen, M.; Laurila, P.; Mizikov, V.; Hübler, M.; Beck, G.; Rietbergen, H.; Nicolayenko, E. A randomized controlled trial comparing sugammadex and neostigmine at different depths of neuromuscular blockade in patients undergoing laparoscopic surgery. *Anaesthesia* **2012**, *67*, 991–998. [CrossRef]
8. Paton, F.; Paulden, M.; Chambers, D.; Heirs, M.; Duffy, S.; Hunter, J.M.; Sculpher, M.; Woolacott, N. Sugammadex compared with neostigmine/glycopyrrolate for routine reversal of neuromuscular block: A systematic review and economic evaluation. *Br. J. Anaesth.* **2010**, *105*, 558–567. [CrossRef]
9. Luo, J.; Chen, S.; Min, S.; Peng, L. Reevaluation and update on efficacy and safety of neostigmine for reversal of neuromuscular blockade. *Ther. Clin. Risk Manag.* **2018**, *14*, 2397–2406. [CrossRef]
10. Kamine, T.H.; Papavassiliou, E.; Schneider, B.E. Effect of Abdominal Insufflation for Laparoscopy on Intracranial Pressure. *JAMA Surg.* **2014**, *149*, 380. [CrossRef]
11. Cerantola, Y.; Valerio, M.; Persson, B.; Jichlinski, P.; Ljungqvist, O.; Hübner, M.; Kassouf, W.; Müller, S.; Baldini, G.; Carli, F.; et al. Guidelines for perioperative care after radical cystectomy for bladder cancer: Enhanced Recovery After Surgery (ERAS®) society recommendations. *Clin. Nutr.* **2013**, *32*, 879–887. [CrossRef]
12. Simone, G.; Papalia, R.; Misuraca, L.; Tuderti, G.; Minisola, F.; Ferriero, M.; Vallati, G.E.; Guaglianone, S.; Gallucci, M. Robotic Intracorporeal Padua Ileal Bladder: Surgical Technique, Perioperative, Oncologic and Functional Outcomes. *Eur. Urol.* **2018**, *73*, 934–940. [CrossRef]
13. Yağan, Ö.; Taş, N.; Mutlu, T.; Hancı, V.; Hanci, V. Comparison of the effects of sugammadex and neostigmine on postoperative nausea and vomiting. *Braz. J. Anesthesiol.* **2017**, *67*, 147–152.
14. Løvstad, R.Z.; Thagaard, K.S.; Berner, N.S.; Raeder, J.C. Neostigmine 50 microg kg(−1) with glycopyrrolate increases postoperative nausea in women after laparoscopic gynecological surgery. *Acta Anaesthesiol. Scand.* **2001**, *45*, 495–500. [CrossRef]
15. Law, N.-M.; Bharucha, A.E.; Undale, A.S.; Zinsmeister, A.R. Cholinergic stimulation enhances colonic motor activity, transit, and sensation in humans. *Am. J. Physiol. Gastrointest. Liver Physiol.* **2001**, *281*, G1228–G1237. [CrossRef]
16. Lassen, K.; Soop, M.; Nygren, J.; Cox, P.B.W.; Hendry, P.O.; Spies, C.; von Meyenfeldt, M.F.; Fearon, K.C.; Revhaug, A.; Norderval, S.; et al. Enhanced Recovery After Surgery (ERAS) Group. Consensus review of optimal perioperative care in colorectal surgery: Enhanced Recovery After Surgery (ERAS) Group recommendations. *Arch. Surg.* **2009**, *144*, 961–969. [CrossRef]
17. Paech, M.J.; Kaye, R.; Baber, C.; Nathan, E.A. Recovery characteristics of patients receiving either sugammadex or neostigmine and glycopyrrolate for reversal of neuromuscular block: A randomised controlled trial. *Anaesthesia* **2018**, *73*, 340–347. [CrossRef]
18. Koyuncu, O.; Turhanoglu, S.; Akkurt, C.O.; Karcıoğlu, M.; Ozkan, M.; Ozer, C.; Sessler, D.I.; Turan, A. Comparison of sugammadex and conventional reversal on postoperative nausea and vomiting: A randomized, blinded trial. *J. Clin. Anesth.* **2015**, *27*, 51–56. [CrossRef]
19. Goetz, B.; Benhaqi, P.; Müller, M.H.; Kreis, M.E.; Kasparek, M.S. Changes in beta-adrenergic neurotransmission during postoperative ileus in ratcircular jejunal muscle. *Neurogastroenterol. Motil.* **2013**, *25*, 154-e84. [CrossRef]
20. Neunlist, M.; Rolli-Derkinderen, M.; Latorre, R.; Van Landeghem, L.; Coron, E.; Derkinderen, P.; De Giorgio, R. Enteric Glial Cells: Recent Developments and Future Directions. *Gastroenterology* **2014**, *147*, 1230–1237. [CrossRef]
21. Rasmussen, L.S.; Larsen, K.; Houx, P.; Skovgaard, L.T.; Hanning, C.D.; Moller, J.T. The assessment of postoperative cognitive function. *Acta Anaesthesiol. Scand.* **2001**, *45*, 275–289. [CrossRef] [PubMed]
22. KUŞKU, A.; Demir, G.; Çukurova, Z.; Eren, G.; Hergünsel, O. Monitorization of the effects of spinal anaesthesia on cerebral oxygen saturation in elder patients using near-infrared spectroscopy. *Braz. J. Anesthesiol.* **2014**, *64*, 241–246. [PubMed]
23. Adam, J.M.; Bennett, D.J.; Bom, A.; Clark, J.K.; Feilden, H.; Hutchinson, E.J.; Palin, R.; Prosser, A.; Rees, D.C.; Rosair, G.M.; et al. Cyclodextrin-Derived Host Molecules as Reversal Agents for the Neuromuscular Blocker Rocuronium Bromide: Synthesis and Structure-Activity Relationships. *J. Med. Chem.* **2002**, *45*, 1806–1816. [CrossRef] [PubMed]
24. Sparr, H.J.; Vermeyen, K.M.; Beaufort, A.M.; Rietbergen, H.; Proost, J.H.; Saldien, V.; Velik-Salchner, C.; Wierda, J.M. Early reversal of profound rocuronium-induced neuromuscular blockade by sugammadex in a randomized multicenter study: Efficacy, safety, and pharmacokinetics. *Anesthesiology* **2007**, *106*, 935–943. [CrossRef]

25. Amorim, P.; Lagarto, F.; Gomes, B.; Esteves, S.; Bismarck, J.; Rodrigues, N.; Nogueira, M. Neostigmine vs. sugammadex: Observational cohort study comparing the quality of recovery using the Postoperative Quality Recovery Scale. *Acta Anaesthesiol. Scand.* **2014**, *58*, 1101–1110. [CrossRef]
26. Chazot, T.; Dumont, G.; Le Guen, M.; Hausser-Hauw, C.; Liu, N.; Fischler, M. Sugammadex administration results in arousal from intravenous anaesthesia: A clinical and electroencephalographic observation. *Br. J. Anaesth.* **2011**, *106*, 914–916. [CrossRef]
27. Lanier, W.L.; Laizzo, P.A.; Milde, J.H.; Sharbrough, F.W. The Cerebral and Systemic Effects of Movement in Response to a Noxious Stimulus in Lightly Anesthetized Dogs Possible Modulation of Cerebral Function by Muscle Afferents. *Anesthesiology* **1994**, *80*, 392–401. [CrossRef]
28. Illman, H.; Antila, H.; Olkkola, K.T. Reversal of neuromuscular blockade by sugammadex does not affect EEG derived indices of depth of anesthesia. *J. Clin. Monit. Comput.* **2010**, *24*, 371–376. [CrossRef]
29. Sadhasivam, S.; Ganesh, A.; Robison, A.; Kaye, R.; Watcha, M.F. Validation of the Bispectral Index Monitor for Measuring the Depth of Sedation in Children. *Anesth. Analg.* **2006**, *102*, 383–388. [CrossRef]
30. Abulrob, A.; Tauskela, J.S.; Mealing, G.; Brunette, E.; Faid, K.; Stanimirovic, D. Protection by cholesterol-extracting cyclodextrins: A role for N-methyl-d-aspartate receptor redistribution. *J. Neurochem.* **2005**, *92*, 1477–1486. [CrossRef]

Stroma Transcriptomic and Proteomic Profile of Prostate Cancer Metastasis Xenograft Models Reveals Prognostic Value of Stroma Signatures

Sofia Karkampouna [1], Maria R. De Filippo [1], Charlotte K. Y. Ng [2], Irena Klima [1], Eugenio Zoni [1], Martin Spahn [3], Frank Stein [4], Per Haberkant [4], George N. Thalmann [1,5,†] and Marianna Kruithof-de Julio [1,5,*,†]

1 Urology Research Laboratory, Department for BioMedical Research, University of Bern, Murtenstrasse 35, 3008 Bern, Switzerland; sofia.karkampouna@dbmr.unibe.ch (S.K.); mariarosaria.defilippo@unibas.ch (M.R.D.F.); irena.klima@dbmr.unibe.ch (I.K.); eugenio.zoni@dbmr.unibe.ch (E.Z.); george.thalmann@insel.ch (G.N.T.)
2 Oncogenomics Laboratory, Department for BioMedical Research, University of Bern, Murtenstrasse 40, 3008 Bern, Switzerland; charlotte.ng@dbmr.unibe.ch
3 Lindenhofspital Bern, Prostate Center Bern, 3012 Bern, Switzerland; martin.spahn@hin.ch
4 Proteomics Core Facility, EMBL Heidelberg, Meyerhofstraße 1, 69117 Heidelberg, Germany; frank.stein@embl.de (F.S.); per.haberkant@embl.de (P.H.)
5 Department of Urology, Inselspital, Anna Seiler Haus, Bern University Hospital, 3010 Bern, Switzerland
* Correspondence: marianna.kruithofdejulio@dbmr.unibe.ch
† These authors contributed equally to this work.

Simple Summary: Currently, there is a need for prognostic tools that can stratify patients, who present with primary disease, based on whether they are at low or high risk for drug resistant and hormone-independent lethal metastatic prostate cancer. The aim of our study was to assess the potentially added value of tumor microenvironment (stroma) components for the characterisation of prostate cancer. By utilising patient derived-xenograft models we show that the molecular properties of the stroma cells are highly responsive to androgen hormone levels, and considerable ECM remodelling processes take place not only in androgen-dependent but also in androgen-independent tumor models. Transcriptomic mechanisms linked to osteotropism are conserved in bone metastatic xenografts, even when implanted in a different microenvironment. A stroma-specific gene list signature was identified, which highly correlates with Gleason score, metastasis progression and progression-free survival, and thus could potentially complement current patient stratification methods.

Abstract: Resistance acquisition to androgen deprivation treatment and metastasis progression are a major clinical issue associated with prostate cancer (PCa). The role of stroma during disease progression is insufficiently defined. Using transcriptomic and proteomic analyses on differentially aggressive patient-derived xenografts (PDXs), we investigated whether PCa tumors predispose their microenvironment (stroma) to a metastatic gene expression pattern. RNA sequencing was performed on the PCa PDXs BM18 (castration-sensitive) and LAPC9 (castration-resistant), representing different disease stages. Using organism-specific reference databases, the human-specific transcriptome (tumor) was identified and separated from the mouse-specific transcriptome (stroma). To identify proteomic changes in the tumor (human) versus the stroma (mouse), we performed human/mouse cell separation and subjected protein lysates to quantitative Tandem Mass Tag labeling and mass spectrometry. Tenascin C (TNC) was among the most abundant stromal genes, modulated by androgen levels in vivo and highly expressed in castration-resistant LAPC9 PDX. The tissue microarray of primary PCa samples (n = 210) showed that TNC is a negative prognostic marker of the clinical progression to recurrence or metastasis. Stroma markers of osteoblastic PCa bone metastases seven-up signature were induced in the stroma by the host organism in metastatic xenografts, indicating conserved mechanisms of tumor cells to induce a stromal premetastatic signature. A 50-gene list stroma signature was identified based on androgen-dependent responses, which shows a linear association with the Gleason score, metastasis progression and progression-free survival. Our data show that metastatic PCa PDXs, which differ in androgen sensitivity, trigger differential stroma responses, which show the metastasis risk stratification and prognostic biomarker potential.

Keywords: prostate cancer; stroma signature; patient-derived xenografts

---

1. Introduction

Bone metastases are detected in 10% of patients already at the initial diagnosis of prostate cancer (PCa) or will develop in 20–30% of the patients subjected to radical prostatectomy and androgen deprivation therapy and will progress to an advanced disease called castration-resistant prostate cancer [1]. Metastases are established when disseminated cancer cells colonize a secondary organ site. An important component of tumor growth is the supportive stroma: the extracellular matrix (ECM) and the nontumoral cells of the matrix microenvironment (e.g., endothelial cells, smooth muscle cells and cancer-associated fibroblasts). Upon interaction of the stroma compartment and tumor cells, the stroma responds by the secretion of growth factors, proteases and chemokines, thereby facilitating the remodeling of the ECM and, thus, tumor cell migration and invasion [2]. Therefore, tumor cell establishment requires an abnormal microenvironment. It is unclear whether the stroma is modulated by the tumor cells or by intrinsic gene expression alterations. Understanding the mechanisms of tumor progression to the metastatic stage is necessary for the design of therapeutic and prognostic schemes.

The bone microenvironment is favorable for the growth of PCa, as well as breast cancer, indicated by the high frequency of bone metastasis in these tumors. Studies have shown that cancer cell growth competes for the hematopoietic niche in the bone marrow with the normal residing stem cells [3], and depending on the cancer cell phenotype, this may lead to either osteoblastic or osteolytic lesions. The stroma signature of osteolytic PCa cells (PC-3) xenografted intraosseously in immunocompromised mice induce a vascular/axon guidance signature [4]. The stroma signature of osteoblastic lesions from human VCap and C4-2B PCa cell lines indicated an enrichment of the hematopoietic and prostate epithelial stem cell niche. A curated prostate-specific bone metastasis signature (Ob-BMST) implicated seven highly upregulated genes (*Aspn, Pdgrfb, Postn, Sparcl1, Mcam, Fscn1* and *Pmepa1)* [5], among which, *Postn* and *Fscn1* are bone-specific. Furthermore, *Aspn* and *Postn* expression is also increased in primary PCa cases [5], indicative of osteomimicry processes. The induction of osteoblastic genes in the stroma of primary tumors (PCa and breast), such as osteopontin and osteocalcin, has been suggested as a mechanism termed osteomimicry [6] to explain why the bone microenvironment is the preferential metastasis site. High stromal differences between benign, indolent and lethal PCa, combined with the enrichment of bone remodeling genes in high Gleason score cases [7], suggest that the stroma is an active player in PCa. During androgen deprivation, androgen-dependent epithelial cells will undergo apoptosis, while the supporting stroma is largely maintained or replaces the necrotic tissue areas [8]. Stromal cells do express androgen receptors (AR) and have active downstream signaling, while the absence of stromal AR expression is used as a prognostic factor of disease progression [9]. Furthermore, AR binds to different genomic sites in prostate fibroblasts compared to the epithelium [10] and to cancer-associated fibroblasts (CAFs) [11], indicating different roles of AR in epithelial or stroma cellular contexts. Prostate CAFs have tumor-promoting effects on marginally tumorigenic cells (LNCaP), irreversibly altering their phenotype and influencing their progression to androgen independence and metastasis [12,13].

In this study, we investigated whether metastatic PCa patient-derived xenograft models (PDXs) that differ in androgen sensitivity are triggering a differential stroma response. To elucidate the mechanisms of stroma contribution to tumor growth later on, we determined the unique gene expression profile of the stroma compared to the tumor compartment, the proteome changes of the tumor versus stroma. We identified androgen-dependent stroma gene expression signatures with potential disease progression prognostic values for primary PCa.

2. Results

2.1. Simultaneous Transcriptome Analysis of Human and Murine Signatures in PDXs Can Distinguish Androgen-Dependent Expression Changes in Tumor and Host-Derived Stroma

We analyzed the transcriptome of bulk PDX tumors grown subcutaneously in immunocompromised murine hosts by next-generation RNA-sequencing (RNA-Seq). Bone metastasis (BM)18 and LAPC9 PDXs were used in three different states: intact, post-castration (day 8 LAPCa9 and day 14 BM18) and androgen replacement (24 h) (Figure 1A). Tumor growth kinetics revealed the androgen-dependent phenotype of BM18, which regressed completely in two weeks post-castration (Figure 1B), and the androgen-independent phenotype of LAPC9 PDX tumors, which grew exponentially even after castration (Figure 1C), thus confirming the differential aggressiveness of the two models. The reduction of epithelial glands and proliferating Ki67+ cells in the BM18 castrated conditions (Figure 1D) was in contrast to the LAPC9 tumors (Figure 1E), which were morphologically indistinguishable among intact and castrated hosts. Bulk tumor tissues, which contain human tumor cells and mouse infiltrating stroma cells, were simultaneously analyzed from the same samples by RNA-Seq. To distinguish the transcriptome of the different organisms, the mouse and human reads were separated by alignment to a mouse and a human reference genome, respectively. Principal component analysis (PCA) of the human (tumor) 500 most variable genes showed that both castrated and replaced groups have altered expression profiles among each other and compared to the intact tumors. This was the case for the BM18 (Figure 2A) and the LAPC9 human transcriptomes (Figure 2B). The response to short-term androgen replacement showed a larger degree of variability in the BM18 (Figure 2A). However, the expression levels of direct AR target genes (*KLK3, NKX3.1* and *FKBP5*) identified by the RNA-Seq confirmed that androgen levels affected the activation of androgen receptor signaling in both BM18 (Figure 2C) and LAPC9 (Figure 2D, *KLK3* and *NKX3.1*). Differential expression analysis of the most variable human (tumor) genes, showed high variability among the castrated and intact groups, for both BM18 (Figure S1A) and LAPC9 (Figure S1B) transcript levels, while the LAPC9 replaced and castrated groups had similar profile among each other, discriminating them from the intact condition (Figure S1B).

PCA analysis of the BM18 mouse (stroma) transcriptome indicated that the majority of castrated samples (with and without 24-h androgen replacement) diverged from the intact tumor (Figure 2E). The LAPC9 mouse (stroma) transcriptome instead did not show specific clustering within or between the sample groups when plotting the top 500 most variably expressed genes (Figure 2F). The Ob-BMST signature of all seven genes (*Aspn, Pdgrfb, Postn, Aspn, Sparcl1, Mcam, Fscn1* and *Pmepa1),* which were upregulated in the bone stroma, as previously identified [5], were indeed expressed in the primary PCa TCGA cohort, as well as in both BM18 and LAPC9 PDXs (Figure S2A). *Pdgrfb, Postn, Aspn* and Sparcl1, specifically in the mouse RNA-Seq data, thus, are stroma-specific. Collectively, the Ob-BMST gene signature is expressed at equal levels in the BM18 and LAPC9 (intact) (Figure S2A). Some of these genes were differentially expressed upon castration in the BM18 (Figure 2G) but not in the LAPC9 (Figure 2H). A bone microenvironment-specific stroma signature induced by osteoblastic cell lines was conserved in bone metastasis PDXs maintained in other microenvironments and found in primary prostatic tissues.

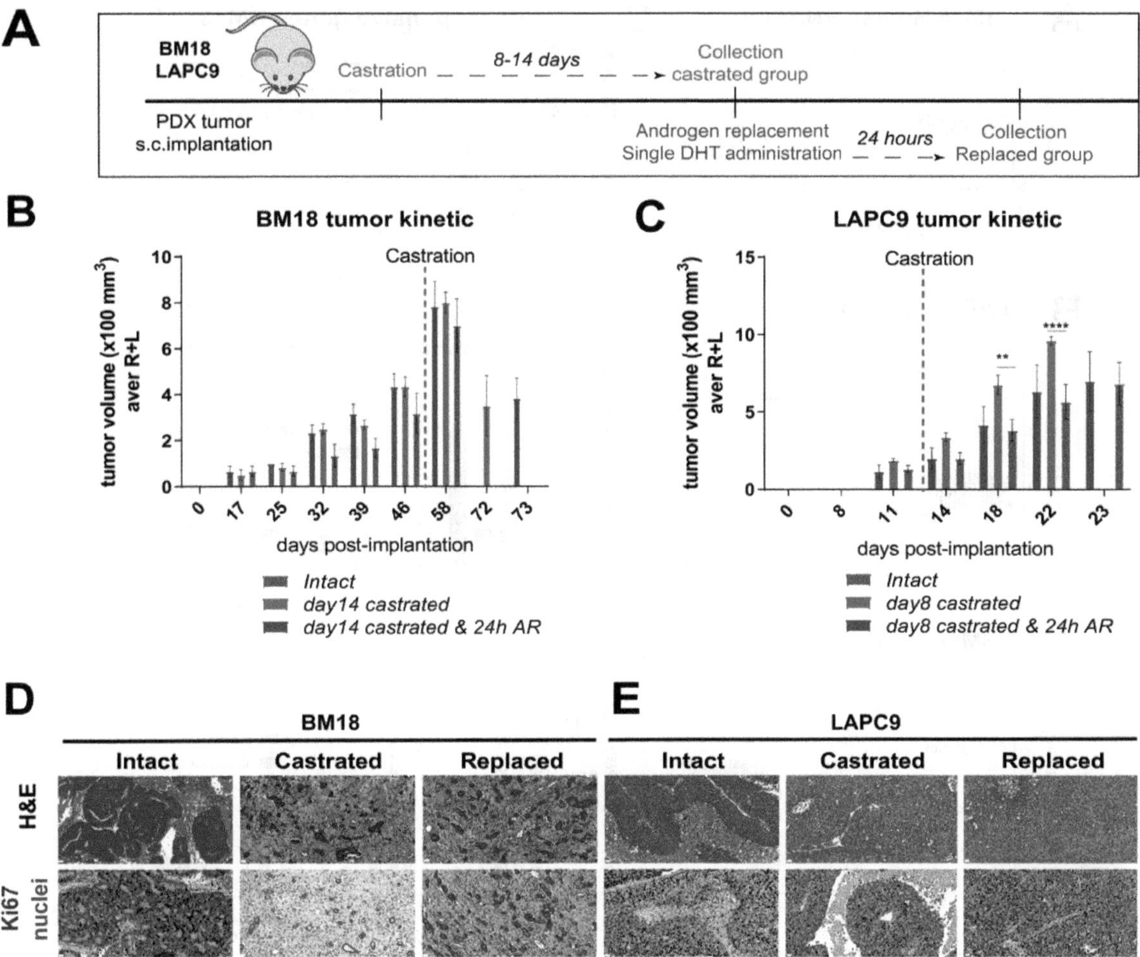

Figure 1. In vivo tumor growth properties of androgen-dependent BM18 versus androgen-independent patient-derived xenograft (PDX) models. (**A**) Scheme of in vivo BM18 and LAPC9 experiments, including the timeline of castration, androgen replacement (single dihydrotestosterone (DHT) administration) and collection of material for transcriptomic analysis. (**B**) BM18 PDX tumor growth progression in time. Groups: (1) intact tumors (collected at max size, $n = 3$), (2) castrated (day 14, $n = 4$) and (3) castrated, followed by testosterone readministration (castrated-testosterone) (day 15 since castration and 24 h since the androgen receptor (AR), $n = 3$). R; right tumor, L; left tumor per animal. (**C**) LAPC9 PDX tumor growth progression in time. Groups: (1) intact tumors (collected at max size, $n = 3$), (2) castrated (day 8, $n = 4$) and (3) castrated, followed by testosterone readministration (castrated-testosterone) (day 9 since castration and 24 h since AR, $n = 3$). Tumor scoring was performed weekly by routine palpation; values represent average calculations of the tumors of all animals per group (considering 2 tumors, left, L, and right, R, of each animal). Error bars represent SEM, calculated considering the no. of animals for each time point. Ordinary two-way ANOVA with Tukey's multiple comparison correction was performed, $p < 0.01$ (**) and $p < 0.0001$ (****). (**D**) Histological morphology of BM18 and (**E**) LAPC9 (from intact, castrated and androgen-replaced hosts), as assessed by Hematoxylin and Eosin staining (H&E, top). Scale bars: 20 μm, and proliferation marker Ki67 protein expression (bottom panel).

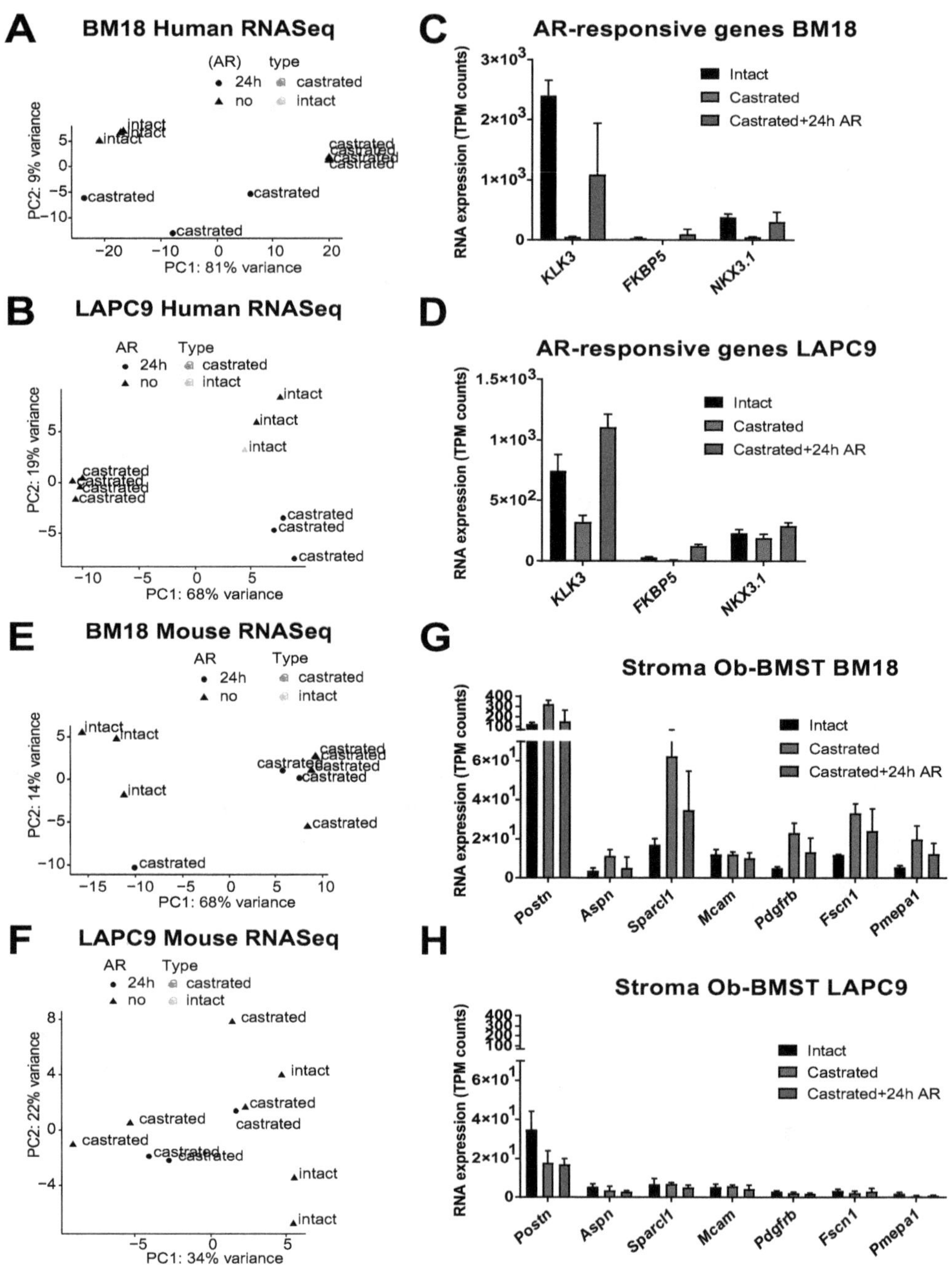

Figure 2. Separation of human (tumor) and mouse (stroma) transcriptomes of BM18 and LAPC9 tumors. (**A**,**B**) Principal component analysis plot of the gene expression of the 500 most variable genes on all samples; BM18 human transcripts (**A**) and LAPC9 human (**B**) at intact, castrated and replaced (castrated + 24 h AR) conditions. (**C**,**D**) Expression values of AR direct target genes as detected by RNA-Seq (transcript per million (TPM) counts) in the BM18 (**C**) or LAPC9 (**D**) tumors as confirmation of the effective repression of AR downstream signaling by castration. Intact ($n = 3$), castrated ($n = 4$) and replaced ($n = 3$). (**E**,**F**) Principal component analysis plot of the gene expression of the 500 most variable genes on all samples, BM18 mouse (**E**) and LAPC9 mouse (**F**) at intact, castrated and replaced (castrated + 24 h AR) conditions. (**G**,**H**) Expression values of the prostate-specific bone metastasis signature (Ob-BMST) seven upregulated stroma signature genes, as detected by RNA-Seq (TPM normalized counts) in the mouse transcriptome of BM18 (**E**) or LAPC9 (**F**) tumors.

2.2. Proteomic Analysis Provides Functional Information over the Identified Human/Mouse-Specific Transcriptome

To study the proteome of the tumor versus the stroma, human and mouse cell fractions were isolated by the magnetic cell sorting (MACS) mouse depletion method from tumor sample preparations: BM18 and LAPC9 each at the intact, castrated and replaced states. Protein lysates of either mouse or human origins (single replicate from a pool of $n = 3$ to 4 biological replicates per condition) were subjected to an in-solution tryptic digest following Tandem Mass Tag (TMT)-labeling of the resulting peptides and their mass spectrometric analysis (Figure 3A).

In addition to the initial experimental separation of the protein lysates, we further explored the species homologs of the identified proteins by computational analysis using a combined human and mouse protein sequence database. We identified 4198 proteins in the sample that were enriched for human cells. Thereof, 3154 were human-specific proteins, with 996 revealing a high homology shared among human and mouse, and only a fraction of 48 mouse-specific, peptides. (Figure 3B, left plot). For samples enriched in mouse cells, we identified, in total, 5192 proteins; thereof, 2486 mouse-specific proteins, 2379 shared homologs and 247 human-specific (Figure 3B, right plot). We searched for prostate specific markers such as KLK3, a prostate-specific antigen that is secreted by luminal cells. In the proteomic data, the human-specificity was confirmed, and the secreted protein was found also in the mouse fraction (Figure 3C). To further ensure that the proteomic data were indeed identifying real stromal-specific candidates, we searched specifically for the seven-gene Ob-BMST signature found also to be expressed in both BM18 and LAPC9. POSTN, PDGFRB and MCAM (Figure 3C) were indeed detected at the protein level, thus might have a functional role, and were found exclusively in the mouse fraction (Figure 3C, right plot) and hybridizing with mouse-specific sequences (Figure 3C, triangle indicates Mus Musculus species specificity).

2.3. Differential Expression Analysis Reveals Androgen-Dependent Stromal Gene Modulation in Androgen-Independent PDX Model

The relative ratio of human and mouse transcript reads reflected a higher stroma content in the BM18 compared to LAPC9 and significantly reduced human tumor content with enriched stroma content in the BM18 castrated group (Figure S2B). No major differences were observed in the LAPC9 castrated group (Figure S2C). We demonstrated that the human (tumor), as well as the mouse (stroma), transcriptomes follow androgen-dependent transcriptomic changes in the BM18 groups (intact versus castrated versus replaced) (Figure 2A,E). Venn Euler diagrams illustrate androgen level-dependent stromal gene expression modulation not only in the BM18 (Figure S2D and Table S1) but, also, in the androgen-independent (in terms of tumor growth) LAPC9 model (Figure S2E,F and Table S1). To identify the top-most significant AR-regulated stromal genes, we performed a differential expression analysis of BM18 tumors (Figure 4A) from castrated hosts and compared it to BM18 intact (the replaced tumors were not included here due to higher variability). Of the top-most variable genes, 50 were highly upregulated in BM18 tumors (z-score >1) and downregulated upon castration (Figure 4A). A differential expression analysis of LAPC9 tumors from castrated/replaced tumors versus intact tumors revealed the top-most differentially regulated genes: the 27 most upregulated genes in intact, which were downregulated in the castrated groups (Figure 4B). Among the 50 mouse genes that were highly upregulated in the intact BM18, and significantly modulated by castration, were 23 genes implicated in cell cycle/mitosis, 10 implicated in ECM and 3 related to spermatogenesis/hormone regulation, according to the Gene Ontology terms (Figure 4C). Two of these genes, *Tnc* and *Crabp1*, were also detected in the proteomic data (Figure 4C, highlighted in bold) and in both PDXs (Figure 4C,D, highlighted in red). Among the 27 mouse genes that were highly upregulated in the intact LAPC9, and significantly modulated by castration, seven genes were implicated in ECM/cell adhesion/smooth muscle function, and 14 were implicated in non-smooth muscle function and metabolism based on the Gene Ontology terms (Figure 4D). In the LAPC9 proteomic data, we detected 14 genes out of the 27 to be expressed in the mouse fractions (Figure 4D, bold), indicative of potential functional values. Of interest in potentially mediating tumor stroma extracellular interactions are a neural adhesion protein (*CD56*), implicated in cell–cell adhesion and migration by homotypic signaling, as well as Tenascin C (*Tnc*), an extracellular protein that is found abundantly in the reactive stroma of various cancer types, yet not expressed in normal stroma. Both genes were expressed at the protein level, exclusively in the mouse compartment of the BM18 and LAPC9, at all states (intact, castrated and replaced). Furthermore, Tnc was detected in both BM18 and LAPC9 at the transcriptional and proteomic levels and was reactivated after 24 h of androgen replacement (Figure 4B), indicative of AR-direct target gene modulation.

2.4. Cross Comparison of Stromal Transcriptome among Different PDXs Identifies ECM and Cell Adhesion Pathways in the LAPC9 Androgen-Independent Model

To assess the similarity between the stromal transcriptome of the androgen-independent LAPC9 and the BM18, a differential expression analysis was performed. In a panel of the 50 top-most variable genes comparing the tumors at their intact conditions, we identified several genes that follow the same pattern of modulation in intact tumors (Figure 5A) and in castrated tumors (Figure 5B). Of interest were the ECM-related genes downregulated in LAPC9 versus BM18; the Fibroblast Growth Factor receptor (*Fgfr4*), elastin microfibril interface (*Emilin3*) and upregulated collagen type 2 chain a1 (*Col2a1*).

The differential expression of LAPC9 castrated versus BM18 castrated highlighted genes that were identified in the analysis among LAPC9 castrated, replaced versus LAPC9 intact, such as Apelin (*Apln*), *Col2a1* and Tenascin C (*Tnc*).

To identify the biological processes ongoing in the LAPC9 compared to BM18, a pathway analysis was performed on the differentially expressed murine genes of the LAPC9 versus the BM18. Enrichment maps of the top 20 enriched GO biological pathways highly overlap pathways, such as ECM, focal tadhesion and cell adhesion/migration in the intact and castrated LAPC9 (Figure S3A,B). Similarly, among the KEGG pathway sets, there was an enrichment of stroma regulation (e.g., actin cytoskeleton, focal adhesion and cell adhesion) and bone and immune-related processes (e.g., osteoclast differentiation) (Figure S3C–F and Table S2). The enrichment of cancer-related pathways (e.g., PI3K/AKT, proteoglycans in cancer, pathways in cancer) was commonly found in the LAPC9 intact and castrated stroma transcriptomes (Figure S3E,F and Table S2).

Given that genes activated in a castrated state might be indicative of androgen resistance mechanism activation, we postulated that genes upregulated in the androgen-resistant LAPC9 over the androgen-dependent BM18 might be relevant for understanding the aggressive phenotype of LAPC9 and, therefore, of the advanced metastatic phenotype of similar tumors. One of those genes, Tenascin, is an ECM protein that is produced at the (myo)fibroblasts that is virtually absent in normal stroma in the prostate and other tissues and has been associated with the cancerous reactive stroma response in different cancers. We interrogated the expression of *Tnc* in the RNA-Seq data and found that it was highly upregulated in LAPC9 compared to BM18 both in intact ($\log_{FC}$ 4.23, $p < 0.001$) and among the castrated conditions ($\log_{FC}$ 6.9, $p < 0.001$) (Figure 5C). However, in both models, the *Tnc* levels significantly decreased upon castration (BM18, $p < 0.001$ and LAPC9, $p < 0.05$), indicating the potentially AR-mediated regulation of *Tnc* expression. In LAPC9 tumors, the TNC protein is expressed in the tumor-adjacent ECM and in the proximity of vessels (Figure 5D, intact and castrated) and co-expressed by smooth muscle actin (αSMA)- and collagen type I-positive myofibroblasts (Figure 5E). Instead, the intact BM18 tumors show TNC and collagen type I deposition in the ECM, but there is no overlap with αSMA-positive myofibroblasts (Figure 5D,E, BM18 intact). Castrated BM18 tumors have minimal TNC expression, found only in cells proximal to the remaining epithelial glands, yet with no typical fibroblast/stromal morphology (Figure 5D,E, BM18 intact), suggesting an altered phenotype of TNC upon androgen deprivation.

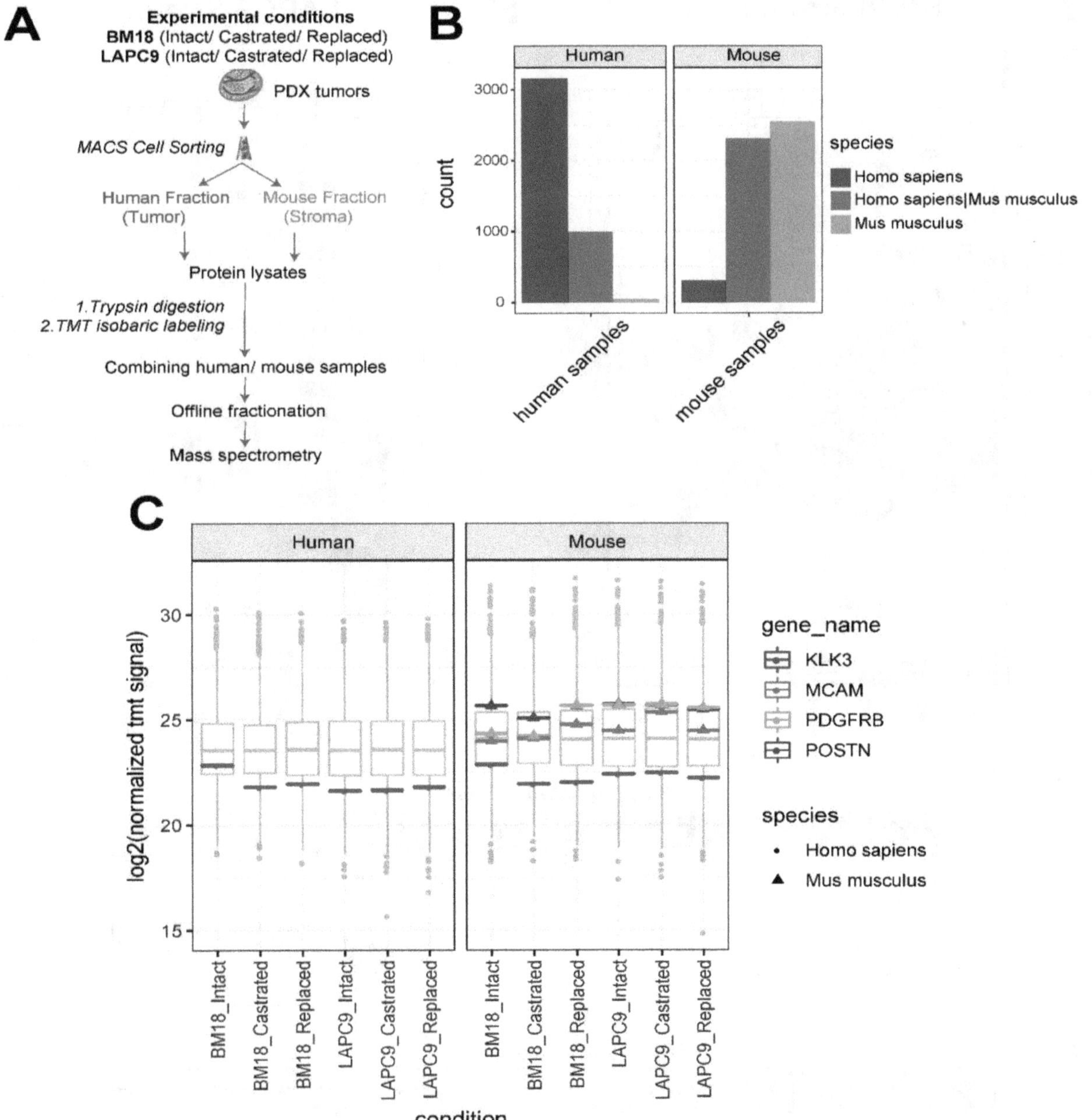

Figure 3. Proteomic analysis of human (tumor) versus mouse (stroma) of BM18 and LAPC9 tumors. (**A**) Experimental separation of human from mouse cell suspensions from fresh tumor isolations by MACS mouse depletion sorting. Cell fractions from intact/replaced ($n = 3$ each), castrated ($n = 4$) biological replicates were pooled into a single replicate ($n = 1$) to achieve an adequate cell number for the proteomic analysis (1×10^6 cells). Protein lysates from the different fractions of BM18/LAPC9 (intact, castrated and replaced) were subjected to Tandem Mass Tag (TMT) labeling (all-mouse or all-human samples were multiplexed in one TMT experiment each), followed by mass spectrometry. (**B**) Detected peptides from human and mouse fractions were searched against a combined human and mouse protein database. Number of species specific or shared proteins is indicated in different colors. (**C**) KLK3 (PSA; Prostate Serum Antigen) protein levels ($\log_2$ normalized TMT signal sum values) in human cell isolations (left) and in mouse cell isolations (right), and the protein sequence was predicted as human-specific (spheres indicate Homo Sapiens sequence). Seven-up Ob-BMST signature markers POSTN, PDGFRB and MCAM protein levels were absent in human cell isolations (left) and present in mouse cell isolations (right), while all the protein sequences were mouse-specific (triangles indicate Mus Musculus sequences).

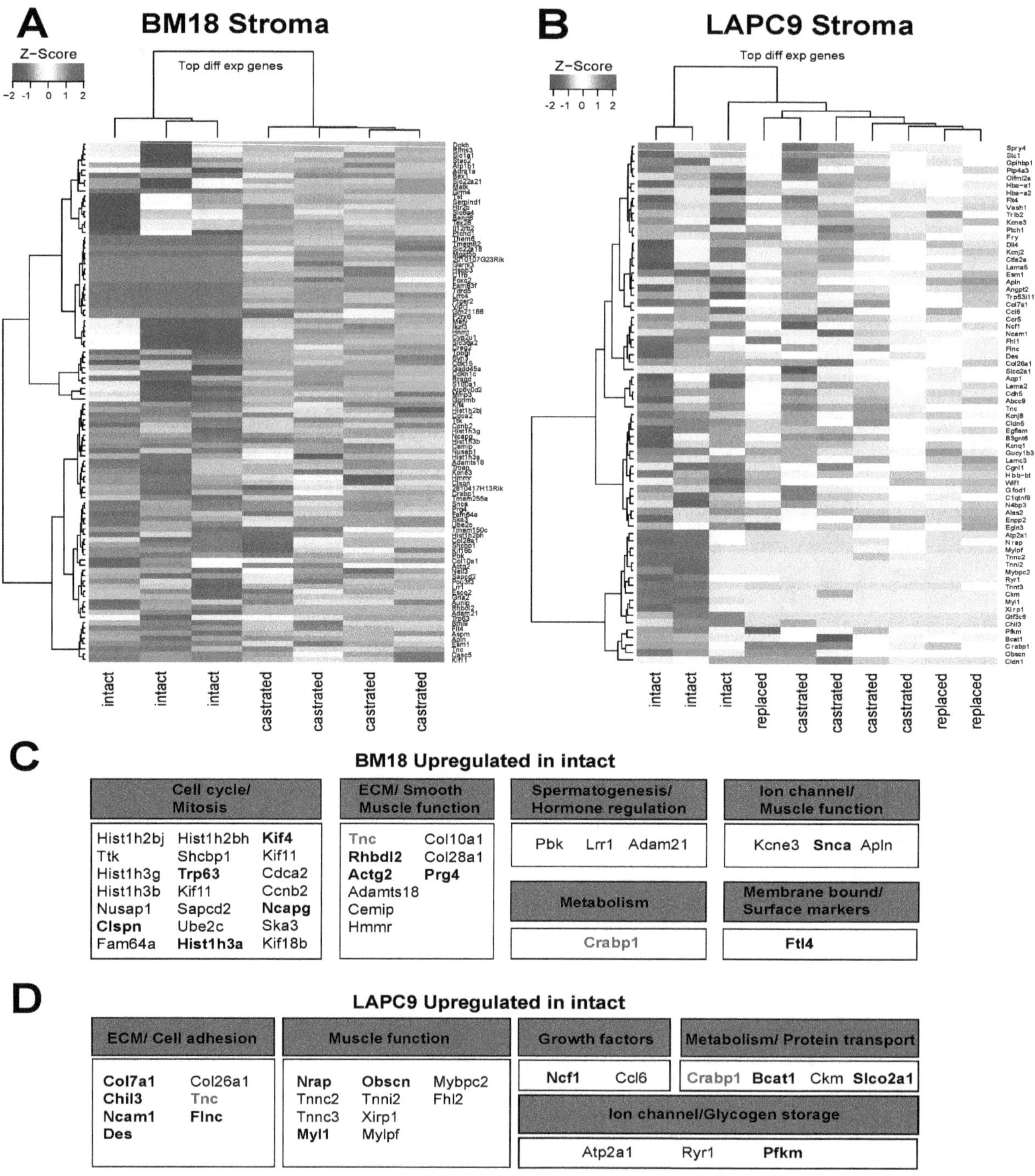

Figure 4. Differential expression analysis of the transcriptome indicates different expression profiles of stromal genes as response to androgen deprivation. (**A**) Heatmap represents a differential expression analysis of the most variable genes from the mouse transcriptome of BM18 castrated compared to BM18 intact tumors. Genes modulated by androgen deprivation due to castration in the up/downregulation compared to intact tumors are indicated in red or blue colors, respectively. (**B**) Heatmap represents Z-score of the differential expression analysis of most variable genes in the mouse transcriptome of LAPC9 castrated (with and without androgen replacement) compared to LAPC9 intact tumors. (**C**) Description of mouse genes found upregulated in BM18 intact tumors and the biological processes they are involved in, according to the Gene Ontology (GO) terms. (**D**) Description of the mouse genes found upregulated in LAPC9 intact tumors and the biological processes they are involved in, according to the GO terms.

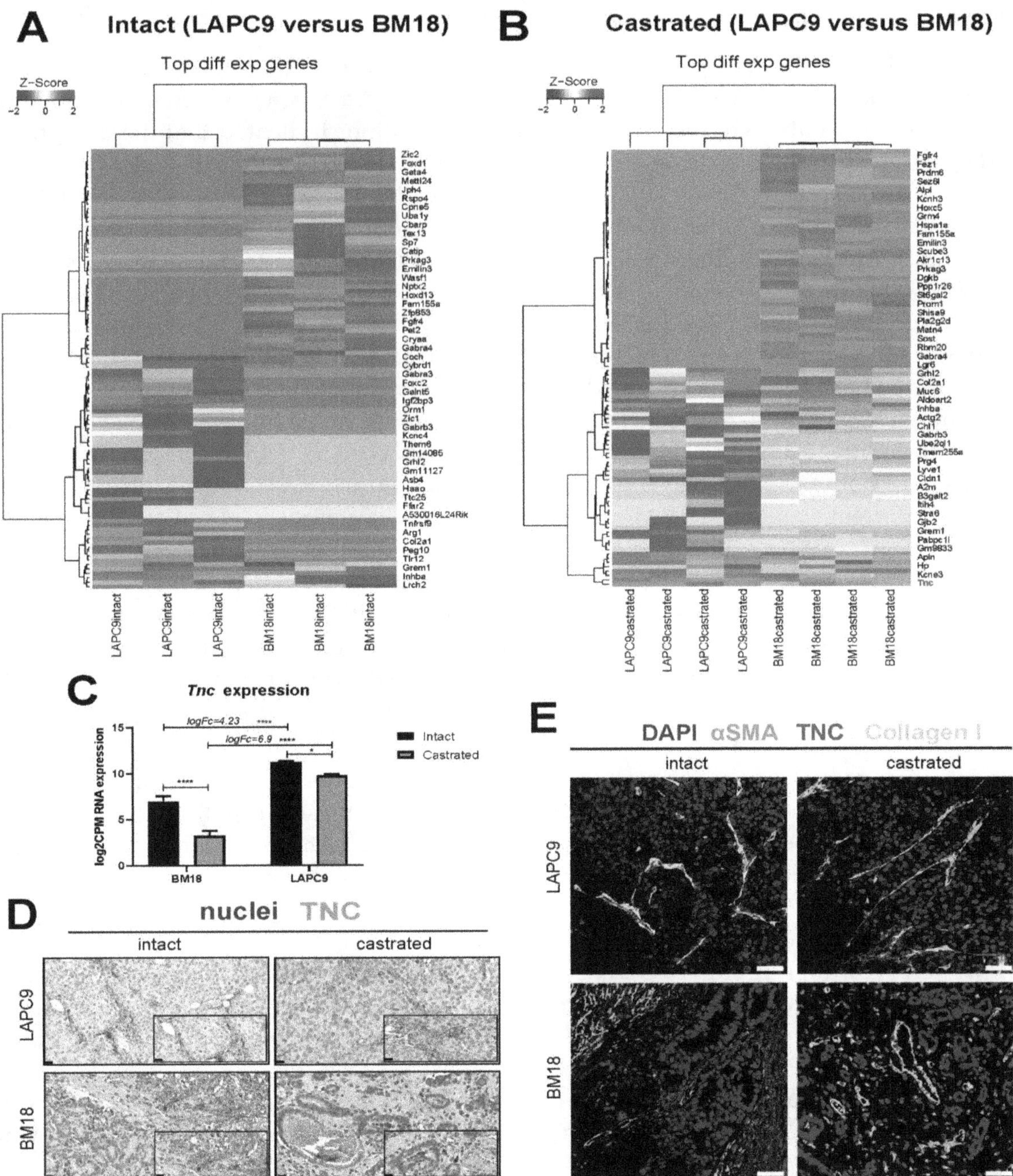

Figure 5. Cross-comparison of LAPC9 versus BM18 suggests stromal gene Tenascin C expression being associated with advanced PCa and regulated by androgen levels. (**A**) Heatmap represents the differential expression analysis of the top 100 most variable genes from the mouse transcriptome of LAPC9 intact tumors compared to BM18 intact tumors and (**B**) of LAPC9 castrated tumors compared to BM18 castrated tumors. (**A**) Subset of genes in LAPC9 samples have zero counts, leading to the same z-score, while the same genes are highly expressed in BM18 samples. (**C**) *Tnc* RNA expression (log_2CMP counts) in the stroma transcriptome. Log_{FC} (fold change) enrichment of *Tnc* in LAPC9 over BM18 is indicated. Ordinary two-way ANOVA with Tukey's multiple comparison correction was performed, $p < 0.05$ (*) and $p < 0.0001$ (****). (**D**) Tenascin protein expression and stromal specificity assessed by immunohistochemistry in LAPC9 and BM18 tumors, both at the intact and castrated states. Scale bars: 20 μm. (**E**) Tenascin protein (indicated in red) colocalization with stromal markers, smooth muscle actin (αSMA, green) and collagen type I (gray) assessed by immunofluorescence in LAPC9 and BM18 tumors, both at the intact and castrated states. DAPI marks the nuclei. Scale bars: 50 μm.

2.5. Protein Expression of Tenascin and Its Interaction Partners

To assess whether the transcriptomic changes of *Tnc* in the PDX models corresponds to the functional protein and, thus, a relevant role in bone metastatic PCa, we performed a proteomic analysis. A mass spectrometry analysis of the human and mouse fractions indicated that the Tnc protein was expressed specifically in the mouse (stromal) fractions in BM18 and LAPC9 (Figure 6A). The isoform Tenascin X was also expressed at the protein level (Figure 6B). The interaction network of the mouse protein Tnc is based on experimental observations and prediction tools (STRING) and consists of laminins (Lamc1 and Lamb2); fibronectin (Fb1); integrins (Itga2, a7, a8 and a9) and proteoglycans (Bcan and Vcan) (Figure 6C). The human interactome is less-characterized, yet most of the interactome is conserved: laminins (LAMC1 and LAMB2); proteoglycans (NCAN and ACAN) and others such as interleukin 8 (IL-8), BMP4, ALB and SDC4 (Figure 6D). However, integrin interaction-binding partners in a human setting have not been confirmed. Given the importance of integrins for cell adhesion and migration known to be found in mesenchymal/stromal and epithelial tumor cells, we focused on the expression of human- and mouse-derived integrins. The *ITGA9*, *ITGA6* and *ITGA2* were all found to be expressed in both the RNA-Seq and proteomic data (Figure 6E, ITGA6, respectively); however, only the *ITGA2* protein was specifically found in the human counterpart and not overlapping with the mouse stroma (Figure 6F). Co-labeling both proteins indicated adjacent spatial localization with TNC deposition in close proximity to ITGA2-positive epithelial cells (Figure 6G); however, whether those cell populations acquired different properties compared to other epithelial cells has yet to be investigated. Overall, the tumor *ITGA2* and stromal *Tnc* is a potential molecular interaction, possibly part of the dual cellular communication among a tumor and its microenvironment cellular types and ECM.

2.6. Stromal Tenascin Expression as a Prognostic Factor of Disease Progression in High-Risk PCa

The detection of key mouse stromal genes in PCa PDXs gives the opportunity to evaluate the role and potential prognostic value of the human orthologs of these stromal genes. To validate the localization and stromal specificity of TNC protein expression, we performed immunohistochemistry on the primary PCa tissue sections. TNC is localized in the extracellular space (Figure 7A, primary cases). Next, we evaluated the TNC expression in a tissue microarray of 210 primary prostate tissues, part of the European Multicenter High Risk Prostate Cancer Clinical and Translational research group (EMPaCT) [14–16] (Figure 7B–G). Based on the preoperative clinical parameters of the TMA patient cases (Table 1, Table 2) and the D'Amico classification system [17], they represent intermediate (clinical T2b or Gleason $n = 7$ and PSA >10 and ≤ 20) and high-risk (clinical T2c-3a or Gleason score (GS) = 8 and PSA ≥ 20) PCa. The number of TNC-positive cells (Figure 7B) were quantified and averaged for all cores (four cores per patient case) in an automated way, including tissue selection, core annotation and equal staining parameters set. To investigate the association between the number of TNC-positive cells and patient survival or disease progression, we calculated the optimal cut-point for the number of TNC-positive cells by estimation of the maximally selected rank statistics [18]. Association between TNC-expressing cells and pT Stage indicated that the majority of cases cluster towards stages 3a and 3b (Figure 7C). A multiple comparison test among all groups showed no statistically significant association between the TNC expression and pathological stage (Table S3, $p > 0.05$). The overall survival probability between two patient groups with, respectively, high and low numbers of TNC-positive cells was indifferent ($p = 0.29$, Log-rank test) (Figure 7D). We focused on the probability of TNC expression in primary tumors to be a deterministic factor for clinical progression to local or metastasis recurrence. Clinical progression probability was higher in the TNC-low group compared the TNC-high group ($p = 0.04$ *, Log-rank test) (Figure 7E). Next, we examined the clinical progression in patients with pT Stage ≥3 (groups 3a, 3b and 4). The high T-Stage cases did separate into two groups based on the TNC expression, with the TNC low-expressing group exhibiting earlier a clinical progression (local or metastatic recurrence, $p = 0.013$ *, Log-rank test) (Figure 7F). The PSA progression probability in patients with pT Stage ≥3 indicated an association trend of a TNC-low group with earlier biochemical relapse events ($p = 0.07$, Log-rank test) (Figure 7G). Similarly, the TNC-low group correlated with a higher probability for PSA progression after radical prostatectomy among cases with carcinoma-containing (positive) surgical margins (Figure S4A, $p = 0.031$ *, Log-rank test) or positive lymph nodes (Figure S4B, $p = 0.092$, Log-rank test). A low number of TNC-expressing cells coincides with a poor prognosis in terms of metastasis progression, similarly to its downregulation upon castration in the bone metastasis PDXs (Figure 4B) based on the RNA-Seq analysis. To further evaluate the clinical relevance of this finding, in multiple clinical cohorts with available transcriptomic data and clinical information, a CANCERTOOL analysis was performed [19]. Similar to the protein TMA data (Figure 7), the *TNC* mRNA levels were significantly downregulated during the disease progression from primary to PCa metastasis, compared to the expression in the normal prostatic tissues in all five datasets tested (Figure 8A). The *TNC* expression shows a pattern of inverse correlations, with the Gleason score among GS6 to GS9; however, it significantly discriminated patient groups for the Gleason score in one out of three datasets tested (Figure 8B, TCGA dataset * $p = 0.049$, Glinsky $p = 0.06$, Taylor $p = 0.192$), with the highest expression found in a high GS10 group and indifferent among GS6-GS9. A disease-free survival analysis indicated that a low TNC expression is associated with a worse prognosis based on the Glinsky dataset (Q1 Glinsky et al. [20], * $p = 0.02$), while no statistically significant association was observed in the Taylor and TCGA dataset (Figure 8C). Overall, the TNC expression in tumor samples, both at the RNA and protein levels, becomes progressively less abundant in primary and metastasis PCa specimens, while a low TNC expression is significantly associated with the disease progression and poor disease-free survival (DFS) outcome.

2.7. *Stroma Signatures from Androgen-Dependent and -Independent States Correlate with Disease Progression*

In order to comprehensively map the stroma responses related to the disease severity, we analyzed the stroma gene signature lists associated to androgen dependency and aggressive androgen-independent states. The stroma signatures are categorized in clusters (C1–C4, Table S4) based on a differential expression analysis (Figures 4 and 5): C1 (50 highly upregulated genes in BM18 intact that get downregulated upon castration), C2 (27 highly upregulated genes in LAPC9 intact that get downregulated upon castration), C3 (32 highly upregulated genes in LAPC9 intact compared to BM18 intact) and C4 (24 highly upregulated genes in LAPC9 castrated compared to BM18 intact). Clusters C1 and C2 aim to identify the most responsive genes to androgen deprivation. C3 and C4 are designated to identify the genes/pathways enriched in the stroma of castration-resistant prostate cancer (CRPC) compared to the androgen-dependent tumor model. The TNC gene was among the signature list: C1, C3 and C4. The prognostic potential of the C1-C4 signatures in comparison to the bone signature Ob-BMST was tested on the TCGA cohort based on the Gleason score, gene expression and outcome data (Figure 9 and Table S5). The high signature scores of Ob-BMST, C1, C2 and C4 had statistically significant positive correlations with the high GS groups (Figure 9A, Ob-BMST and C1 ($p < 0.001$), C2 and C4 ($p < 0.01$)). In terms of gene expression, the C1 signature was significantly higher in primary tumors versus normal tissues (Figure 9B, $p < 0.001$), while the C2, C3 and C4 have lower signature scores in the tumor samples compared to normal (Figure 9B, C2 and C3 ($p < 0.001$) and C4 ($p < 0.01$)). Kaplan-Meier plots of progression-free survival (PFS) stratified as the bottom 25% (Q1), middle 50% (Q2 and 3) and top 25% (Q4) showed significant correlations among the high signature scores (Q4) of the C1 gene set and PFS (Figure 9C, $p < 0.001$), while none of the other gene lists showed significant correlations.

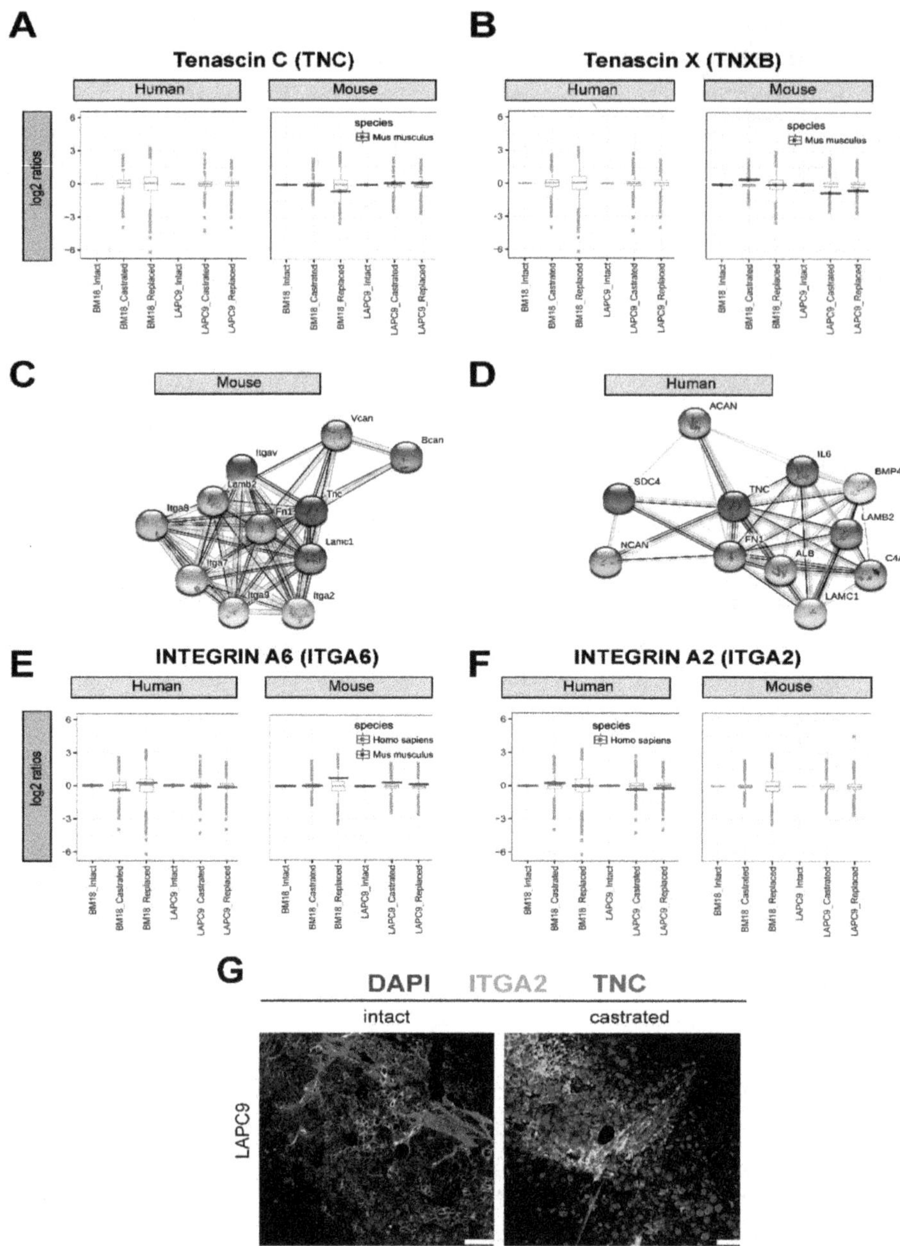

Figure 6. Tenascin C and its predicted interaction partners analyzed by mass spectrometry. (**A**) Tenascin C (TNC) and (**B**) alternative isoform Tenascin X (TNXB) protein relative abundance ($\log_2$ ratios; single replicates per sample from a pool of $n = 3$ to 4) in human cell isolations (left) and present in mouse cell isolations (right). The variance stabilization normalization (vsn)-corrected TMT reporter ion signals were normalized by the intact conditions of either BM18 or LAPC9. The protein sequences were predicted as mouse-specific (green). (**C**) Protein interaction network of the mouse TNC protein based on the STRING association network (https://string-db.org/). (**D**) Protein interaction network of the human TNC protein based on the STRING association network https://string-db.org/. (**E**) Predicted TNC-binding partner integrin A6 (ITGA6) was detected by mass spectrometry in both the human and mouse protein lysates and matching the organism-specific protein sequence based on the bioinformatics analysis (red for human and green for mouse). (**F**) Predicted TNC-binding partner integrin A2 (ITGA2) was detected by mass spectrometry, specifically in the human protein lysates, and matched the human-specific protein sequence. (**G**) Spatial localization of the Tenascin protein (TNC, indicated in red) and integrin A2 (ITGA2, green) assessed by immunofluorescent co-labeling in LAPC9 intact and castrated tumors. DAPI marks the nuclei. Scale bars: 50 μm.

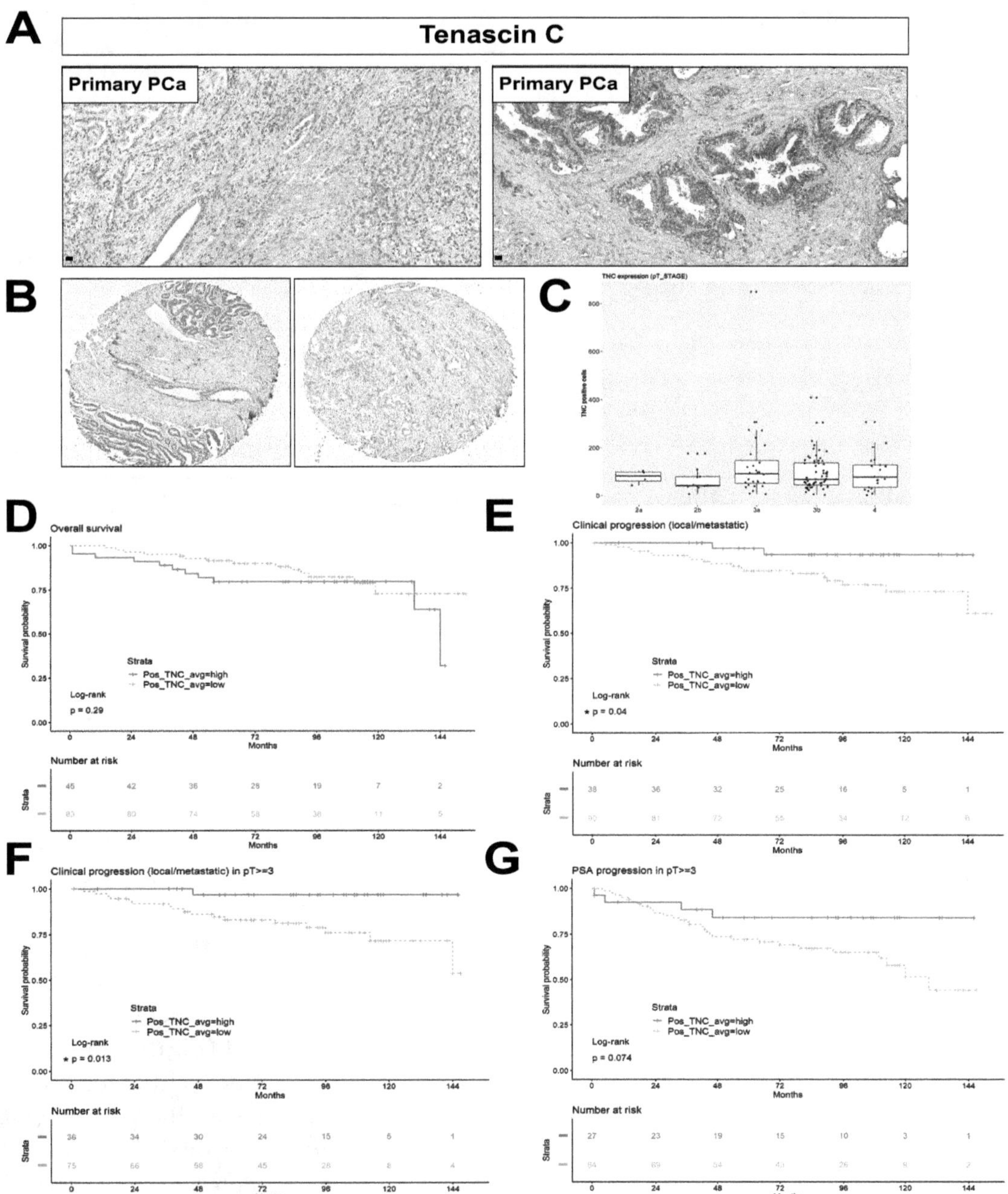

Figure 7. TNC protein expression is a negative metastasis prognostic factor in primary, high-risk PCa. (**A**) Validation of the protein expression and stromal specificity of TNC by immunohistochemistry in primary PCa cases. (**B**) Representative cases of TNC staining on primary PCa Tissue Microarray (TMA) from European Multicenter Prostate Cancer Clinical and Translational Research Group (EMPaCT). (**C**) TNC expression levels in terms of the no. of positive cells in the pT Stage classification. Statistical multiple comparison test, the Wilcoxon rank sum test, was performed; $p > 0.05$ (**D**) Overall survival probability in patient groups of TNC-high and TNC-low (no. of positive, TNC-expressing cells) ($p = 0.29$, ns—non significant). Average value represents the mean of four cores per patient case. (**E**) Clinical progression to the local recurrence or metastasis probability in patient groups of TNC-high and TNC-low expressions ($p = 0.04$ and * < 0.05). (**F**) Clinical progression to the local recurrence or metastasis probability among patients of pT Stages 3a, 3b and 4 based on TNC-high and TNC-low expressions ($p = 0.013$ and * < 0.05). (**G**) PSA progression probability among patients of pT Stages 3a, 3b and 4 based on the TNC-high and TNC-low expressions ($p = 0.074$, ns).

Table 1. Clinical parameters of the EMPaCT TMA patient cases.

Descriptive Statistics	Age at Surgery	PSA at Surgery	PSA Progression Time (Months)	Clinical Progression Time (Months)
Min	43	20	1	1
1st quartile	62	25.33	29.5	40.5
Median quartile	67	36.99	63.5	75.5
Mean quartile	66.18	50.56	63.47	70.89
3rd quartile	71	61.9	90	95.75
Max quartile	81	597	151	153

Table 2. Pathological staging, PSA and Clinical Progression of the EMPaCT TMA patient cases.

PSA Progression	Clinical Progression	Pathological Staging (No. of Patient Cases)				
		2a	**2b**	**3a**	**3b**	**4**
no	no	6	15	37	63	26
	yes	0	0	0	1	0
yes	no	0	5	7	11	7
	yes	1	7	9	9	6

To further assess the prognostic performance of the signatures, we correlated the C1-C4 gene signatures with PCa-specific stroma signatures identified by Tyekucheva et al. [7] and Mo et al. [21] (Table S4) across two cohorts containing both primary and metastatic PCa that were used [22,23]. The C3 and C4 showed the strongest linear correlations with the Tyekucheva and the Mo_up (upregulated in metastases) signatures when tested across the Grasso dataset (Figure S5A, $r > 0.64$), while the C4 signature also had positive correlations when tested across the Taylor et al. dataset (Figure S5B, $r > 0.6$). The C1 signature did not significantly correlate with the gene lists tested (Figure S5A, C1 $p > 0.05$). The low signature score of the C2 and C3 were significantly associated with metastatic disease progression (Figure S5B, $p < 0.001$) in both cohorts tested, and C4 showed a similar pattern (Figure S5B, C4 $p = 0.062$). A common pattern of the stroma signatures is a similar or enriched signature score at the primary stage compared to benign/normal tissue, and lower/depleted signature scores at the metastasis stage (Figure S5C,D; C2, C3 and C4, Tyekucheva and Mo and Figure 9B; C2-C4). Only a significant correlation with the Gleason score was observed by the C1 signature list, with a high signature score found at the high GS patient groups (Figure S5E, $p \leq 0.001$), which is in concordance to the linear correlation with metastatic disease in all clinical cohorts tested (Figure S5C,D, $p \leq 0.001$ and Figure 9, TCGA).

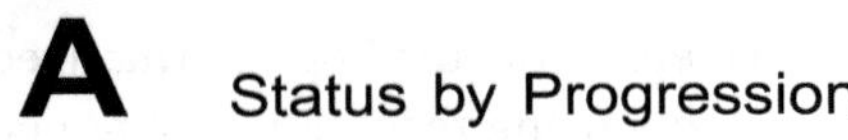

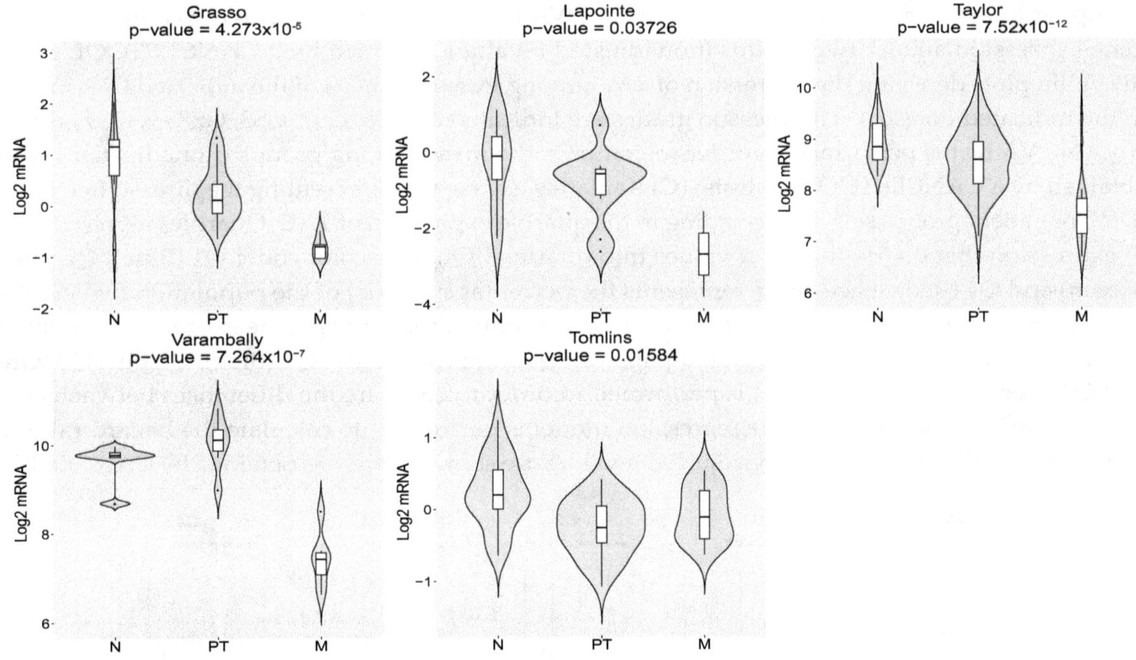

B Status by Gleason Grade

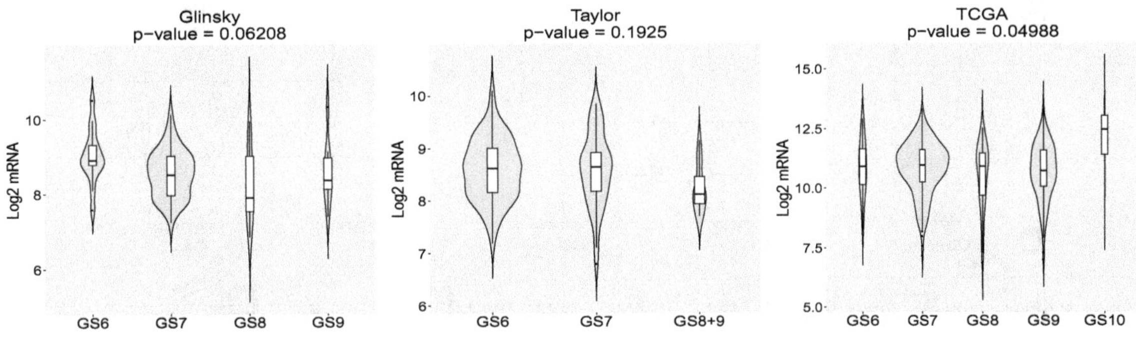

C Disease-Free Survival

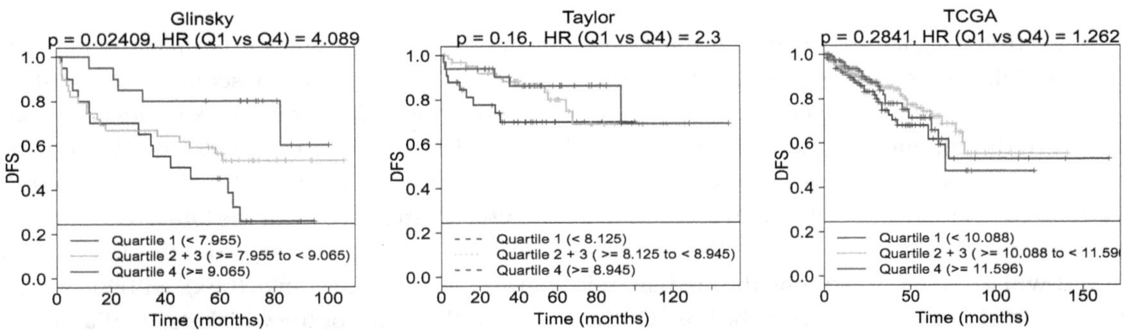

Figure 8. *TNC* RNA expression is inversely correlated with the disease progression, Gleason score and survival. (**A**) Violin plots depicting the expression of *TNC* among nontumoral (N), primary tumor (PT)

and metastatic (M) PCa specimens in the indicated datasets. The Y-axis represents the Log_2-normalized gene expression (fluorescence intensity values for microarray data or sequencing read values obtained after gene quantification with RNA-Seq Expectation Maximization (RSEM) and normalization using the upper quartile in case of RNA-seq). An ANOVA test is performed in order to compare the mean gene expression among two groups (nonadjusted *p*-value), obtained by a CANCERTOOL analysis. (**B**) Violin plots depicting the expression of *TNC* among PCa specimens of the indicated Gleason grade in the indicated datasets. The Gleason grades are indicated as GS6, GS7, GS8, GS8+9, GS9 and GS10. An ANOVA test is performed in order to compare the mean among groups (nonadjusted *p*-value), obtained by a CANCERTOOL analysis. (**C**) Kaplan-Meier curves representing the disease-free survival (DFS) of patient groups selected according to the quartile expression of *TNC*. Quartiles represent ranges of expression that divide the set of values into quarters. Quartile color code: Q1 (Blue), Q2 plus Q3 (Green) and Q4 (Red). Each curve represents the percentage (Y-axis) of the population that exhibits a recurrence of the disease along the time (X-axis, in months) for a given gene expression distribution quartile. Vertical ticks indicate censored patients. Quartile color code: Q1 (Blue), Q2 plus Q3 (Green) and Q4 (Red). A Mantel-Cox test is performed in order to compare the differences between curves, while a Cox proportional hazards regression model is performed to calculate the hazard ratio (HR) between the indicated groups. Nonadjusted *p*-values are shown. Analysis obtained by CANCERTOOL.

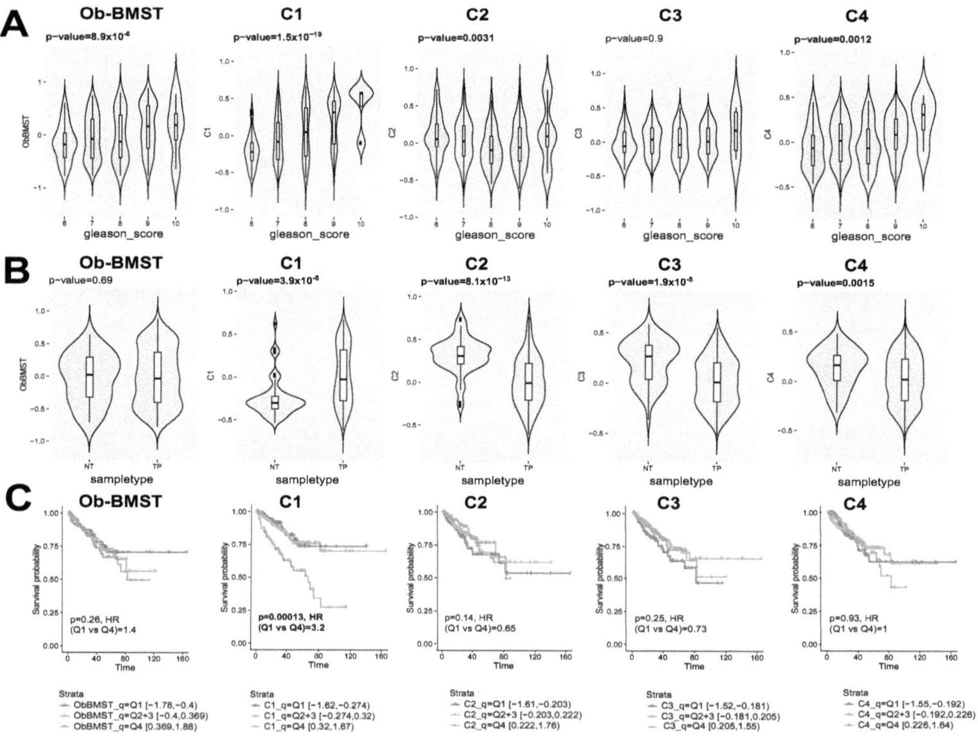

Figure 9. Stroma signatures identified from bone metastatic PDXs as prognostic biomarkers in primary PCa. (**A**) Violin plots showing Gene Set Variation Analysis (GSVA) signature scores of the Ob-BMST, C1-C4 gene sets, stratified by Gleason score from the TCGA cohort. Box-and-whisker plots illustrating median (midline), inter-quartile range (box), with the whiskers extending to at most 1.5 IQR from the box. Outliers beyond the range of the whiskers are illustrated as dots. P-values computed by Spearman correlation tests. (**B**) Violin plots showing GSVA signature scores of the Ob-BMST and C1-C4 gene sets stratified by sample types (NT: nontumor and TP: primary tumor) from the TCGA cohort. Box-and-whisker plots illustrating the median (midline) and interquartile range (box), with the whiskers extending to at most 1.5 IQR from the box. Outliers beyond the range of the whiskers are illustrated as dots. *P*-values computed by Mann-Whiney U tests. (**C**) Kaplan-Meier plots of progression-free survival (PFS) stratified as the bottom 25% (Q1), middle 50% (Q2 and 3) and top 25% (Q4) of the signature scores of the Ob-BMST and C1-C4 gene sets. *P*-values and hazard ratios computed by Cox proportional hazard regression.

3. Discussion

The role of the microenvironment upon cancer formation and progression to metastasis is supported by numerous studies [24,25]; however, the current knowledge is not sufficient to reconstruct the chain events from primary to secondary tumor progression. The normal stroma microenvironment is considered to halt tumor formation; however, after interactions with tumor cells, it also undergoes a certain "transformation" at the transcriptomic, and even at the genetic, levels [26–29]. The processes by which PCa tumor cells affect stroma and, in turn, stroma impacts primary PCa tumor growth or metastasis are complex and remain largely unclear.

We utilized well-established bone metastasis PDX models, which can be propagated subcutaneously and have different aggressiveness in terms of androgen dependency: the CRPC model LAPC9 representing complete androgen-independent advanced disease [30] and the BM18 that mimics human luminal PCa [31,32] and uniquely retains androgen sensitivity, typically seen in the primary and treatment-naïve stages. The androgen-independent stem cell populations that survive castration are well characterized in both models [31,33,34]; yet, the contribution of the stroma in those district tumor phenotypes has not been investigated. In vivo PDX models grafted in immunocompromised mice, although they lack the complexity of a complete immune system, represent the stroma compartment (endothelial cells, smooth muscle cells, myofibroblasts and cancer-associated fibroblasts). Due to the subcutaneous growth of BM PCa PDXs, the human stroma is replaced by mouse-infiltrating stromal cells and vasculature [35,36]. Mouse cell infiltration allows the discrimination of organism-specific transcripts, human-derived transcripts representing the tumor cells and mouse-derived transcripts representing the mouse stroma compartment. Using next-generation RNA-Seq, MACS-based human and mouse cell sorting, mass spectrometry and organism-specific reference databases, we have identified the tumor-specific (human) from the stroma-specific (mouse) transcriptomes and proteomes of bone metastasis PCa PDXs. The dynamics of AR signaling in the stroma are best represented in an in vivo setting [11]; therefore, to specifically examine the stroma changes dictated by PCa cells, we subjected the PDXs in androgen and androgen-deprived conditions. By imposing this selection pressure, we could identify androgen-dependent gene expression patterns.

We demonstrated that the human (tumor), as well as the mouse (stroma), transcriptomes follow androgen-dependent transcriptomic changes in the BM18 groups (intact versus castrated versus replaced). Despite the androgen-independent tumor growth of LAPC9, at the gene expression level, the LAPC9 tumor cells do follow AR-responsive patterns (human transcriptomes). However, the principal component analysis showed that, although castrated and replaced LAPC9 groups separate adequately based on the human transcriptome, they appear to have overall uniform stromal transcriptomes.

We report that transcriptomic mechanisms linked to osteotropism were conserved in bone metastatic PDXs, even in nonbone environments, and differential stroma gene expressions are induced by different tumors, indicating the tumor specificity of stroma reactivity. The Ob-BMST signature of all seven genes (*Aspn, Pdgrfb, Postn, Sparcl1, Mcam, Fscn1* and *Pmepa1*), which were upregulated in bone stroma previously identified [5], were indeed expressed in both BM18 and LAPC9 PDXs, specifically in the mouse RNA-Seq and, also, expressed at the protein level, as identified by mass spectrometry. The gene expression modulation of mouse stroma is, ultimately, an important evidence of the effects of tumor cells in their microenvironment, where they induce favorable conditions for their growth.

The differential expression analysis of the LAPC9 stroma signature from intact, castrated and replaced hosts highlighted the most significantly variable genes, which were modulated by androgen levels, despite the androgen-independent tumor growth phenotype. Focusing on the genes that were highly activated in intact but strongly modulated by castration, we categorized these genes based on Gene Ontology terms. We found that LAPC9 stromal genes were ECM remodeling components and genes involved in smooth muscle function or even in striated muscle function. Of interest are *CD56, Tnc* and *Flnc*. Among the BM18 most abundant stromal transcripts are genes involved in cell cycle regulation and cell division. Interrogating the differences among the two models, we focused on the transcriptome of LAPC9 normalized versus the less aggressive, androgen-dependent BM18. In particular, *Tnc* is expressed in both PDXs, higher in LAPC9, yet downregulated upon castration, suggesting a direct AR gene regulation. The differential expression analysis among both the PDXs after castration indicated that *Tnc* is upregulated more in LAPC9 than BM18, suggesting an association with disease aggressiveness. Genes that become upregulated in castrated conditions are likely to be linked to androgen resistance; thus, we studied *Tnc* for its potential role in metastasis progression.

TNC is an extracellular glycoprotein absent in normal prostates and postnatally silenced in most tissues. TNC is re-expressed in reactive stroma in human cancers, and there is evidence of its expression in low-grade tumors (Gleason 3) of human PCa [37] and, possibly, already activated at the prostatic intraepithelial neoplasia (PIN) stage [38,39]. In particular, high molecular weight TNC isoforms are expressed in cancer due to alternative mRNA splicing [38]. We examined whether an abundance of TNC-positive cells in primary PCa TMA can predict the metastatic progression and overall survival (12 years follow-up after radical prostatectomy). A high number of TNC-positive cells did not correlate with the overall survival or histological grade, in agreement with previous data [38]. The PSA progression after radical prostatectomy occurred earlier in the TNC-low group compared to the TNC-high group when high stage cases (pT ≥ 3), surgical margin-positive or lymph node-positive cases were investigated. In terms of clinical progression, the TNC-low group in the total number of cases and among the high stage (pT ≥ 3) cases showed a worse prognosis in terms of local recurrence/metastasis. This finding is in contrast to the study of Ni et al., showing that high levels of TNC are significantly linked to lymph node metastasis and the clinical stage [40] but in agreement with another study that reported a weak TNC expression in high-grade PCa [39]. No low-risk cases or metastasis tissues were used in our study, and we focused on TNC-producing cells, not the overall TNC expression in the matrix. Therefore we can only conclude that the TNC is indeed expressed in intermediate- and high-risk primary PCa as assessed at the preoperative diagnosis based on the D´Amico criteria [17] and that a high number of TNC-positive cells is inversely correlated with clinical progression.

More evidence points to the direction that the TNC might be degraded upon local recurrence in lung cancer [41,42], while high TNC is found in lymph and bone metastases sites [38] or even in certain types of bone metastasis [43]. In the TMA of PCa bone metastasis, San Martin et al. demonstrated a high TNC expression in trabeculae endosteum, the site of osteoblastic metastasis, and yet, a low TNC expression in the adjacent bone marrow sites [43]. Osteoblastic PCa cell lines proliferate rapidly in vitro and adhere to TNC protein, while osteolytic PC3 or lymph node-derived PCa lines do not show this phenotype, suggesting an association of TNC with osteoblastic but not osteolytic metastases. One of the ligands of TNC highly upregulated in VCap cells was $\alpha9$ integrin, which binds directly TNC and a modulate expression of collagen [43], providing evidence for TNC-integrins in human PCa. Our RNA-Seq data indicate, also, the expression of $\alpha9$ integrin, along with $\alpha6$ and $\alpha2$, and based on the proteomic human–mouse separation, we found integrin $\alpha2$ to be the only one human-specific and, thus, tumor-specific for the PDXs used in this study. Although the molecular mechanism among TNC-ITGA2 should be further characterized, evidence on the correlation among $\alpha2$ and $\alpha6$ expressions in primary PCa and bone metastasis occurrence has been previously reported [44].

The reactivation of TNC expression is relevant for reactive stroma regulation, while TNC downregulation might be relevant for recurrence or metastasis initiation, which remains to be further investigated. Indeed, TNC is known to have pleiotropic functions in different cellular contexts, with both autocrine TNC expression in tumor cells and paracrine TNC from stroma in different stages of metastasis [45]; however, the cellular source of TNC in primary PCa was not addressed in our study. Our data demonstrate that androgens regulate stromal TNC expression, evident by the reduced TNC expression upon castration (even in the castration-resistant LAPC9) and immediate increased expression upon androgen replacement; thus, the TNC expression should be further evaluated in CRPC samples. Genomic amplification in the TNC gene associated with highly aggressive neuroendocrine PCa occurrence [46]. In a multi-omics approach study, the TNC protein was one of the panels of four markers detected in preoperative serum samples and, collectively, predict the biochemical relapse events with high accuracy [47].

In summary, we identified the stroma signature of bone metastatic PDXs, and by analyzing androgen-dependent versus androgen-independent tumors, we could demonstrate that the tumor-specific stroma gene expression changes. We could show that there are AR-regulated stromal genes modulated upon castration, even in the androgen-independent, for tumor growth, like the LAPC9 model. The osteoblastic bone metastasis stromal seven-gene signature was induced in the mouse-derived stroma compartment of BM18 and LAPC9, indicating conserved tumor mechanisms that can induce the transcriptomic "transformation" of mouse-infiltrating stroma (even in subcutaneous sites) to bone microenvironment-like stroma. The prognostic value of stroma signatures has been also demonstrated by another study utilizing PDXs associated with the metastasis prognosis from different lesions from a single PCa case and demonstrated the strong predictability of 93-gene stroma signatures to metastasis phenotypes in different clinical cohorts [21]. We identified androgen-dependent Tenascin C expression in the stroma of PDX models, which is downregulated in the conditions mimicking an aggressive disease (upon castration), similarly to the high clinical progression probability of a low TNC group in the primary PCa TMA. The higher stromal *Tnc* mRNA levels in the aggressive LAPC9 compared to BM18 may suggest that it would be relevant to examine the TNC mRNA and protein expressions in human bone metastasis or ideally matched primary metastasis cases in order to understand the kinetics of TNC in terms of disease progression. Given that TNC expression was found elevated from 0% in benign prostatic hyperplasia (BPH) stroma to 47% in tumor-associated stroma [29], its detection in circulation [47] and its immunomodulatory role [48] indicate TNC as a promising drug target and disease-determining factor. The TNC clinical progression predictive value performs best in an earlier stage, low-risk PCa, while our data show that, in high-risk PCa, a low number of TNC-producing cells were associated with poor prognosis, possibly due to changes in tissue remodeling and, thus, variable TNC levels.

These findings were corroborated by the external clinical cohorts of patients [22,23,49,50] (Grasso et al., Lapointe et al., Taylor et al. and Varambally et al.) showing that TNC levels are downregulated during the disease progression from primary to metastasis. Based on differential expression analysis, we identified clusters of stroma signatures based on androgen-(in)dependent responses (C1-C4). TNC is a component of the C1, C3 and C4 signatures. In silico validation of the identified prostate cancer-specific stroma expression signatures on additional clinical cohorts showed the potential for patient stratification. A common feature of the majority of the four clusters of gene lists tested indicated a low stroma signature score in the advanced disease stage and a correlation with disease progression (metastasis). This was the case also for previously published stroma signatures [7,21] (Tyekucheva et al. 2017 and Mo et al. 2017) when compared to our gene sets, perhaps due to the reduced stroma content in low-differentiated, advanced PCa stage. The signature most related to the androgen-independent stage (C4) positively correlated with the Gleason score in primary tissues from TCGA but not in the metastatic cohort of the Taylor dataset. Instead, we identified a 50-gene stroma signature (C1, derived from the most androgen-responsive stroma genes), which positively correlates with the disease progression, Gleason score and poor prognosis survival, consistently on all patient cohorts evaluated, both the primary and metastasis stages.

The regime that a metastatic, stroma-specific molecular signature may be detectable in the PCa site either prior to or during metastasis will most likely require not a single marker approach but a combination of biochemical and histological markers, taking into consideration dual tumor–stroma interactions in order to provide prognostic tools for improved patient stratification after the initial PCa diagnosis and preventive surveillance for metastasis risk.

4. Materials and Methods

4.1. Tumor Sample Preparation and Xenograft Surgery Procedure

LAPC9 and BM18 xenografts were maintained subcutaneously in 6-week-old CB17 SCID male mice under anesthesia (Domitor® 0.5 mg/kg, Dormicum 5 mg/kg and Fentanyl 0.05 mg/kg). All animal experiments were approved by the Ethical Committee of Canton Bern (animal licenses BE55/16 and BE12/17). Castration was achieved by bilateral orchiectomy. For androgen replacement, testosterone propionate dissolved in castor oil (86541-5G, Sigma-Aldrich, Buchs, Switzerland) was administered by single subcutaneous injection (2 mg per dosage, 25-G needle).

4.2. RNA Isolation from Tissue Samples

Tissue RNA was extracted using the standard protocol of Qiazol (79306, Qiagen AG, Hombrechtikon, Switzerland) tissue lysis by TissueLyser (2 min, 20 Hz). Quality of RNA was assessed by Bioanalyzer 2100 (Agilent Technologies, Basel, Switzerland). RNA from formalin-fixed-paraffin embedded (FFPE) material was extracted using the Maxwell® 16 LEV RNA FFPE Purification Kit (AS1260, Promega AG, Dübendorf, Switzerland).

4.3. RNA Sequencing

RNA extracted from BM18, and LAPC9 whole PDX tumor extracts (300 ng) were subjected to RNA sequencing. Specimens were prepared for RNA sequencing using Tru-Seq RNA Library Preparation Kit v2 or riboZero, as previously described [51]. RNA integrity was verified using the Bioanalyzer 2100 (Agilent Technologies, Basel, Switzerland). Complementary cDNA was synthesized from total RNA using Superscript III reverse transcriptase (18080093, Thermo Fisher Scientific, Basel, Switzerland). Sequencing was then performed on GAII, Hi-Seq 2000 or Hi-Seq 2500. The sample preparation was performed according to the protocol "NEBNext Ultra II Directional RNA Library Prep Kit (NEB #E7760S/L, Illumina GmbH, Zürich, Switzerland). Briefly, mRNA was isolated from total RNA using the oligo-dT magnetic beads. After fragmentation of the mRNA, a cDNA synthesis was performed. This was used for ligation with the sequencing adapters and PCR amplification of the resulting product. The quality and yield after sample preparation was measured with the Fragment Analyzer. The size of the resulting products was consistent with the expected size distribution (a broad peak between 300–500 bp). Clustering and DNA sequencing using the NovaSeq6000 was performed according to manufacturer's protocols. A concentration of 1.1 nM of DNA was used. Image analysis, base calling and quality check was performed with the Illumina (Illumina GmbH, Zürich, Switzerland) data analysis pipeline RTA3.4.4 and Bcl2fastq v2.20.

Sequence reads were aligned using STAR two-pass to the human reference genome GRCh37 [52] and mouse reference genome GRCm38. Gene counts were quantified using the "GeneCounts" option. Per-gene counts-per-million (CPM) were computed and $\log_2$-transformed, adding a pseudo-count of 1 to avoid transforming 0. Genes with $\log_2$ CPM <1 in more than three samples were removed. Differential expression analysis was performed using the edgeR package [53]. Normalization was performed using the "TMM" (weighted trimmed mean) method, and differential expression was assessed using the quasi-likelihood F test. Genes with false discovery rate FDR <0.05 and >2-fold were considered significantly differentially expressed. RNA-Seq Expectation Maximization (RSEM) was used to obtain TPM (transcripts per million) counts.

Pathway analysis (over-representation analysis) was performed using clusterProfiler R package [54] for Gene Ontology biological processes and KEGG. For Venn Euler diagram analysis, expressed genes were identified using the zFPKM transformation [55]. For the comparison between the states of the BM18 and LAPC9 models, genes were considered expressed if a gene had zFPKM values > -3 [55] in all samples.

4.4. *Signature Validation on TCGA and Other Publically Available Datasets*

TCGA gene expression, Gleason scores and outcome data were obtained from the PanCanAtlas publications supplemental data site (https://gdc.cancer.gov/about-data/publications/pancanatlas) [56,57]. For the Gene Set Variation Analysis (GSVA) analysis, RSEM expected counts in the upper quartile normalized to 1000 (i.e., the same normalization as TCGA) were used for BM18/LAPC9 gene expression. Mouse genes in gene signature lists were mapped to human homologs using the biomaRt R package (Table S5), using the "mmusculus_gene_ensembl" dataset and selecting only homologs with hsapiens_homolog_orthology_confidence = 1. Signature scores were calculated using the GSVA R package using the GSVA method [58].

Validation of the C1-C4 stroma signatures on publicly availably cohorts was performed using the Taylor (GSE21034) and the Grasso (GSE35988) datasets. Gene expression and sample information, including Gleason scores, were obtained via the GEOquery Bioconductor package. Mouse genes in the C1-C4 gene signature lists were mapped to human homologs using the biomaRt R package, using the "mmusculus_gene_ensembl" dataset and selecting only homologs with hsapiens_homolog_orthology_confidence = 1. Other gene sets are either human genes or include info on human homologs. Signature scores were calculated using the GSVA R package using the GSVA method [58].

4.5. *Tissue Dissociation and MACS*

Tumor tissue was collected in a basis medium (advanced Dulbecco Modified Eagle Medium F12 serum-free medium (12634010, Thermo Fisher Scientific, Basel, Switzerland) containing 10-mM Hepes (15630080, Thermo Fisher Scientific, Basel, Switzerland), 2-mM GlutaMAX supplement (35050061, Thermo Fisher Scientific, Basel, Switzerland) and 100 µg/mL Primocin (ant-pm-1, InVivoGen, LabForce AG, Muttenz, Switzerland). After mechanical disruption, the tissue was washed in the basis medium (220 relative centrifugal force (rcf), 5 min) and incubated in the enzyme mix for tissue dissociation (collagenase type II enzyme mix (17101-015, Gibco, Thermo Fisher Scientific, Basel, Switzerland) 5 mg/mL dissolved in the basis medium and DNase: 15 µg/mL (10104159001, Sigma-Aldrich, Buchs, Switzerland) and 10-µM Y-27632-HCl rock inhibitor (S1049, Selleckchem, Zürich, Switzerland). Enzyme mix volume was adjusted so that the tissue volume did not exceed 1/10 of the total volume, and tissue was incubated at 37 °C for 1 to 2 h, with mixing every 20 min. After the digestion of large pieces was complete, the suspension was passed through a 100-µm cell strainer (21008-950, Falcon®, VWR International GmbH, Dietikon, Switzerland) attached to a 50-mL Falcon tube, then using a rubber syringe to crash tissue against the strainer and wash in 5-mL basic medium (220 rcf, 5 min). Cell pellet was incubated in 5-mL precooled red blood cell lysis buffer (150-mM NH_4Cl, 10-mM $KHCO_3$ and 0.1-mM EDTA), incubated for 10 min and washed in equal volume of basis medium, followed by centrifugation (220 rcf, 5 min). Pellet was resuspended in 2–5 mL accutase™ (StemCell Technologies, 07920), depending on the sample amount; biopsies versus tissue and incubated for 10 min at room temperature. The cell suspension was passed through a 40-µm pore size strainer (21008-949, Falcon®, International GmbH, Dietikon, Switzerland), and the strainer was washed by adding 2 mL of accutase on the strainer. Single-cell suspension was counted to determine the seeding density and washed in 5 mL of basis medium and spun down 220 rcf, 5 min. Magnetic cell sorting was performed to separate purified human versus mouse cell fractions using the Mouse Cell Depletion Kit (130-104-694, Miltenyi Biotek, Solothurn, Switzerland). For the proteomic experiments, cell fractions from tumor tissues ($n = 3$ to 4 per condition) were pooled together in order to suffice for 10^6 cells, representing one technical replicate per sample.

4.6. Proteomics

4.6.1. Sample Preparation

Approx. 10^6 cell pellets ($n = 1$ technical replicate per condition deriving from $n = 3$ to 4 biological replicate samples) were resuspended in 50 μL PBS following the addition of 50 μL 1% SDS in 100-mM Hepes/NaOH, pH 8.5 supplemented with protease inhibitor cocktail EDTA-free (11836170001, Sigma-Aldrich, Buchs, Switzerland). Samples were heated to 95 °C for 5 min, transferred on ice, and benzonase (71206-3, Merck AG, Zug, Switzerland) was added to degrade DNA at 37 °C for 30 min. Samples were reduced by the addition of 2 μL of a 200-mM DTT solution in 200-mM Hepes/NaOH, pH 8.5 and, subsequently, alkylated by the addition of 4 μL of a 400-mM chloroacetamide (CAA, #C0267, Sigma-Aldrich, Buchs, Switzerland) solution in 200 mM Hepes/NaOH, pH 8.5. Samples were incubated at 56 °C for 30 min. Access CAA was quenched by the addition of 4 μl of a 200-mM DTT solution in 200 mM Hepes/NaOH, pH 8.5. Lysate were subjected to an in-solution tryptic digest using the single-pot solid phase-enhanced sample preparation (SP3) protocol [59,60]. To this end, 20 μL of Sera-Mag Beads (#4515-2105-050250 and 6515-2105-050250, Thermo Fisher Scientific, Basel, Switzerland) were mixed, washed with H_2O and resuspended in 100 μL H_2O. Two microliters of freshly prepared bead mix and 5 μl of an aqueous 10% formic acid were added to 40 μL of lysates to achieve an acidic pH. Forty-seven microliters of acetonitrile were added, and samples were incubated for 8 min at room temperature. Beads were captured on a magnetic rack and washed three times with 70% ethanol and once with acetonitrile. Sequencing grade-modified trypsin (0.8 μg; V5111, Promega AG, Dübendorf, Switzerland) in 10 μL 50 mM Hepes/NaOH, pH 8.5 were added. Samples were digested overnight at 37 °C. Beads were captured and the supernatant transferred and dried down. Peptides were reconstituted in 10 μL of H_2O and reacted with 80 μg of TMT10plex (#90111, Thermo Fisher Scientific, Basel, Switzerland) [61] label reagent dissolved in 4 μL of acetonitrile for 1 h at room temperature. Excess TMT reagent was quenched by the addition of 4 μL of an aqueous solution of 5% hydroxylamine (438227, Sigma-Aldrich, Buchs, Switzerland). Mixed peptides were subjected to a reverse-phase clean-up step (OASIS HLB 96-well μElution Plate, 186001828BA, Waters Corporation, Milford, MA, USA) and analyzed by LC-MS/MS on a Q Exactive Plus (Thermo Fisher Scientific, Basel, Switzerland), as previously described [62].

4.6.2. Mass Spectrometric Analysis

Briefly, peptides were separated using an UltiMate 3000 RSLC (Thermo Scientific, Basel, Switzerland) equipped with a trapping cartridge (Precolumn; C18 PepMap 100, 5 Lm, 300 Lm i.d. × 5 mm, 100 A°) and an analytical column (Waters nanoEase HSS C18 T3, 75 Lm × 25 cm, 1.8 Lm, 100 A°). Solvent A: aqueous 0.1% formic acid and Solvent B: 0.1% formic acid in acetonitrile (all solvents were of LC-MS grade). Peptides were loaded on the trapping cartridge using solvent A for 3 min with a flow of 30 μL/min. Peptides were separated on the analytical column with a constant flow of 0.3 μL/min applying a 2 h gradient of 2–28% of solvent B in A, followed by an increase to 40% B. Peptides were directly analyzed in positive ion mode, applied with a spray voltage of 2.3 kV and a capillary temperature of 320°C using a Nanospray-Flex ion source and a Pico-Tip Emitter 360 Lm OD × 20 Lm ID;, 10 Lm tip (New Objective, Littleton, MA, USA). MS spectra with a mass range of 375–1.200 m/z were acquired in profile mode using a resolution of 70,000 (maximum fill time of 250 ms or a maximum of 3×10^6 ions (automatic gain control, AGC)). Fragmentation was triggered for the top 10 peaks with 2–4 charges on the MS scan (data-dependent acquisition), with a 30 s dynamic exclusion window (normalized collision energy was 32). Precursors were isolated with a 0.7 m/z window and MS/MS spectra were acquired in profile mode with a resolution of 35,000 (maximum fill time of 120 ms or an AGC target of 2×10^5 ions).

4.6.3. Raw MS Data Analysis

Acquired data were analyzed using IsobarQuant [63] and Mascot V2.4 (Matrix Science, Chicago, IL, USA) using either a reverse-UniProt FASTA Mus musculus (UP000000589) or Homo sapiens (UP000005640) database. Moreover, a combined database thereof was generated and used for the analysis. These databases also included common contaminants. The following modifications were taken into account: Carbamidomethyl (C, fixed), TMT10plex (K, fixed), Acetyl (N-term, variable), Oxidation (M, variable) and TMT10plex (N-term, variable). The mass error tolerance for full-scan MS spectra was set to 10 ppm and for MS/MS spectra to 0.02 Da. A maximum of 2 missed cleavages were allowed. A minimum of 2 unique peptides with a peptide length of at least seven amino acids and a false discovery rate below 0.01 were required on the peptide and protein levels [64].

4.6.4. MS Data Analysis

The raw output files of IsobarQuant (protein.txt files) were processed using the R programming language (ISBN 3-900051-07-0). As a quality filter, only proteins were allowed that you were quantified with at least two unique peptides. Human and mouse samples were searched against a combined human and mouse database and annotated as unique for human or mouse or mixed. Raw signal-sums (signal_sum columns) were normalized using vsn (variance stabilization normalization) [65]. In order to try to annotate each observed ratio with a p-value, each ratio distribution was analyzed with the locfdr function of the locfdr package [66] to extract the average and the standard deviation (using the maximum likelihood estimation). Then, the ratio distribution was transformed into a z-distribution by normalizing it by its standard deviation and mean. This z-distribution was analyzed with the fdrtool function of the fdrtool package [67] in order to extract p-values and false discovery rates (fdr, q-values).

4.7. Tissue Microarray

Tissue microarray core annotations and quantification of positive staining were performed by QuPath software version v0.2.0-m8 [68] using the TMA map function. Kaplan–Meier curves to calculate the association between TNC-positive cells and disease progression were calculated using the "survfit" function and the global Log-Rank test using the Survival R package [69,70]. To estimate the survival, we used the function "surv_cutpoint", which employs maximally selected rank statistics (maxstat) to determine the optimal cut-point for continuous variables [18]. For pairwise comparison, the p-value was estimated by the Log-Rank test and adjusted with the Benjamini–Hochberg (BH) method. If no information on patient outcome was available, information at the last follow-up was used for all parameters. Clinical progression was defined as metastasis or local recurrence. Disease progression was defined by combining any form of recurrence (PSA and clinical progression). Data representation and graphical plots were generated using the ggplot2 R package [71]. Data analyses were done using RStudio version 1.1.463 [72] and R version 3.5.3 [73].

4.8. Immunohistochemistry

FFPE sections (4 μm) were deparaffinized and used for heat-mediated antigen retrieval (citrate buffer, pH 6, Vector Labs). Sections were blocked for 10 min in 3% H_2O_2, followed by 30 min, RT incubation in 1% BSA in PBS–0.1%Tween 20. The following primary antibodies were used (Table 3):

Table 3. Primary antibodies used for Immunohistochemistry

Dilution	Antibody	Company	Catalog No.
1 to 500	Ki67	Gene Tex	GTX16667
1 to 100	Tnc	R&D	MAB2138

Secondary anti-rabbit antibody Envision HRP (DAKO, Agilent Technologies, Basel, Switzerland) for 30 min or anti-rat HRP (Thermo Scientific, Basel, Switzerland). Signal detection with AEC substrate

(DAKO, Agilent Technologies, Basel, Switzerland). Sections were counterstained with Hematoxylin and mounted with Aquatex.

4.9. Immunofluorescence

After deparaffinization, heat-mediated antigen retrieval (citrate buffer, pH 6, Vector Labs) was performed. Sections were blocked in 1% BSA in PBS–0.1% Tween 20 for 30 min, RT incubation. The primary antibodies used (Table 4), were incubated overnight in blocking solution at 4 °C:

Table 4. Primary antibodies used for Immunofluorescence

Dilution	Antibody	Company	Catalog No.
1 to 500	αSMA	Sigma	A2547
1 to 500	ITGA2	Abcam	ab181548
1 to 500	Collagen type I	Southern Biotech	1310-01
1 to 50	Tnc	R&D	MAB2138

Secondary anti-rabbit/mouse/goat/rat antibodies coupled to Alexa Fluor®-488, 555 or 647 fluorochrome conjugates (Invitrogen, Thermo Scientific, Basel, Switzerland) were incubated for 90 min at 1:250 dilution in PBS. Sections were counterstained with DAPI solution (Thermo Scientific, Basel, Switzerland, final concentration 1 µg/mL in PBS, 10 min), washed and mounted with prolonged diamond antifade reagent (Invitrogen, Thermo Scientific, Basel, Switzerland).

5. Conclusions

In this proof-of-concept study, the molecular profile of the stroma in prostate cancer was shown to be responsive to androgen deprivation even in advanced, androgen-independent bone metastasis prostate cancer. We identified a stroma-specific gene expression signature that correlates with the Gleason score and metastatic disease progression of prostate cancer. Given the inevitable drug resistance to androgen deprivation therapies, stroma biomarker identification associated with resistance acquisition may complement standard histopathology and genomic evaluations for improved stratification of patients at high risk.

Author Contributions: Conceptualization, S.K. and M.K.d.J.; formal analysis, S.K., M.R.D.F., C.K.Y.N., E.Z., F.S. and P.H.; funding acquisition, S.K., G.N.T. and M.K.d.J.; investigation, S.K. and I.K.; methodology, E.Z. and P.H.; project administration, M.K.d.J.; resources, M.S., G.N.T. and M.K.d.J.; software, P.H.; supervision, M.K.d.J.; writing—original draft, S.K., F.S. and M.K.d.J. and writing—review and editing, M.R.D.F., C.K.Y.N., E.Z. and G.N.T. All authors have read and agreed to the published version of the manuscript.

Acknowledgments: The authors would like to thank the Microscopy Facility of the University of Bern, Francesco Bonollo, Peter C Gray, Salvatore Piscuoglio and all the members of the DBMR Urology laboratory for critical discussions and technical support.

References

1. Heidenreich, A.; Bastian, P.J.; Bellmunt, J.; Bolla, M.; Joniau, S.; van der Kwast, T.; Mason, M.; Matveev, V.; Wiegel, T.; Zattoni, F.; et al. EAU guidelines on prostate cancer. Part II: Treatment of advanced, relapsing, and castration-resistant prostate cancer. *Eur. Urol.* **2014**, *65*, 467–479. [CrossRef] [PubMed]
2. Malanchi, I.; Santamaria-Martinez, A.; Susanto, E.; Peng, H.; Lehr, H.A.; Delaloye, J.F.; Huelsken, J. Interactions between cancer stem cells and their niche govern metastatic colonization. *Nature* **2011**, *481*, 85–89. [CrossRef] [PubMed]
3. Shiozawa, Y.; Pedersen, E.A.; Havens, A.M.; Jung, Y.; Mishra, A.; Joseph, J.; Kim, J.K.; Patel, L.R.; Ying, C.; Ziegler, A.M.; et al. Human prostate cancer metastases target the hematopoietic stem cell niche to establish footholds in mouse bone marrow. *J. Clin. Invest.* **2011**, *121*, 1298–1312. [CrossRef] [PubMed]

4. Hensel, J.; Wetterwald, A.; Temanni, R.; Keller, I.; Riether, C.; van der Pluijm, G.; Cecchini, M.G.; Thalmann, G.N. Osteolytic cancer cells induce vascular/axon guidance processes in the bone/bone marrow stroma. *Oncotarget* **2018**, *9*, 28877–28896. [CrossRef] [PubMed]
5. Ozdemir, B.C.; Hensel, J.; Secondini, C.; Wetterwald, A.; Schwaninger, R.; Fleischmann, A.; Raffelsberger, W.; Poch, O.; Delorenzi, M.; Temanni, R.; et al. The molecular signature of the stroma response in prostate cancer-induced osteoblastic bone metastasis highlights expansion of hematopoietic and prostate epithelial stem cell niches. *PLoS ONE* **2014**, *9*, e114530. [CrossRef] [PubMed]
6. Rucci, N.; Teti, A. Osteomimicry: How the seed grows in the soil. *Calcif. Tissue Int.* **2018**, *102*, 131–140. [CrossRef]
7. Tyekucheva, S.; Bowden, M.; Bango, C.; Giunchi, F.; Huang, Y.; Zhou, C.; Bondi, A.; Lis, R.; Van Hemelrijck, M.; Andrén, O.; et al. Stromal and epithelial transcriptional map of initiation progression and metastatic potential of human prostate cancer. *Nat. Commun.* **2017**, *8*, 420. [CrossRef]
8. Setlur, S.R.; Rubin, M.A. Current thoughts on the role of the androgen receptor and prostate cancer progression. *Adv. Anat. Pathol.* **2005**, *12*, 265–270. [CrossRef]
9. Leach, D.A.; Need, E.F.; Toivanen, R.; Trotta, A.P.; Palenthorpe, H.M.; Tamblyn, D.J.; Kopsaftis, T.; England, G.M.; Smith, E.; Drew, P.A.; et al. Stromal androgen receptor regulates the composition of the microenvironment to influence prostate cancer outcome. *Oncotarget* **2015**, *6*, 16135–16150. [CrossRef]
10. Leach, D.A.; Panagopoulos, V.; Nash, C.; Bevan, C.; Thomson, A.A.; Selth, L.A.; Buchanan, G. Cell-lineage specificity and role of AP-1 in the prostate fibroblast androgen receptor cistrome. *Mol. Cell. Endocrinol.* **2017**, *439*, 261–272. [CrossRef]
11. Nash, C.; Boufaied, N.; Mills, I.G.; Franco, O.E.; Hayward, S.W.; Thomson, A.A. Genome-wide analysis of AR binding and comparison with transcript expression in primary human fetal prostate fibroblasts and cancer associated fibroblasts. *Mol. Cell. Endocrinol.* **2018**, *471*, 1–14. [CrossRef] [PubMed]
12. Thalmann, G.N.; Rhee, H.; Sikes, R.A.; Pathak, S.; Multani, A.; Zhau, H.E.; Marshall, F.F.; Chung, L.W.K. Human prostate fibroblasts induce growth and confer castration resistance and metastatic potential in LNCaP Cells. *Eur. Urol.* **2010**, *58*, 162–171. [CrossRef]
13. Thalmann, G.N.; Anezinis, P.E.; Chang, S.M.; Zhau, H.E.; Kim, E.E.; Hopwood, V.L.; Pathak, S.; von Eschenbach, A.C.; Chung, L.W. Androgen-independent cancer progression and bone metastasis in the LNCaP model of human prostate cancer. *Cancer Res.* **1994**, *54*, 2577–2581. [PubMed]
14. Briganti, A.; Spahn, M.; Joniau, S.; Gontero, P.; Bianchi, M.; Kneitz, B.; Chun, F.K.; Sun, M.; Graefen, M.; Abdollah, F.; et al. Impact of age and comorbidities on long-term survival of patients with high-risk prostate cancer treated with radical prostatectomy: A multi-institutional competing-risks analysis. *Eur. Urol.* **2013**, *63*, 693–701. [CrossRef] [PubMed]
15. Tosco, L.; Laenen, A.; Briganti, A.; Gontero, P.; Karnes, R.J.; Bastian, P.J.; Chlosta, P.; Claessens, F.; Chun, F.K.; Everaerts, W.; et al. The EMPaCT classifier: A validated tool to predict postoperative prostate cancer-related death using competing-risk analysis. *Eur. Urol. Focus.* **2018**, *4*, 369–375. [CrossRef] [PubMed]
16. Chys, B.; Devos, G.; Everaerts, W.; Albersen, M.; Moris, L.; Claessens, F.; De Meerleer, G.; Haustermans, K.; Briganti, A.; Chlosta, P.; et al. Preoperative risk-stratification of high-risk prostate cancer: A multicenter analysis. *Front. Oncol.* **2020**, *10*, 246. [CrossRef] [PubMed]
17. D'Amico, A.V.; Whittington, R.; Malkowicz, S.B.; Schultz, D.; Blank, K.; Broderick, G.A.; Tomaszewski, J.E.; Renshaw, A.A.; Kaplan, I.; Beard, C.J.; et al. Biochemical outcome after radical prostatectomy, external beam radiation therapy, or interstitial radiation therapy for clinically localized prostate cancer. *JAMA* **1998**, *280*, 969–974.
18. Kassambara, A. Survminer: Drawing Survival Curves Using 'ggplot2'. 2018. Available online: http://www.sthda.com/english/rpkgs/survminer/ (accessed on 1 January 2016).
19. Cortazar, A.R.; Torrano, V.; Martín-Martín, N.; Caro-Maldonado, A.; Camacho, L.; Hermanova, I.; Guruceaga, E.; Lorenzo-Martín, L.F.; Caloto, R.; Gomis, R.R.; et al. CANCERTOOL: A visualization and representation interface to exploit cancer datasets. *Cancer Res.* **2018**, *78*, 6320–6328. [CrossRef]
20. Glinsky, G.V.; Glinskii, A.B.; Stephenson, A.J.; Hoffman, R.M.; Gerald, W.L. Gene expression profiling predicts clinical outcome of prostate cancer. *J. Clin. Invest.* **2004**. [CrossRef]
21. Mo, F.; Lin, D.; Takhar, M.; Ramnarine, V.R.; Dong, X.; Bell, R.H.; Volik, S.V.; Wang, K.; Xue, H.; Wang, Y.; et al. Stromal gene expression is predictive for metastatic primary prostate cancer. *Eur. Urol.* **2018**, *73*, 524–532. [CrossRef]

22. Grasso, C.S.; Wu, Y.M.; Robinson, D.R.; Cao, X.; Dhanasekaran, S.M.; Khan, A.P.; Quist, M.J.; Jing, X.; Lonigro, R.J.; Brenner, J.C.; et al. The mutational landscape of lethal castration-resistant prostate cancer. *Nature* **2012**, *487*, 239–243. [CrossRef] [PubMed]
23. Taylor, B.S.; Schultz, N.; Hieronymus, H.; Gopalan, A.; Xiao, Y.; Carver, B.S.; Arora, V.K.; Kaushik, P.; Cerami, E.; Reva, B.; et al. Integrative genomic profiling of human prostate cancer. *Cancer Cell.* **2010**, *18*, 11–22. [CrossRef] [PubMed]
24. Sahai, E.; Astsaturov, I.; Cukierman, E.; DeNardo, D.G.; Egeblad, M.; Evans, R.M.; Fearon, D.; Greten, F.R.; Hingorani, S.R.; Hunter, T.; et al. A framework for advancing our understanding of cancer-associated fibroblasts. *Nat. Rev. Cancer* **2020**, *20*, 174–186. [CrossRef] [PubMed]
25. Corn, P.G. The tumor microenvironment in prostate cancer: Elucidating molecular pathways for therapy development. *Cancer Manag. Res.* **2012**, *4*, 183–193. [CrossRef]
26. Bissell, M.J.; Hines, W.C. Why don't we get more cancer? A proposed role of the microenvironment in restraining cancer progression. *Nat. Med.* **2011**, *17*, 320–329. [CrossRef]
27. Petersen, O.W.; Rønnov-Jessen, L.; Howlett, A.R.; Bissell, M.J. Interaction with basement membrane serves to rapidly distinguish growth and differentiation pattern of normal and malignant human breast epithelial cells. *Proc. Natl. Acad. Sci. USA.* **1992**, *89*, 9064–9068. [CrossRef]
28. Weaver, V.M.; Petersen, O.W.; Wang, F.; Larabell, C.A.; Briand, P.; Damsky, C.; Bissell, M.J. Reversion of the malignant phenotype of human breast cells in three-dimensional culture and in vivo by integrin blocking antibodies. *J. Cell. Biol.* **1997**, *137*, 231–245. [CrossRef]
29. Sung, S.-Y.; Hsieh, C.-L.; Law, A.; Zhau, H.E.; Pathak, S.; Multani, A.S.; Lim, S.; Coleman, I.M.; Wu, L.-C.; Figg, W.D.; et al. Coevolution of prostate cancer and bone stroma in three-dimensional coculture: Implications for cancer growth and metastasis. *Cancer Res.* **2008**, *68*, 9996–10003. [CrossRef]
30. Craft, N.; Chhor, C.; Tran, C.; Belldegrun, A.; DeKernion, J.; Witte, O.N.; Said, J.; Reiter, R.E.; Sawyers, C.L. Evidence for clonal outgrowth of androgen-independent prostate cancer cells from androgen-dependent tumors through a two-step process. *Cancer Res.* **1999**, *59*, 5030–5036.
31. Germann, M.; Wetterwald, A.; Guzman-Ramirez, N.; van der Pluijm, G.; Culig, Z.; Cecchini, M.G.; Williams, E.D.; Thalmann, G.N. Stem-like cells with luminal progenitor phenotype survive castration in human prostate cancer. *Stem Cells* **2012**, *30*, 1076–1086. [CrossRef]
32. McCulloch, D.R.; Opeskin, K.; Thompson, E.W.; Williams, E.D. BM18: A novel androgen-dependent human prostate cancer xenograft model derived from a bone metastasis. *Prostate* **2005**, *65*, 35–43. [CrossRef] [PubMed]
33. Li, Q.; Deng, Q.; Chao, H.-P.; Liu, X.; Lu, Y.; Lin, K.; Liu, B.; Tang, G.W.; Zhang, D.; Tracz, A.; et al. Linking prostate cancer cell AR heterogeneity to distinct castration and enzalutamide responses. *Nat. Commun.* **2018**, *9*, 3600. [CrossRef] [PubMed]
34. Chen, X.; Li, Q.; Liu, X.; Liu, C.; Liu, R.; Rycaj, K.; Zhang, D.; Liu, B.; Jeter, C.; Calhoun-Davis, T.; et al. Defining a population of stem-like human prostate cancer cells that can generate and propagate castration-resistant prostate cancer. *Clin. Cancer Res.* **2016**, *22*, 4505–4516. [CrossRef] [PubMed]
35. Cutz, J.-C.; Guan, J.; Bayani, J.; Yoshimoto, M.; Xue, H.; Sutcliffe, M.; English, J.; Flint, J.; LeRiche, J.; Yee, J.; et al. Establishment in severe combined immunodeficiency mice of subrenal capsule xenografts and transplantable tumor lines from a variety of primary human lung cancers: Potential models for studying tumor progression–related changes. *Clin. Cancer Res.* **2006**, *12*, 4043–4054. [CrossRef] [PubMed]
36. Hidalgo, M.; Amant, F.; Biankin, A.V.; Budinská, E.; Byrne, A.T.; Caldas, C.; Clarke, R.B.; de Jong, S.; Jonkers, J.; Mælandsmo, G.M.; et al. Patient-derived xenograft models: An emerging platform for translational cancer research. *Cancer Discov.* **2014**, *4*, 998–1013. [CrossRef] [PubMed]
37. Tuxhorn, J.A.; Ayala, G.E.; Smith, M.J.; Smith, V.C.; Dang, T.D.; Rowley, D.R. Reactive stroma in human prostate cancer. Induction of myofibroblast phenotype and extracellular matrix remodeling. *Clin. Cancer Res.* **2002**, *8*, 2912–2923. [PubMed]
38. Ibrahim, S.N.; Lightner, V.A.; Ventimiglia, J.B.; Ibrahim, G.K.; Walther, P.J.; Bigner, D.D.; Humphrey, P.A. Tenascin expression in prostatic hyperplasia, intraepithelial neoplasia, and carcinoma. *Hum. Pathol.* **1993**, *24*, 982–989. [CrossRef]
39. Xue, Y.; Smedts, F.; Latijnhouwers, M.A.; Ruijter, E.T.; Aalders, T.W.; de la Rosette, J.J.; Debruyne, F.M.; Schalken, J.A. Tenascin-C expression in prostatic intraepithelial neoplasia (PIN): A marker of progression? *Anticancer Res.* **1998**, *18*, 2679–2684.

40. Ni, W.-D.; Yang, Z.-T.; Cui, C.-A.; Cui, Y.; Fang, L.-Y.; Xuan, Y.-H. Tenascin-C is a potential cancer-associated fibroblasts marker and predicts poor prognosis in prostate cancer. *Biochem. Biophys. Res. Commun.* **2017**, *486*, 607–612. [CrossRef]
41. Cai, M.; Onoda, K.; Takao, M.; Kyoko, I.-Y.; Shimpo, H.; Yoshida, T.; Yada, I. Degradation of tenascin-C and activity of matrix metalloproteinase-2 are associated with tumor recurrence in early stage non-small cell lung cancer. *Clin. Cancer Res.* **2002**, *8*, 1152–1156.
42. Kusagawa, H.; Onoda, K.; Namikawa, S.; Yada, I.; Okada, A.; Yoshida, T.; Sakakura, T. Expression and degeneration of tenascin-C in human lung cancers. *Br. J. Cancer* **1998**, *77*, 98–102. [CrossRef] [PubMed]
43. San Martin, R.; Pathak, R.; Jain, A.; Jung, S.Y.; Hilsenbeck, S.G.; Piña-Barba, M.C.; Sikora, A.G.; Pienta, K.J.; Rowley, D.R. Tenascin-C and integrin $\alpha 9$ mediate interactions of prostate cancer with the bone microenvironment. *Cancer Res.* **2017**, *77*, 5977–5988. [CrossRef] [PubMed]
44. Colombel, M.; Eaton, C.L.; Hamdy, F.; Ricci, E.; van der Pluijm, G.; Cecchini, M.; Mege-Lechevallier, F.; Clezardin, P.; Thalmann, G. Increased expression of putative cancer stem cell markers in primary prostate cancer is associated with progression of bone metastases. *Prostate* **2012**, *72*, 713–720. [CrossRef] [PubMed]
45. Lowy, C.M.; Oskarsson, T. Tenascin C in metastasis: A view from the invasive front. *Cell Adh. Migr.* **2015**, *9*, 112–124. [CrossRef]
46. Mishra, P.; Kiebish, M.A.; Cullen, J.; Srinivasan, A.; Patterson, A.; Sarangarajan, R.; Narain, N.R.; Dobi, A. Genomic alterations of Tenascin C in highly aggressive prostate cancer: A meta-analysis. *Genes Cancer* **2019**, *10*, 150–159. [CrossRef]
47. Kiebish, M.A.; Cullen, J.; Mishra, P.; Ali, A.; Milliman, E.; Rodrigues, L.O.; Chen, E.Y.; Tolstikov, V.; Zhang, L.; Panagopoulos, K.; et al. Multi-omic serum biomarkers for prognosis of disease progression in prostate cancer. *J. Transl. Med.* **2020**, *18*, 1–10. [CrossRef]
48. Jachetti, E.; Caputo, S.; Mazzoleni, S.; Brambillasca, C.S.; Parigi, S.M.; Grioni, M.; Piras, I.S.; Restuccia, U.; Calcinotto, A.; Freschi, M.; et al. Tenascin-C protects cancer stem–like cells from immune surveillance by arresting T-cell activation. *Cancer Res.* **2015**, *75*, 2095–2108. [CrossRef]
49. Lapointe, J.; Li, C.; Higgins, J.P.; van de Rijn, M.; Bair, E.; Montgomery, K.; Ferrari, M.; Egevad, L.; Rayford, W.; Bergerheim, U.; et al. Gene expression profiling identifies clinically relevant subtypes of prostate cancer. *Proc. Natl. Acad. Sci. USA* **2004**. [CrossRef]
50. Varambally, S.; Yu, J.; Laxman, B.; Rhodes, D.R.; Mehra, R.; Tomlins, S.A.; Shah, R.B.; Chandran, U.; Monzon, F.A.; Becich, M.J.; et al. Integrative genomic and proteomic analysis of prostate cancer reveals signatures of metastatic progression. *Cancer Cell.* **2005**. [CrossRef]
51. Beltran, H.; Eng, K.; Mosquera, J.M.; Sigaras, A.; Romanel, A.; Rennert, H.; Kossai, M.; Pauli, C.; Faltas, B.; Fontugne, J.; et al. Whole-exome sequencing of metastatic cancer and biomarkers of treatment response. *JAMA Oncol.* **2015**, *1*, 466–474. [CrossRef]
52. Dobin, A.; Davis, C.A.; Schlesinger, F.; Drenkow, J.; Zaleski, C.; Jha, S.; Batut, P.; Chaisson, M.; Gingeras, T.R. STAR: Ultrafast universal RNA-seq aligner. *Bioinformatics* **2013**, *29*, 15–21. [CrossRef] [PubMed]
53. Nikolayeva, O.; Robinson, M.D. Edger for differential RNA-seq and ChIP-seq analysis: An application to stem cell biology. *Methods Mol. Biol.* **2014**, *1150*, 45–79.
54. Yu, G.; Wang, L.G.; Han, Y.; He, Q.Y. clusterProfiler: An R package for comparing biological themes among gene clusters. *OMICS: J. Integr. Biol.* **2012**, *16*, 284–287. [CrossRef]
55. Hart, T.; Komori, H.K.; LaMere, S.; Podshivalova, K.; Salomon, D.R. Finding the active genes in deep RNA-seq gene expression studies. *BMC Genom.* **2013**, *14*, 778. [CrossRef]
56. Cancer Genome Atlas Research, N. The molecular taxonomy of primary prostate cancer. *Cell* **2015**, *163*, 1011–1025.
57. Hoadley, K.A.; Yau, C.; Hinoue, T.; Wolf, D.M.; Lazar, A.J.; Drill, E.; Shen, R.; Taylor, A.M.; Cherniack, A.D.; Thorsson, V.; et al. Cell-of-origin patterns dominate the molecular classification of 10,000 tumors from 33 types of cancer. *Cell* **2018**, *173*, 291–304.e6. [CrossRef] [PubMed]
58. Hänzelmann, S.; Castelo, R.; Guinney, J. GSVA: Gene set variation analysis for microarray and RNA-seq data. *BMC Bioinform.* **2013**, *14*, 7. [CrossRef]
59. Hughes, C.S.; Foehr, S.; Garfield, D.A.; Furlong, E.E.; Steinmetz, L.M.; Krijgsveld, J. Ultrasensitive proteome analysis using paramagnetic bead technology. *Mol. Syst. Biol.* **2014**, *10*, 757. [CrossRef]
60. Moggridge, S.; Sorensen, P.H.; Morin, G.B.; Hughes, C.S. Extending the compatibility of the SP3 paramagnetic bead processing approach for proteomics. *J. Proteome. Res.* **2018**, *17*, 1730–1740. [CrossRef]

61. Werner, T.; Sweetman, G.; Savitski, M.F.; Mathieson, T.; Bantscheff, M.; Savitski, M.M. Ion coalescence of neutron encoded TMT 10-plex reporter ions. *Anal. Chem.* **2014**, *86*, 3594–3601. [CrossRef]
62. Becher, I.; Andres-Pons, A.; Romanov, N.; Stein, F.; Schramm, M.; Baudin, F.; Helm, D.; Kurzawa, N.; Mateus, A.; Mackmull, M.T.; et al. Pervasive protein thermal stability variation during the cell cycle. *Cell* **2018**, *173*, 1495–1507.e18. [CrossRef] [PubMed]
63. Franken, H.; Mathieson, T.; Childs, D.; Sweetman, G.M.; Werner, T.; Togel, I.; Doce, C.; Gade, S.; Bantscheff, M.; Drewes, G.; et al. Thermal proteome profiling for unbiased identification of direct and indirect drug targets using multiplexed quantitative mass spectrometry. *Nat. Protoc.* **2015**, *10*, 1567–1593. [CrossRef] [PubMed]
64. Savitski, M.M.; Wilhelm, M.; Hahne, H.; Kuster, B.; Bantscheff, M. A scalable approach for protein false discovery rate estimation in large proteomic data sets. *Mol. Cell. Proteomics.* **2015**, *14*, 2394–2404. [CrossRef] [PubMed]
65. Huber, W.; von Heydebreck, A.; Sultmann, H.; Poustka, A.; Vingron, M. Variance stabilization applied to microarray data calibration and to the quantification of differential expression. *Bioinformatics* **2002**, *18* (Suppl. S1), S96–S104. [CrossRef]
66. Efron, B. Large-scale simultaneous hypothesis testing. *J. Am. Statist. Assoc.* **2004**, *99*, 96–104. [CrossRef]
67. Strimmer, K. fdrtool: A versatile R package for estimating local and tail area-based false discovery rates. *Bioinformatics* **2008**, *24*, 1461–1462. [CrossRef]
68. Bankhead, P.; Loughrey, M.B.; Fernández, J.A.; Dombrowski, Y.; McArt, D.G.; Dunne, P.D.; McQuaid, S.; Gray, R.T.; Murray, L.J.; Coleman, H.G.; et al. QuPath: Open source software for digital pathology image analysis. *Sci. Rep.* **2017**, *7*, 16878. [CrossRef]
69. Therneau, T. A Package for Survival Analysis in S. 2015. Available online: https://www.mayo.edu/research/documents/tr53pdf/doc-10027379 (accessed on 28 September 2020).
70. Therneau, T. *PMG: Modeling Survival Data: Extending the Cox Model*; Springer: New York, NY, USA, 2000.
71. Wickham, H. *ggplot2: Elegant Graphics for Data Analysis*; Springer: New York, NY, USA, 2016.
72. RStudio Team. *RStudio: Integrated Development for R.*; RStudio: Boston, MI, USA, 2016.
73. R Core Team. *R: A language and Environment for Statistical Computing*; ARFfSC: Vienna, Austria, 2019.

14

Analysis of CXCL9, PD1 and PD-L1 mRNA in Stage T1 Non-Muscle Invasive Bladder Cancer and their Association with Prognosis

Jennifer Kubon [1,†], Danijel Sikic [1,†,‡], Markus Eckstein [2,‡], Veronika Weyerer [2,‡], Robert Stöhr [2,‡], Angela Neumann [1], Bastian Keck [1,‡], Bernd Wullich [1,‡], Arndt Hartmann [2,‡], Ralph M. Wirtz [3,‡], Helge Taubert [1,*,‡,§] and Sven Wach [1,‡,§]

1. Department of Urology and Pediatric Urology, University Hospital Erlangen, Friedrich-Alexander Universität Erlangen-Nürnberg, 91054 Erlangen, Germany; jennifer.kubon@fau.de (J.K.); danijel.sikic@uk-erlangen.de (D.S.); Angela.Neumann@uk-erlangen.de (A.N.); bastian.keck@web.de (B.K.); Bernd.Wullich@uk-erlangen.de (B.W.); sven.wach@uk-erlangen.de (S.W.)
2. Institute of Pathology, University Hospital Erlangen, Friedrich-Alexander Universität Erlangen-Nürnberg, 91054 Erlangen, Germany; Markus.Eckstein@uk-erlangen.de (M.E.); veronika.weyerer@uk-erlangen.de (V.W.); robert.stoehr@uk-erlangen.de (R.S.); arndt.hartmann@uk-erlangen.de (A.H.)
3. STRATIFYER Molecular Pathology GmbH, 50935 Cologne, Germany; ralph.wirtz@stratifyer.de

* Correspondence: helge.taubert@uk-erlangen.de

† These authors share equal contribution.

‡ Authors belong to Bridge Consortium, 12049 Berlin, Germany.

§ These authors share equal senior authorship.

Simple Summary: Non-muscle invasive bladder cancer (NMIBC) patients possess a high rate of recurrences and very long treatment times, which remains a major unresolved problem for them and the health care system. We analyzed the mRNA of three immune markers, *CXCL9, PD1* and *PD-L1*, in 80 NMIBC by qRT-PCR. Lower *CXCL9* mRNA appeared to be an independent prognostic parameter for reduced OS and RFS. Furthermore, low *PD-L1* mRNA was an independent prognostic factor for DSS and RFS. In univariate Cox's regression analysis, the stratification of patients revealed that low *CXCL9* or *PD1* mRNA was associated with reduced RFS in the patient group younger than 72 years. Low *CXCL9* or *PD-L1* was associated with shorter RFS in patients with higher tumor cell proliferation or without instillation therapy. In conclusion, the characterization of mRNA levels of the immune markers *CXCL9*, *PD1* and *PD-L1* differentiates NIMBC patients with respect to prognosis.

Abstract: Non-muscle invasive bladder cancer (NMIBC), which is characterized by a recurrence rate of approximately 30% and very long treatment times, remains a major unresolved problem for patients and the health care system. The immunological interplay between tumor cells and the immune environment is important for tumor development. Therefore, we analyzed the mRNA of three immune markers, *CXCL9*, *PD1* and *PD-L1*, in NMIBC by qRT-PCR. The results were subsequently correlated with clinicopathological parameters and prognostic data. Altogether, as expected, higher age was an independent prognostic factor for overall survival (OS) and disease-specific survival (DSS), but not for recurrence-free survival (RFS). Lower *CXCL9* mRNA was observed in multivariate Cox's regression analysis to be an independent prognostic parameter for reduced OS (relative risk; RR = 2.08; $p = 0.049$), DSS (RR = 4.49; $p = 0.006$) and RFS (RR = 2.69; $p = 0.005$). In addition, *PD-L1* mRNA was an independent prognostic factor for DSS (RR = 5.02; $p = 0.042$) and RFS (RR = 2.07; $p = 0.044$). Moreover, in univariate Cox's regression analysis, the stratification of patients revealed that low *CXCL9* or low PD1 mRNA was associated with reduced RFS in the younger patient group (≤71 years), but not in the older patient group (>71 years). In addition, low *CXCL9* or low *PD-L1* was associated with shorter RFS in patients with higher tumor cell proliferation and in patients without instillation therapy. In conclusion, the characterization of mRNA levels of immune markers differentiates NIMBC patients with respect to prognosis.

Keywords: *CXCL9*; *PD1*; *PD-L1*; stage T1 NMIBC; prognosis

---

1. Introduction

Urothelial bladder cancer (BCa) accounts for approximately 3% of global cancer diagnoses. It was recently reported to be the 10th most commonly diagnosed cancer and the 13th leading cause of cancer-related death worldwide [1]. Approximately 25% of BCas are categorized as muscle-invasive BCa (MIBC) and 75% as non-muscle invasive BCa (NMIBC) [2]. NMIBC treatment comprises transurethral resection of the bladder (TURB) and, depending on the risk of progression, instillation with bacillus Calmette-Guerin (BCG) or mitomycin [3–5]. However, high-risk NMIBC remains a challenge because 30% to 60% of patients with stage pT1 NMIBC develop local recurrence, and up to 20% experience disease progression to MIBC [6–8]. There is heterogeneity in stage pT1 NMIBC, and its risk stratification is based only on clinicopathological parameters that necessitate lifelong follow-up [9]. Altogether, bladder cancers, including NMIBC, impose the highest costs on society among cancers per patient from diagnosis to death [10]. However, bladder tumor markers cannot yet definitively replace cystoscopy in surveillance regimens [10]. Therefore, the continued search for biomarkers in bladder cancer is necessary.

The tumor biology of BCa, including NMIBC, is related to cell lineage and cell proliferation [11–13]. Therefore, we included an analysis of the mRNA of keratin 5 (*KRT5*; basal-like lineage), keratin 20 (*KRT20*; luminal-like lineage) and marker of proliferation KI67 (*MKI67*, *KI67*) in this study. Furthermore, studies conducted by other groups, as well as our own previous studies, showed that gene expression can differentiate NMIBCs into subsets that possess different risk profiles, and may impact treatment decisions in the future [14,15].

In the current study, we investigated the expression of genes associated with tumor immune status and their association with prognosis in stage pT1 NMIBC. Recently, we reported that a cytotoxic T-cell-related gene expression signature containing three genes (*CXCL9*, *CD3 Z*, *CD8*) correlates with immune cell infiltration, and predicts improved survival in MIBC patients after radical cystectomy and adjuvant chemotherapy [16]. All three immune signature genes were strongly associated with each other, which is why we chose only *CXCL9* for the current analysis. Additionally, we chose programmed cell death 1 gene (*PD1/PDCD1*) and programmed cell death ligand 1 (*PD-L1/CD274/B7-H1*) since they are also very prominent in the immune response of MIBC, and represent therapeutic targets for MIBC [16–18]. *CXCL9* (*SCYB9/MIG*) and *CXCL10* (*SCYB10*) genes are located in chromosome band 4 q21 [19], and belong to the CXC family of chemokines [20]. *CXCL9* encodes a T-cell chemoattractant that is significantly induced by interferon gamma, which mediates a T-cell-driven antitumoral immune response [21]. *CXCL9* has not been previously studied in NMIBC. The *PD1* gene has been mapped to the chromosome region 2 q37.3 by the Honyo group [22]. It encodes a cell surface receptor on T-cells and tumor-associated macrophages (TAMs), and is a member of the B7 superfamily involved in immunomodulation. PD1 acts as an inhibitory molecule on T-cells/TAMs after interacting with its ligand PD-L1 [23,24]. The *PD-L1* gene is located on chromosome 9 p24.1 and codes for a costimulatory molecule that negatively regulates cell-mediated immune responses [23,25]. PD-L1 is expressed by both tumor cells and tumor-associated antigen-presenting cells [26]. Le Goux et al. [27] did not find an association between *PD1* or *PD-L1* gene expression and prognosis (RFS and progression-free survival) in NMIBC. We recently demonstrated in an NMIBC cohort that increased *PD-L1* mRNA was an independent prognostic indicator for both RFS and DSS [28]. However, in that study, *PD1* mRNA was not associated with prognosis [28].

In this study, we analyzed a new independent cohort of NMIBC patients with extended follow-up periods to reassess the long-term association of *PD-L1* mRNA with disease prognosis, and to determine whether the two immune markers *CXCL9* and *PD1* are associated with survival.

2. Results

2.1. Correlations of CXCL9, PD1, PD-L1, KRT5 and KRT20 mRNA with Each Other and with Clinicopathological Parameters

CXCL9 mRNA negatively correlated with the incidence of recurrence (correlation coefficient; $r_s = -0.374$; $p = 0.001$) and with mRNA of *KRT20* ($r_s = -0.305$; $p = 0.006$) and *KRT5* ($r_s = -0.230$; $p = 0.040$), and is positively correlated with mRNA of *PD1* ($r_s = 0.639$; $p < 0.001$) and *PD-L1* ($r_s = 0.601$; $p < 0.001$) (Table 1). *PD1* mRNA was negatively correlated with mRNA of *KRT20* ($r_s = -0.253$; $p = 0.024$) and *KI67* ($r_s = -0.222$; $p = 0.047$), and positively correlated with time of RFS ($r_s = 0.298$; $p = 0.007$) and *PD-L1* mRNA ($r_s = 0.459$; $p < 0.001$). *PD-L1* mRNA negatively correlated with *KRT20* ($r_s = -0.233$; $p = 0.038$) (Table 1).

Table 1. Bivariate correlations for mRNA of *CXCL9, KRT20, KRT5, PD1, PD-L1* and *KI67* with clinicopathological parameters.

Bivariate Correlations		*KRT20*	*KRT5*	*PD1*	*PD-L1*	*KI67*	Fu_Recurr	Recurr
CXCL9	Correlation coefficient	−0.305	−0.230	0.639	0.601	−0.136	0.208	−0.374
	Sig. (2-sided)	**0.006**	0.040	**<0.001**	**<0.001**	0.228	0.065	**0.001**
KRT20	Correlation coefficient		−0.042	−0.253	−0.233	0.356	−0.152	0.116
	Sig. (2-sided)		0.714	0.024	0.038	**0.001**	0.178	0.304
KRT5	Correlation coefficient			−0.212	0.036	−0.070	0.039	0.067
	Sig. (2-sided)			0.059	0.753	0.537	0.733	0.557
PD1	Correlation coefficient				0.459	−0.222	0.298	−0.204
	Sig. (2-sided)				**<0.001**	0.047	**0.007**	0.070
PD-L1	Correlation coefficient					0.001	0.096	−0.215
	Sig. (2-sided)					0.994	0.397	0.055
KI67	Correlation coefficient						−0.152	0.138
	Sig. (2-sided)						0.177	0.222
fu_recurr	Correlation coefficient							−0.562
	Sig. (2-sided)							**<0.001**

Abbreviation: fu recur—follow-up recurrence (time until occurrence of recurrence); recur.—recurrence. Bonferroni correction results in $\alpha = 0.00714$. Significance at the α level is marked in bold.

2.2. Association of CXCL9, PD1, PD-L1, KRT5 and KRT20 mRNA with NMIBC Prognosis

The association of mRNA in the 80 tumor samples with patient survival was examined by Kaplan–Meier analysis. As expected, age was associated with both OS and DSS ($p = 0.019$ and $p = 0.025$). However, *CXCL9, PD1* and *PD-L1* mRNA was not associated with OS or DSS (Table 2).

Interestingly, higher *CXCL9* ($p < 0.001$), *PD1* ($p = 0.023$) or *PD-L1* ($p = 0.007$) mRNA were associated with increased RFS (all Kaplan–Meier analyses, Table 2; Figure 1).

Table 2. Kaplan–Meier analysis of the association of age, *CXCL9*, *PD1* and *PD-L1* mRNA with prognosis.

Parameter	Kaplan–Meier Analysis								
	n	OS Months	*p*	*n*	DSS Months	*p*	*n*	RFS Months	*p*
Age									
≤71 vs. >71 year	40 vs. 40	124.8 vs. 84.5	**0.019**	40 vs. 40	170.2 vs. 108.3	**0.025**	40 vs. 40	n.s.	n.s.
CXCL9									
low vs. high	32 vs. 48	n.s.	n.s.	25 vs. 55	n.s.	n.s.	32 vs. 48	38.7 vs. 87.4	**<0.001**
PD1									
low vs. high	40 vs. 40	n.s.	n.s.	40 vs. 40	n.s.	n.s.	53 vs. 27	62.0 vs. 99.5	**0.023**
PD-L1									
low vs. high	24 vs. 56	n.s.	n.s.	46 vs. 34	n.s.	n.s.	46 vs. 34	58.6 vs. 102.7	**0.007**

Significant values are in bold face. Abbreviation: n.s., not significant.

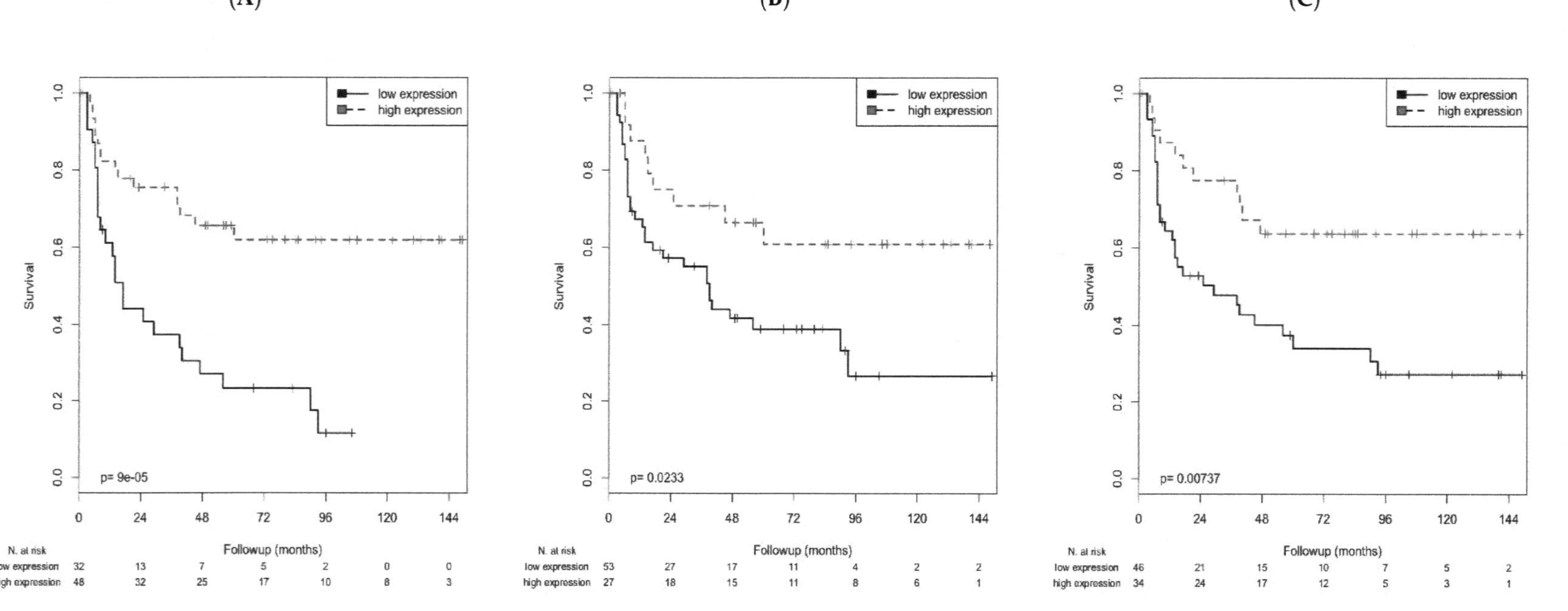

Figure 1. Kaplan–Meier analysis of the association of *CXCL9*, *PD1* or *PD-L1* mRNA with RFS. Gene expression was significantly associated with RFS for the genes. (**A**): *CXCL9* ($p < 0.001$). (**B**): *PD1* ($p = 0.023$). (**C**): *PD-L1* ($p = 0.007$).

In univariate Cox's regression analysis, the clinicopathological parameters of histological grade, tumor stage (pT1 with/without presence of cis), intravesical therapy and gender, and the molecular parameters *KI67*, *KRT5* and *KRT20*, were not associated with prognosis (OS, DSS, RFS), and therefore were not included in further multivariate Cox's regression analysis (data not shown).

As expected, in univariate Cox's regression analysis, higher age (RR = 2.29; p = 0.022) was associated with an increased risk of shorter OS. Furthermore, higher age (RR = 3.44; p = 0.034) was associated with increased risk of shorter DSS (Table 3).

Table 3. Univariate Cox's regression analysis for the association of age and *CXCL9, PD1* and *PD-L1* mRNA with prognosis.

	Univariate Cox's Regression Analysis								
Parameter	*n*	**OS RR**	*p*	*n*	**DSS RR**	*p*	*n*	**RFS RR**	*p*
Age ≤71 vs. >71 year	40 vs. 40	2.29	**0.022**	40 vs. 40	3.44	**0.034**	40 vs. 40	n.s.	n.s.
CXCL9						n.s.			
low vs. high	32 vs. 48	n.s.	n.s.	25 vs. 55	n.s.	n.s.	21 vs. 59	3.30	**<0.001**
PD1 low vs. high	40 vs. 40	n.s.	n.s.	40 vs. 40	n.s.	n.s.	53 vs. 27	2.31	**0.027**
PD-L1 low vs. high	24 vs. 56	n.s.	**n.s.**	46 vs. 34	n.s.	n.s.	46 vs. 34	2.51	**0.009**

Significant values are in bold face. Abbreviation: n.s., not significant.

In univariate Cox's regression analysis, lower *CXCL9* (RR = 3.30; $p < 0.001$), lower *PD1* (RR = 2.31; p = 0.027) and lower *PD-L1* (RR = 2.51; p = 0.009) mRNA showed an increased risk for shorter RFS. However, age was not associated with an increased risk of shorter RFS (Table 3).

In multivariate Cox's regression analysis (adjusted for age and the molecular parameters *PD1*, *PD-L1* and *CXCL9*), an association with OS was found for higher age (RR = 2.31; p = 0.021) and lower *CXCL9* (RR = 2.08; p = 0.049) mRNA (Table 4). Multivariate analysis (adjusted for age and the molecular parameters *PD1*, *PD-L1* and *CXCL9*) revealed associations with DSS for higher age (RR = 4.47; p = 0.014), lower *CXCL9* (RR = 4.49; p = 0.006) and lower *PD-L1* (RR = 5.02; p = 0.042) mRNA (Table 4).

Table 4. Multivariate Cox's regression analysis for the association of age and *CXCL9, PD1* and PD-L1 mRNA with prognosis.

	Multivariate Cox's Regression Analysis								
Parameter	*n*	**OS RR**	*p*	*n*	**DSS RR**	*p*	*n*	**RFS RR**	*p*
Age ≤71 vs. >71 year	40 vs. 40	2.31	**0.021**	40 vs. 40	4.47	**0.014**	40 vs. 40	*n.s.*	*n.s.*
CXCL9 low vs. high	32 vs. 48	2.08	**0.049**	25 vs. 55	4.49	**0.006**	21 vs. 59	2.69	**0.005**
PD1 low vs. high	40 vs. 40	*n.s*	*n.s*	40 vs. 40	*n.s.*	*n.s.*	53 vs. 27	*n.s.*	*n.s.*
PD-L1 low vs. high	24 vs. 56	*n.s.*	*n.s.*	46 vs. 34	5.02	**0.042**	46 vs. 34	2.07	**0.044**

Significant values are in bold face. Abbreviation: n.s., not significant.

Furthermore, in the multivariate Cox's regression analysis, associations with shorter RFS were found for lower *CXCL9* (RR = 2.69; p = 0.005) and lower *PD-L1* (RR = 2.07; p = 0.044) mRNA (Table 4).

Altogether, as expected, higher age was an independent prognostic factor for OS and DSS, but not for RFS. *CXCL9* mRNA was as independent prognostic parameter for OS, DSS and RFS. In addition, *PD-L1* mRNA was an independent prognostic factor for DSS and RFS.

2.3. *Association of CXCL9, PD1, PD-L1, KRT5 and KRT20 mRNA with RFS Stratified by Clinicopathological Parameters or mRNA*

2.3.1. Stratification by Age

Using the median age of 71 years as a cut-off to define the two age groups (≤71 vs. >71 years), age itself was not associated with RFS (Table 4). In the univariate Cox's regression analysis in the younger age group, low *CXCL9* (RR = 6.21; $p = < 0.001$) was associated with an increased risk of recurrence (Table 5). This finding is in accordance with the above mentioned results for all patients, but it indicates the greater relevance of *CXCL9* mRNA in younger patients. Low *PD1* mRNA was only associated with a risk of shorter RFS in the younger patient group (RR = 4.93; $p = 0.035$). Altogether, the higher risks of recurrence for *CXCL9* and low *PD1* levels were only relevant to the younger age group (Table 5).

Table 5. Univariate Cox's regression analysis for stratification by clinicopathological or molecular parameters: the association of *CXCL9, PD1* and *PD-L1* mRNA with RFS.

Parameter by Stratification	Univariate Cox's Regression Analysis		
	n	RFS RR	*p*
Strata age: young patients	40		
CXCL9 low vs. high	15 vs. 25	6.21	**<0.001**
PD1 low vs. high	27 vs.13	4.93	**0.035**
Strata KRT5 low	40		
CXCL9 low vs. high	13 vs. 27	3.76	**0.004**
Strata KRT5 high	40		
CXCL9 low vs. high	19 vs. 21	3.33	**0.013**
PD-L1 low vs. high	22 vs. 18	3.68	**0.012**
Strata KRT20 low	40		
CXCL9 low vs. high	13 vs. 27	3.04	**0.019**
Strata KRT20 high	40		
CXCL9 low vs. high	19 vs. 21	3.28	**0.007**
PD-L1 low vs. high	25 vs. 15	4.23	**0.009**
Strata *KI67* high	40		
CXCL9 low vs. high	19 vs. 21	4.54	**<0.001**
PD-L1 low vs. high	25 vs. 15	7.49	**0.001**
Strata: no intravesical	39		
CXCL9 low vs. high	15 vs. 24	10.33	**<0.001**
PD1 low vs. high	23 vs. 16	5.31	**0.010**
PD-L1 low vs. high	22 vs. 17	4.36	**0.022**

Significant values are in bold face.

2.3.2. Stratification by *KRT5* or *KRT20* Expression

KRT5 or *KRT20* mRNA is considered a characteristic feature for a basal or luminal lineage, respectively, in bladder cancer [11]. We utilized the expressions of both mRNA markers as proxies to define a more basal or more luminal-like gene expression pattern, respectively. The expression of both markers was separated by median expression into two groups with low/high *KRT5* (≤36.78 vs. >36.78) or low/high *KRT20* (≤37.47 vs. >37.47) mRNA level. In low and high *KRT20* groups, *CXCL9* mRNA was associated with a shorter RFS (RR = 3.04; $p = 0.019$ and RR = 3.28, respectively; $p = 0.007$) (Table 5). Similarly, low *CXCL9* mRNA was associated with a shorter RFS in the low and high *KRT5* groups (RR = 3.76; $p = 0.004$ and RR = 3.33; $p = 0.013$, respectively; Table 5). These results were expected since they reflected findings for all patients. In the high *KRT5* and high *KRT20* groups, low *PD-L1* mRNA was associated with shorter RFS (RR = 3.68; $p = 0.012$ and RR = 4.23, respectively; $p = 0.009$; Table 5), but this was not so in the low *KRT5* or low *KRT20* group.

2.3.3. Stratification by *KI67*

KI67 characterizes the proliferation activity of tumor cells [29]. *KI67* expression was separated into two groups (low vs. high expression) by median mRNA (≤33.10 vs. >33.10). In the high *KI67* expression group, low *CXCL9* (RR = 4.54; $p < 0.001$) mRNA and low *PD-L1* (RR = 7.49; $p = 0.001$; Table 5) mRNA were associated with a higher risk of shorter RFS, but these associations were not observed in the low *KI67* group.

2.3.4. Stratification by Intravesical Therapy

Intravesical therapy was not associated with RFS in this study group. In the group with no intravesical therapy, low *CXCL9* (RR = 10.33; $p < 0.001$), low *PD1* (RR = 5.31; $p = 0.010$) and low *PD-L1* (RR = 4.36; $p = 0.022$; Table 5) mRNA was associated with the increased risk of shorter RFS, but no associations were observed with RFS in the intravesical group.

Altogether, *CXCL9* mRNA was associated with RFS in all stratification approaches. Interestingly, the increased risk of shorter RFS in low *CXCL9* mRNA patients was substantiated in the young patient group, the high *KI67* group and in patients without instillation, but it showed no association with RFS in the older patient group, the low *KI67* group or the instillation group.

In addition, the increased risk observed with low *PD1* levels was assigned to the younger patient group and the no instillation group, with no association with RFS being observed in the older patient group or the instillation patient group.

For the third marker, *PD-L1*, an increased risk of shorter RFS with low *PD-L1* mRNA was detected only in the high *KRT5* and high *KRT20* groups, but not in the low *KRT5* or low *KRT20* groups. In addition, this risk was found in the high *KI67* and the no instillation group, but not in the low *KI67* group or the instillation group.

3. Discussion

In this study, we investigated the mRNA of the immune markers CXCL9, PD1 and PD-L1. First, we correlated mRNA data with clinicopathological data and with each other. We observed that *CXCL9* mRNA was positively correlated with transcript levels of *PD1* and *PD-L1*, but negatively correlated with incidence of recurrence, as well as *KRT5* and *KRT20* mRNA. In addition, PD1 was positively correlated with *PD-L1* mRNA and time to RFS, while being negatively correlated with *KRT20* mRNA. *PD-L1* mRNA was additionally negatively correlated with *KRT20* mRNA.

Similar to Huang et al. we showed a correlation between the mRNA of *PD-L1* and *C-C chemokines* (*CCL2, CCL3, CCL8* and *CCL18*) [30,31]. A correlation between *PD1* and *PD-L1* mRNA was previously shown by both Huang et al. [31] and by us [28]. These correlations can all be explained by the common expression of these factors by immune cells, i.e., leukocytes such as T-cells and macrophages.

In this study, multivariate Cox's regression analyses revealed that high *CXCL9* mRNA was associated with longer OS and DSS, and high *PD-L1* mRNA was correlated with longer DSS. In addition, the high mRNA of *CXCL9* or *PD-L1* was significantly associated with longer RFS. Huang and colleagues found that elevated *PD-L1* mRNA was associated with reduced patient survival (OS, DSS), but they studied a mixed cohort of NMIBC and MIBC where the association could have been influenced by MIBC patients, and further, they did not examine RFS [31]. We previously found that increased *PD-L1* mRNA expression was associated with longer DSS and RFS in pT1 NMIBC [28]. In this study, we confirmed the association of high *PD-L1* mRNA with DSS and RFS. However, the impact of *PD-L1* on OS, DSS and RFS need to be evaluated further in prospective studies.

PD1 was previously not described to be associated with RFS [28], but in this study, we observed an association between increased *PD1* mRNA and longer RFS. Although both studies were performed in consecutive patients, in this study, observation time was longer (62 vs. 42 months), and the numbers of recurrences (51.3% vs. 33.4%) were higher than in the previous study, which may explain the differential results.

CXCL9 mRNA level has not been previously described in NMIBC to be associated with OS, DSS or RFS. The effect of an immune intravesical therapy with bacillus Calmette-Guérin (BCG) on *CXCL9* mRNA was controversially discussed. BCG therapy upregulates the mRNA of different chemokines, including *CXCL9*, in an in vivo mouse model [32]. Interestingly, using an in vitro approach in established human BCa cell lines, Özcan et al. demonstrated that BCG treatment reduced *CXCL9* mRNA [33]. This supports the assumption that the tumor microenvironment is responsible for the chemokine reaction following BCG therapy. A recent review reports that the CXCL9/CXCL10/CXCL11/CXCR3 axis is responsible for angiogenesis inhibition, and the activation and migration of immune cells such as cytotoxic lymphocytes and natural killer cells into the tumor microenvironment, to prevent tumor progression in BCa [34].

Next, we were interested in whether the association of *CXCL9*, *PD1* and *PD-L1* mRNA with RFS could be further stratified by clinicopathological parameter (age) or other parameters applied for lineage differentiation, such as *KRT5* or *KRT20* mRNA, proliferation activity (*KI67*), or therapeutic application (instillation therapy). Interestingly, after separating patients by their median age (≤71 vs. >71 years), only in the younger age group (≤71 years) was higher *CXCL9* or higher *PD1* mRNA associated with longer RFS. This finding could be simply related to the fact that the immune system is more active in younger than in older persons, in whom immunosenescence has been reported [35]. Increasing multi morbidity affecting health status in elderly patients may also play a role in shorter RFS, although time to recurrence was not significantly different between the age groups (data not shown).

KRT5 and *KRT20* are considered intrinsic markers for basal and luminal subtypes of muscle-invasive bladder cancer, respectively [11,36,37]. Interestingly, high *PD-L1* mRNA was associated with longer RFS in both high *KRT5* and high *KRT20* groups, but not in the low *KRT5* or low *KRT20* groups. This finding suggests that high *PD-L1* mRNA is favorable for longer RFS in both basal and luminal subtypes of NMIBC. We previously showed that high *KRT20* mRNA was associated with shorter RFS [38]. In this context, *PD-L1* mRNA further distinguishes the unfavorable RFS group (high *KRT20*) in patients with longer RFS (*PD-L1* high) or shorter RFS (*PD-L1* low).

High KI67 expression has been described as a prognostic factor for poor OS, DSS, RFS and PFS in a meta-analysis of NMIBC patients [12]. In the high *KI67* group, high *CXCL9* and high *PD-L1* mRNA were associated with longer RFS, but this association was not observed in the low *KI67* group. In this way, within the unfavorable high *KI67* group, patients with longer RFS (high *CXCL9* or high *PD-L1*) and with shorter RFS (low *CXCL9* or low *PD-L1*) could be distinguished.

Intravesical therapy with either BCG or cytostatic drugs, like mitomycin, is mostly standard therapy for intermediate or high risk NMIBC, but its application differs between several guidelines [3,5]. Interestingly, only in the no instillation group was high *CXCL9*, high *PD1* or high *PD-L1* associated with longer RFS compared to the instillation group. One explanation for this finding could be that BCG therapy affects the immune response of patients, and *CXCL9*, *PD1* and *PD-L1* reflect intrinsic immune status. In this way, both the expression of the immune markers and the intravesical therapy may influence each other. As mentioned above, the BCG exposure of established BCa cell lines devoid of any tumor microenvironment reduced *CXCL9* mRNA in vitro [33]. Furthermore, increases in *PD-L1* protein levels, which are considered a negative prognostic marker, have been reported after BCG therapy compared to before BCG treatment [39].

4. Material and Methods

4.1. Patients and Tumor Material

In this study, we retrospectively analyzed clinical and histopathological data from 80 patients treated with TURB at the Department of Urology and Pediatric Urology of the University Hospital Erlangen between 2000 and 2015 who were initially diagnosed with stage pT1 NMIBC (Table 6). All patients received a Re-TURB within six to eight weeks after the initial TURB. All patients were treated with a bladder-preserving approach. Tissue from formalin-fixed paraffin embedded (FFPE) tumor samples from all patients was evaluated for pathological stage according to the 2010 TNM classification [40], and was graded according to the common grading systems [41,42] by two experienced uropathologists (M.E., A.H.). All specimens contained at least 20% tumor cells. All procedures were performed in accordance with the ethical standards established in the 1964 Declaration of Helsinki and its later amendments. All patients treated after 2008 provided informed consent. For samples collected prior to 2008, the Ethics Committee in Erlangen waived the need for informed individual consent. This study was approved by the Ethics Committee of the University Hospital Erlangen (No. 3755; 2008).

Table 6. Clinicopathological and survival data.

Clinicopathological and Survival Parameters	Patients (Percentage)
Total	80
Gender	
female	19 (23.7)
male	61 (76.3)
Age (years)	
range	46.0–97.0
mean	70.5
median	71.5
Tumor Stage	
pT1	52 (65.0)
pT1 with cis	28 (35.0)
Tumor Grade 1973	
G1	3 (3.7)
G2	28 (35.0)
G3	48 (60.0)
unknown	1 (1.3)
Tumor Grade 2004	
low grade	3 (3.7)
high grade	76 (95.0)
unknown	1 (1.3)
Intravesical Therapy	
yes	41 (51.3)
no	39 (48.7)
Survival/observation Time (months)	
range	0–189.0
mean	71.6
median	62.0
Overall Survival (OS)	
alive	44 (55.0)
dead	36 (45.0)
Disease-Specific Survival (DSS)	
alive	64 (80.0)
dead	16 (20.0)
Recurrence-Free Survival Time (months)	
range	0–149
mean	46.7
median	38.5
Recurrence-Free Survival (RFS)	
without recurrence	39 (48.7)
with recurrence	41 (51.3)

4.2. Assessment of mRNA by qRT-PCR

Tumor specimens were assessed by qRT-PCR as previously described [43]. In short, RNA was extracted from a single 10 µm curl of FFPE tissue and processed according to a commercially available bead-based extraction method (Xtract kit; Stratifyer Molecular Pathology GmbH, Cologne, Germany). RNA was eluted with 100 µL of elution buffer. DNA was digested, and RNA eluates were then stored at −80 °C until use.

The mRNA levels of *CXCL9, PD1, PD-L1, KRT5, KRT20, KI67* and the reference genes *Calmodulin2* (*CALM2*) and *Beta-2 microglobulin* (*B2 M*) were determined by a one-step qRT-PCR using the SuperScript III RT-qPCR system (Invitrogen, Waltham, MA, USA) and gene specific primer-probe combinations (Stratifyer). Each patient sample or control was analyzed in duplicate in an ABI Step One PCR System (ThermoFisher, Darmstadt, Germany) according to the manufacturers' instructions. Gene expression was quantified with a modification of the method by Schmittgen and Livak by calculating 40-ΔCt, whereas ΔCt was calculated as the difference in Ct between the test gene and the mean of the reference genes [38,44].

4.3. Statistical Methods

Correlations between the mRNA of *CXCL9, PD1, PD-L1, KRT5, KRT20* and *KI67* and clinicopathological data were calculated using Spearman's bivariate correlation. Optimized cut-off values for dichotomizing each marker with respect to survival were defined using Youden's index on the receiver operating characteristic (ROC). Detailed information about the calculated optimal cut-off values, the associated area under the ROC curve and internal validation using bootstrapping are provided in Tables S1 and S2. Following standard practice in retrospective survival analysis, the common time point zero for all patients was the date of the first TURB. The associations of mRNA with recurrence-free survival (RFS), overall survival (OS) and cancer-specific survival (CSS) were determined by univariate (Kaplan–Meier analysis and Cox's regression hazard models) and multivariate (Cox's regression hazard models, adjusted for age and the molecular parameters PD1, PD-L1 and CXCL9) analyses. A p-value < 0.05 was considered statistically significant. Statistical analyses were performed with the SPSS 21.0 software package (SPSS Inc., Chicago, IL, USA) and R V3.2.1 (The R foundation for statistical computing, Vienna, Austria).

5. Conclusions

Altogether, we confirmed that high *PD-L1* mRNA is associated with increased DSS and RFS. Furthermore, we demonstrated for the first time that *CXCL9* mRNA is associated with a longer OS, DSS and RFS. Associations with RFS were also identified or further pinpointed to special groups, including the younger age group (*CXCL9, PD1*), the high *KRT5* or high *KRT20* group (*CXCL9, PD-L1*), the high *KI67* group (*CXCL9, PD-L1*) or the no instillation group (*CXCL9, PD-L1*).

An increased mRNA for *PD1, PD-L1* and *CXCL9* being associated with a better prognosis may mirror the host–tumor interaction. In this way, we suggest that the increased mRNA levels of all three genes may reflect the immune response of the host.

Our finding of associations between these immune markers and prognosis may aid in future therapeutic options and decisions.

Author Contributions: D.S., H.T., S.W., R.M.W. and B.K. designed the study. D.S., J.K., S.W., V.W., R.S., A.H. and B.W. acquired the clinical samples and patient information. A.H. and M.E. performed the pathological review of all cases. J.K. and A.N. performed qRT-PCR experiments. H.T., S.W., D.S. and J.K. performed statistical analyses, and H.T., S.W., J.K., D.S., M.E. prepared the tables and figures. H.T., S.W., D.S., B.W., M.E. and A.H. wrote the main manuscript. All authors reviewed the manuscript and approved the final version of the manuscript.

Acknowledgments: The present work was performed in (partial) fulfillment of the requirements for obtaining the degree "Dr. med." (M.D.) of the Friedrich-Alexander-Universität Erlangen-Nürnberg, Medizinische Fakultät for Jennifer Kubon. The authors thank Johannes Breyer (University of Regensburg) and Philipp Erben (Heidelberg University) for helpful discussion. We thank American Journal Experts for editing the manuscript. The authors also acknowledge support from Deutsche Forschungsgemeinschaft and Friedrich-Alexander-Universität Erlangen-Nürnberg within the funding program Open Access Publishing.

Abbreviations

BCa	bladder cancer
CXCL9	Chemokine, CXC motif, ligand 9
DSS	disease-free survival
Fu recur	follow up recurrence
KI67	Proliferation marker KI67
KRT5	Cytokeratin 5
KRT20	Cytokeratin 20
MIBC	muscle invasive bladder cancer
NMIBC	non-muscle invasive bladder cancer
OS	overall survival
n.s.	not significant
n.d.	not determined
PD1	programmed cell death 1
PD-L1	programmed cell death ligand 1
PFS	progression-free survival
pT	pathological tumor stage
pN	pathological lymph node stage
qRT-PCR	quantitative real-time PCR
RFS	recurrence-free survival

References

1. Bray, F.; Ferlay, J.; Soerjomataram, I.; Siegel, R.L.; Torre, L.A.; Jemal, A. Global cancer statistics 2018: GLOBOCAN estimates of incidence and mortality worldwide for 36 cancers in 185 countries. *CA Cancer J. Clin.* **2018**, *68*, 394–424. [CrossRef] [PubMed]
2. Burger, M.; Catto, J.W.; Dalbagni, G.; Grossman, H.B.; Herr, H.; Karakiewicz, P.; Kassouf, W.; Kiemeney, L.A.; La Vecchia, C.; Shariat, S.; et al. Epidemiology and risk factors of urothelial bladder cancer. *Eur. Urol.* **2013**, *63*, 234–241. [CrossRef] [PubMed]
3. Babjuk, M.; Bohle, A.; Burger, M.; Capoun, O.; Cohen, D.; Comperat, E.M.; Hernandez, V.; Kaasinen, E.; Palou, J.; Roupret, M.; et al. EAU Guidelines on Non-Muscle-invasive Urothelial Carcinoma of the Bladder: Update 2016. *Eur. Urol.* **2017**, *71*, 447–461. [CrossRef] [PubMed]
4. Novotny, V.; Froehner, M.; Ollig, J.; Koch, R.; Zastrow, S.; Wirth, M.P. Impact of Adjuvant Intravesical Bacillus Calmette-Guerin Treatment on Patients with High-Grade T1 Bladder Cancer. *Urol. Int.* **2016**, *96*, 136–141. [CrossRef] [PubMed]
5. Zhang, J.; Wang, Y.; Weng, H.; Wang, D.; Han, F.; Huang, Q.; Deng, T.; Wang, X.; Jin, Y. Management of non-muscle-invasive bladder cancer: Quality of clinical practice guidelines and variations in recommendations. *BMC Cancer* **2019**, *19*, 1054. [CrossRef] [PubMed]
6. D'Andrea, D.; Hassler, M.R.; Abufaraj, M.; Soria, F.; Ertl, I.E.; Ilijazi, D.; Mari, A.; Foerster, B.; Egger, G.; Shariat, S.F. Progressive tissue biomarker profiling in non-muscle-invasive bladder cancer. *Expert Rev. Anticancer Ther.* **2018**, *18*, 695–703. [CrossRef]
7. Stein, J.P.; Penson, D.F. Invasive T1 bladder cancer: Indications and rationale for radical cystectomy. *BJU Int.* **2008**, *102*, 270–275. [CrossRef]
8. Thalmann, G.N.; Markwalder, R.; Shahin, O.; Burkhard, F.C.; Hochreiter, W.W.; Studer, U.E. Primary T1G3 bladder cancer: Organ preserving approach or immediate cystectomy? *J. Urol.* **2004**, *172*, 70–75. [CrossRef]

9. van Rhijn, B.W.; Burger, M.; Lotan, Y.; Solsona, E.; Stief, C.G.; Sylvester, R.J.; Witjes, J.A.; Zlotta, A.R. Recurrence and progression of disease in non-muscle-invasive bladder cancer: From epidemiology to treatment strategy. *Eur. Urol.* **2009**, *56*, 430–442. [CrossRef]
10. Hong, Y.M.; Loughlin, K.R. Economic impact of tumor markers in bladder cancer surveillance. *Urology* **2008**, *71*, 131–135. [CrossRef]
11. Choi, W.; Porten, S.; Kim, S.; Willis, D.; Plimack, E.R.; Hoffman-Censits, J.; Roth, B.; Cheng, T.; Tran, M.; Lee, I.L.; et al. Identification of distinct basal and luminal subtypes of muscle-invasive bladder cancer with different sensitivities to frontline chemotherapy. *Cancer Cell* **2014**, *25*, 152–165. [CrossRef] [PubMed]
12. Ko, K.; Jeong, C.W.; Kwak, C.; Kim, H.H.; Ku, J.H. Significance of Ki-67 in non-muscle invasive bladder cancer patients: A systematic review and meta-analysis. *Oncotarget* **2017**, *8*, 100614–100630. [CrossRef] [PubMed]
13. Robertson, A.G.; Kim, J.; Al-Ahmadie, H.; Bellmunt, J.; Guo, G.; Cherniack, A.D.; Hinoue, T.; Laird, P.W.; Hoadley, K.A.; Akbani, R.; et al. Comprehensive Molecular Characterization of Muscle-Invasive Bladder Cancer. *Cell* **2017**, *171*, 540–556. [CrossRef] [PubMed]
14. Dyrskjot, L.; Ingersoll, M.A. Biology of nonmuscle-invasive bladder cancer: Pathology, genomic implications, and immunology. *Curr. Opin. Urol.* **2018**, *28*, 598–603. [CrossRef] [PubMed]
15. Hedegaard, J.; Lamy, P.; Nordentoft, I.; Algaba, F.; Hoyer, S.; Ulhoi, B.P.; Vang, S.; Reinert, T.; Hermann, G.G.; Mogensen, K.; et al. Comprehensive Transcriptional Analysis of Early-Stage Urothelial Carcinoma. *Cancer Cell* **2016**, *30*, 27–42. [CrossRef] [PubMed]
16. Eckstein, M.; Strissel, P.; Strick, R.; Weyerer, V.; Wirtz, R.; Pfannstiel, C.; Wullweber, A.; Lange, F.; Erben, P.; Stoehr, R.; et al. Cytotoxic T-cell-related gene expression signature predicts improved survival in muscle-invasive urothelial bladder cancer patients after radical cystectomy and adjuvant chemotherapy. *J. Immunother. Cancer* **2020**, *8*. [CrossRef]
17. Jiang, Z.; Hsu, J.L.; Li, Y.; Hortobagyi, G.N.; Hung, M.C. Cancer Cell Metabolism Bolsters Immunotherapy Resistance by Promoting an Immunosuppressive Tumor Microenvironment. *Front. Oncol.* **2020**, *10*, 1197. [CrossRef]
18. Pfannstiel, C.; Strissel, P.L.; Chiappinelli, K.B.; Sikic, D.; Wach, S.; Wirtz, R.M.; Wullweber, A.; Taubert, H.; Breyer, J.; Otto, W.; et al. The Tumor Immune Microenvironment Drives a Prognostic Relevance That Correlates with Bladder Cancer Subtypes. *Cancer Immunol. Res.* **2019**, *7*, 923–938. [CrossRef]
19. Lee, H.H.; Farber, J.M. Localization of the gene for the human MIG cytokine on chromosome 4q21 adjacent to INP10 reveals a chemokine "mini-cluster". *Cytogenet. Cell Genet.* **1996**, *74*, 255–258. [CrossRef]
20. Do, H.T.T.; Lee, C.H.; Cho, J. Chemokines and their Receptors: Multifaceted Roles in Cancer Progression and Potential Value as Cancer Prognostic Markers. *Cancers* **2020**, *12*, 287. [CrossRef]
21. Farber, J.M. HuMig: A new human member of the chemokine family of cytokines. *Biochem. Biophys. Res. Commun.* **1993**, *192*, 223–230. [CrossRef] [PubMed]
22. Shinohara, T.; Taniwaki, M.; Ishida, Y.; Kawaichi, M.; Honjo, T. Structure and chromosomal localization of the human PD-1 gene (PDCD1). *Genomics* **1994**, *23*, 704–706. [CrossRef] [PubMed]
23. Freeman, G.J.; Long, A.J.; Iwai, Y.; Bourque, K.; Chernova, T.; Nishimura, H.; Fitz, L.J.; Malenkovich, N.; Okazaki, T.; Byrne, M.C.; et al. Engagement of the PD-1 immunoinhibitory receptor by a novel B7 family member leads to negative regulation of lymphocyte activation. *J. Exp. Med.* **2000**, *192*, 1027–1034. [CrossRef] [PubMed]
24. Gordon, S.R.; Maute, R.L.; Dulken, B.W.; Hutter, G.; George, B.M.; McCracken, M.N.; Gupta, R.; Tsai, J.M.; Sinha, R.; Corey, D.; et al. PD-1 expression by tumour-associated macrophages inhibits phagocytosis and tumour immunity. *Nature* **2017**, *545*, 495–499. [CrossRef] [PubMed]
25. Dong, H.; Zhu, G.; Tamada, K.; Chen, L. B7-H1, a third member of the B7 family, co-stimulates T-cell proliferation and interleukin-10 secretion. *Nat. Med.* **1999**, *5*, 1365–1369. [CrossRef]
26. Bardhan, K.; Anagnostou, T.; Boussiotis, V.A. The PD1:PD-L1/2 Pathway from Discovery to Clinical Implementation. *Front. Immunol.* **2016**, *7*, 550. [CrossRef]
27. Le Goux, C.; Damotte, D.; Vacher, S.; Sibony, M.; Delongchamps, N.B.; Schnitzler, A.; Terris, B.; Zerbib, M.; Bieche, I.; Pignot, G. Correlation between messenger RNA expression and protein expression of immune checkpoint-associated molecules in bladder urothelial carcinoma: A retrospective study. *Urol. Oncol.* **2017**, *35*, 257–263. [CrossRef]

28. Breyer, J.; Wirtz, R.M.; Otto, W.; Erben, P.; Worst, T.S.; Stoehr, R.; Eckstein, M.; Denzinger, S.; Burger, M.; Hartmann, A. High PDL1 mRNA expression predicts better survival of stage pT1 non-muscle-invasive bladder cancer (NMIBC) patients. *Cancer Immunol. Immunother.* **2018**, *67*, 403–412. [CrossRef]
29. Gerdes, J.; Schwab, U.; Lemke, H.; Stein, H. Production of a mouse monoclonal antibody reactive with a human nuclear antigen associated with cell proliferation. *Int. J. Cancer* **1983**, *31*, 13–20. [CrossRef]
30. Eckstein, M.; Epple, E.; Jung, R.; Weigelt, K.; Lieb, V.; Sikic, D.; Stohr, R.; Geppert, C.; Weyerer, V.; Bertz, S.; et al. CCL2 Expression in Tumor Cells and Tumor-Infiltrating Immune Cells Shows Divergent Prognostic Potential for Bladder Cancer Patients Depending on Lymph Node Stage. *Cancers* **2020**, *12*, 1253. [CrossRef]
31. Huang, Y.; Zhang, S.D.; McCrudden, C.; Chan, K.W.; Lin, Y.; Kwok, H.F. The prognostic significance of PD-L1 in bladder cancer. *Oncol. Rep.* **2015**, *33*, 3075–3084. [CrossRef] [PubMed]
32. Seow, S.W.; Rahmat, J.N.; Bay, B.H.; Lee, Y.K.; Mahendran, R. Expression of chemokine/cytokine genes and immune cell recruitment following the instillation of Mycobacterium bovis, bacillus Calmette-Guerin or Lactobacillus rhamnosus strain GG in the healthy murine bladder. *Immunology* **2008**, *124*, 419–427. [CrossRef] [PubMed]
33. Ozcan, Y.; Caglar, F.; Celik, S.; Demir, A.B.; Ercetin, A.P.; Altun, Z.; Aktas, S. The role of cancer stem cells in immunotherapy for bladder cancer: An in vitro study. *Urol. Oncol.* **2020**, *38*, 476–487. [CrossRef] [PubMed]
34. Nazari, A.; Ahmadi, Z.; Hassanshahi, G.; Abbasifard, M.; Taghipour, Z.; Falahati-Pour, S.K.; Khorramdelazad, H. Effective Treatments for Bladder Cancer Affecting CXCL9/CXCL10/CXCL11/CXCR3 Axis: A Review. *Oman Med. J.* **2020**, *35*, e103. [CrossRef] [PubMed]
35. Morgia, G.; Russo, G.I.; Berretta, M.; Privitera, S.; Kirkali, Z. Genito-urological cancers in elderly patients. *Anticancer Agents Med. Chem.* **2013**, *13*, 1391–1405. [CrossRef]
36. Damrauer, J.S.; Hoadley, K.A.; Chism, D.D.; Fan, C.; Tiganelli, C.J.; Wobker, S.E.; Yeh, J.J.; Milowsky, M.I.; Iyer, G.; Parker, J.S.; et al. Intrinsic subtypes of high-grade bladder cancer reflect the hallmarks of breast cancer biology. *Proc. Natl. Acad. Sci. USA* **2014**, *111*, 3110–3115. [CrossRef]
37. Lerner, S.P.; McConkey, D.J.; Hoadley, K.A.; Chan, K.S.; Kim, W.Y.; Radvanyi, F.; Hoglund, M.; Real, F.X. Bladder Cancer Molecular Taxonomy: Summary from a Consensus Meeting. *Bladder Cancer* **2016**, *2*, 37–47. [CrossRef]
38. Breyer, J.; Wirtz, R.M.; Otto, W.; Erben, P.; Kriegmair, M.C.; Stoehr, R.; Eckstein, M.; Eidt, S.; Denzinger, S.; Burger, M.; et al. In stage pT1 non-muscle-invasive bladder cancer (NMIBC), high KRT20 and low KRT5 mRNA expression identify the luminal subtype and predict recurrence and survival. *Virchows Arch.* **2017**, *470*, 267–274. [CrossRef]
39. Hashizume, A.; Umemoto, S.; Yokose, T.; Nakamura, Y.; Yoshihara, M.; Shoji, K.; Wada, S.; Miyagi, Y.; Kishida, T.; Sasada, T. Enhanced expression of PD-L1 in non-muscle-invasive bladder cancer after treatment with Bacillus Calmette-Guerin. *Oncotarget* **2018**, *9*, 34066–34078. [CrossRef]
40. Sobin, L.H.; Gospodarowicz, M.K.; Wittekind, C. *TNM Classification of Malignant Tumours*, 7th ed.; Wiley-Blackwell: Oxford, UK, 2010.
41. Mostofi, F.K.; Sobin, L.H.; Torloni, H. *Histological Typing of Urinary Bladder Tumours;* World Health Organization: Geneva, Switzerland, 1973.
42. Eble, J.N.; Sauter, G.; Epstein, J.I.; Sesterhenn, I.A. *Pathology and Genetics of Tumours of the Urinary System;* IARCPress: Lyon, France, 2004.
43. Sikic, D.; Breyer, J.; Hartmann, A.; Burger, M.; Erben, P.; Denzinger, S.; Eckstein, M.; Stohr, R.; Wach, S.; Wullich, B.; et al. High Androgen Receptor mRNA Expression Is Independently Associated with Prolonged Cancer-Specific and Recurrence-Free Survival in Stage T1 Bladder Cancer. *Transl. Oncol.* **2017**, *10*, 340–345. [CrossRef]
44. Schmittgen, T.D.; Livak, K.J. Analyzing real-time PCR data by the comparative C(T) method. *Nat. Protoc.* **2008**, *3*, 1101–1108. [CrossRef] [PubMed]

15

Cellular and Molecular Progression of Prostate Cancer: Models for Basic and Preclinical Research

Sirin Saranyutanon [1,2], Sachin Kumar Deshmukh [1,2], Santanu Dasgupta [1,2], Sachin Pai [3], Seema Singh [1,2,4] and Ajay Pratap Singh [1,2,4,*]

[1] Cancer Biology Program, Mitchell Cancer Institute, University of South Alabama, Mobile, AL 36604, USA; ss1830@jagmail.southalabama.edu (S.S.); skdeshmukh@health.southalabama.edu (S.K.D.); dasgupta@southalabama.edu (S.D.); seemasingh@health.southalabama.edu (S.S.)
[2] Department of Pathology, College of Medicine, University of South Alabama, Mobile, AL 36617, USA
[3] Department of Medical Oncology, Mitchell Cancer Institute, University of South Alabama, Mobile, AL 36604, USA; spai@health.southalabama.edu
[4] Department of Biochemistry and Molecular Biology, University of South Alabama, Mobile, AL 36688, USA
* Correspondence: asingh@health.southalabama.edu

Simple Summary: The molecular progression of prostate cancer is complex and elusive. Biological research relies heavily on in vitro and in vivo models that can be used to examine gene functions and responses to the external agents in laboratory and preclinical settings. Over the years, several models have been developed and found to be very helpful in understanding the biology of prostate cancer. Here we describe these models in the context of available information on the cellular and molecular progression of prostate cancer to suggest their potential utility in basic and preclinical prostate cancer research. The information discussed herein should serve as a hands-on resource for scholars engaged in prostate cancer research or to those who are making a transition to explore the complex biology of prostate cancer.

Abstract: We have witnessed noteworthy progress in our understanding of prostate cancer over the past decades. This basic knowledge has been translated into efficient diagnostic and treatment approaches leading to the improvement in patient survival. However, the molecular pathogenesis of prostate cancer appears to be complex, and histological findings often do not provide an accurate assessment of disease aggressiveness and future course. Moreover, we also witness tremendous racial disparity in prostate cancer incidence and clinical outcomes necessitating a deeper understanding of molecular and mechanistic bases of prostate cancer. Biological research heavily relies on model systems that can be easily manipulated and tested under a controlled experimental environment. Over the years, several cancer cell lines have been developed representing diverse molecular subtypes of prostate cancer. In addition, several animal models have been developed to demonstrate the etiological molecular basis of the prostate cancer. In recent years, patient-derived xenograft and 3-D culture models have also been created and utilized in preclinical research. This review is an attempt to succinctly discuss existing information on the cellular and molecular progression of prostate cancer. We also discuss available model systems and their tested and potential utility in basic and preclinical prostate cancer research.

Keywords: prostate cancer; research model; oncogenes; tumor suppressor genes

1. Introduction

Prostate cancer (PCa) is the most commonly diagnosed malignancy and the second leading cause of cancer-related death in men in the United States. It is estimated that PCa will afflict approximately

191,930 men and cause nearly 33,330 deaths this year in the United States alone [1]. Notably, PCa incidence and associated mortality are nearly two-thirds and over two times higher, respectively, in African-American (AA) men compared to their Caucasian-American (CA) counterparts [2,3]. PCa follows a defined pattern of cellular progression but exhibits diverse molecular pathobiology making it one of most highly heterogeneous cancers [4,5]. The prostate-specific antigen (PSA) test is the primary detection tool for PCa screening. However, due to the lack of accuracy and specificity, the usefulness of PSA for PCa diagnosis has been questioned [6–8]. Most PCa patients are generally subjected to localized radical prostatectomy, radiation therapy, proton beam therapy, and cryosurgery after the initial diagnosis [9–11]. However, for patients with metastatic disease or recurrent cancer with locoregional and distant metastases, androgen-deprivation therapy (ADT) or castration therapy is considered the primary line of treatment [12]. Unfortunately, despite the initial outstanding therapeutic response, most PCa patients treated with ADT eventually have the relapse of PCa in a highly aggressive and therapy-resistant form leading to poor clinical outcomes [13,14].

To meet the challenges associated with prostate cancer clinical management, research labs across the world have been working tirelessly to understand underlying molecular diversity and biology of PCa. These efforts have resulted in novel therapies that are currently in clinics, while researchers continue to gather more insights to address new hurdles and failures faced in clinical settings. These advances have been possible through the development of several in vitro and in vivo research models, while new models continue to be developed to address the genetic and biological complexities associated with the PCa. In this review, we discuss the cellular and molecular progression of PCa as well as the available in vitro and in vivo models for PCa research. We believe that the information presented herein will be helpful to the researchers, especially those who are new to the field, in understanding the molecular pathobiology of PCa and guide them in choosing the correct model(s) for their laboratory and preclinical research.

2. Cellular and Molecular Progression of Prostate Cancer

The human prostate is a walnut-size glandular organ that develops from the embryonic urogenital sinus [15]. Its primary function is to produce seminal fluid containing zinc, citric acid, and various enzymes, including a protease named prostate-specific antigen (PSA). Histologically, the prostate can be divided into central, peripheral, and transition zones comprised of a secretory ductal-acinar structure located within a fibromuscular stroma [16,17]. The ductal-acinar structure is formed of tall columnar secretory luminal cells, a flattened basal epithelium attached to the basement membrane, and scattered neuroendocrine cells (Figure 1). Luminal epithelial cells express cytokeratins (CK) 8 and 18, NKX3.1, androgen receptor (AR), and PSA, whereas basal epithelial cells express CK5, CK14, glutathione S-transferase Pi 1 (GSTP1), p63, and low levels of AR [18,19].

The cellular origin of prostate cancer is not very clear, partly because of the lack of well-characterized prostate epithelial lineage [20–22]. PCa develops from normal prostate epithelium through a multistep histological transformation process, governed by various underlying molecular changes [23] (Figure 2). Low-grade and high-grade prostate intraepithelial neoplasia (PIN) lesions develop from normal prostate epithelium through the loss of phosphatase and the tensin homolog *(PTEN)*, NK3 Homeobox 1 (*NKX3.1)*, overexpression of *MYC* proto-oncogene, B-cell lymphoma 2 (*BCL-2)*, and the glutathione S-transferase pi 1 gene (*GSTP1)*, accompanied with Speckle Type BTB/POZ Protein (*SPOP)* mutation and Transmembrane Serine Protease 2- ETS-related gene (*TMPRSS2-ERG)* fusion [24–36]. Further loss of the retinoblastoma protein *(RB1)*, along with telomerase activation and frequent Forkhead Box A1 *(FOXA1)* mutation, leads to the development of prostate adenocarcinoma from the advanced PIN lesion [37–43]. Further molecular aberrations including the loss of SMAD Family Member 4 (*SMAD4)*, AR corepressors, mutations in AR, *FOXA1*, *BRCA1/2*, *ATM*, *ATR*, and *RAD51* accompanied with the gain of function of the AR coactivator, *CXCL12*, *CXCR4*, *RANK-RANKL*, EMT, *BAI1*, and *EZH2* lead to the development of metastatic prostate cancer [44–59].

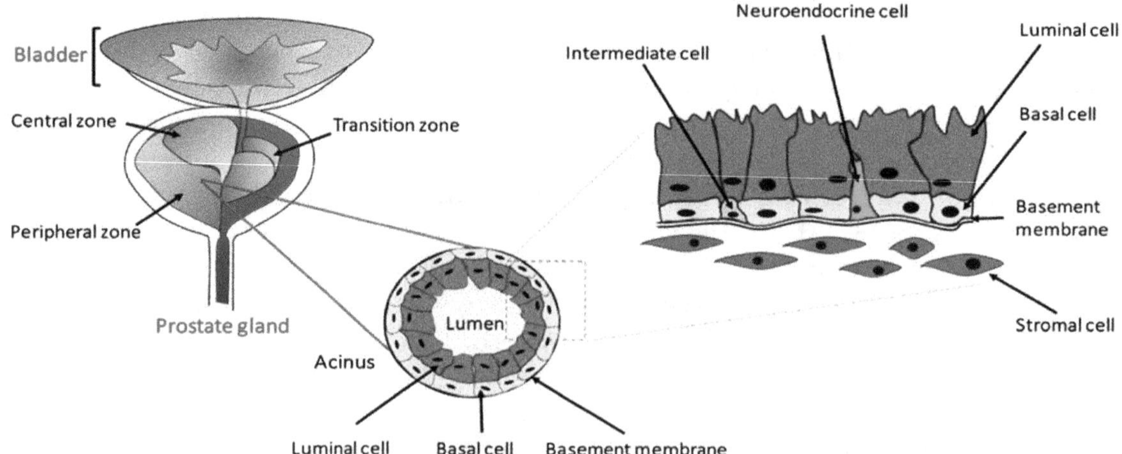

Figure 1. The location and architecture of the human prostate gland. The prostate gland is located below the bladder and consists of a central, a peripheral, and a transition zone. Histologically, it is comprised of secretary luminal, basal, and rare intermediate and neuroendocrine cells. The prostatic epithelium is separated from the stromal cells by the basement membrane as indicated. Preneoplastic or neoplastic cellular transformation can initiate from either basal or luminal cells.

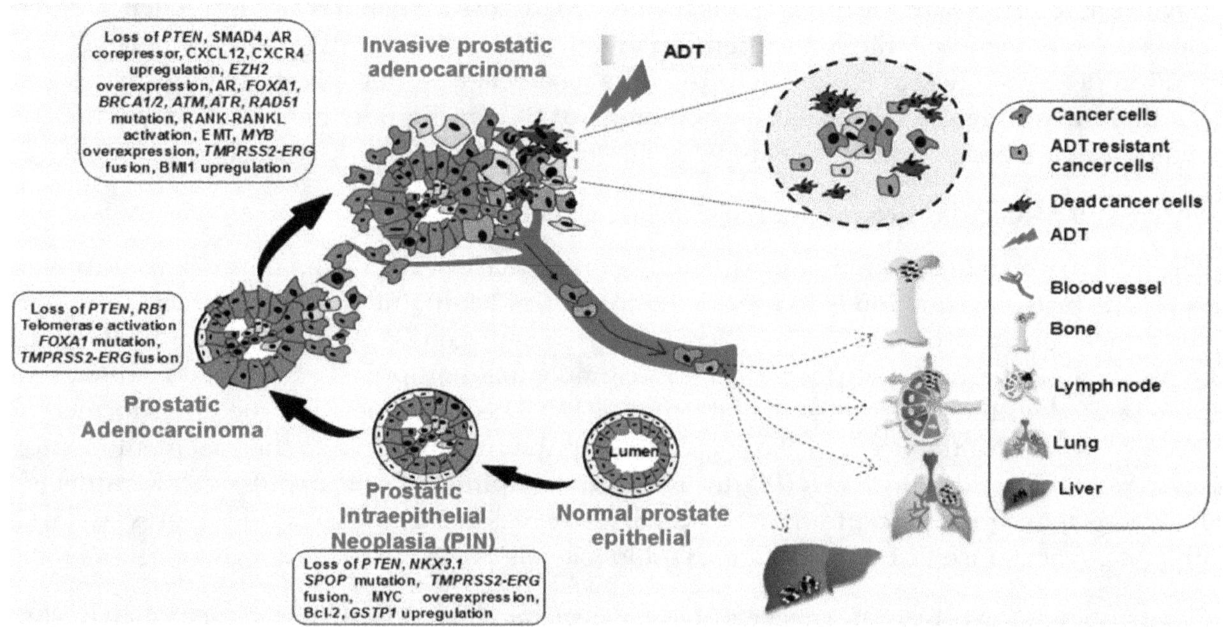

Figure 2. Histopathological and molecular progression of human prostate cancer. Metastatic prostate cancer develops via progression through prostate intraepithelial neoplasia (PIN) and invasive adenocarcinoma through the acquirement of various molecular alterations as depicted. The invasive adenocarcinoma cells and androgen-deprivation therapy resistant cancer cells metastasize to the bone, lymph node, lung, and liver.

As evident from the PCa progression model (Figure 2), inactivation of *PTEN* appears to be a critical event in PCa carcinogenesis and associated with aggressive disease manifestation. *PTEN* alterations occur in various ways in prostate cancer, such as genomic deletion and rearrangement, intragenic breakage, or translocation. The loss of *PTEN* is linked with an upregulation of PI3K/AKT/mTOR signaling that regulates cell survival, proliferation, and energy metabolism [60,61]. Another critical determinant of PCa tumorigenesis is *SMAD4*, a tumor suppressor gene (18q21.1), which mediates the transforming growth factor β (TGF-β) signaling pathway and suppresses epithelial cell growth. Transcriptome analysis revealed significantly lower levels of *SMAD4* in PCa tissues compared to adjacent non-cancerous tissues [46]. Of note, in a mouse model, prostate specific ablation of *Smad4* and *Pten* leads to the development of an invasive and metastatic potential of PCa (discussed below) [45].

In the PCa initiation and progression cascade, tumor suppressor *NKX3.1* (8p21) plays a pivotal role and found to be frequently lost due to the loss of heterozygosity (LOH) [62,63]. Of note, LOH at 8p21 appears to be an early event in PCa tumorigenesis [63–65]. Thus, it is likely that the genes that reside within these frequently deleted regions are associated with PCa initiation. Under the normal condition, *NKX3.1* drives growth-suppressing and differentiating effects on the prostatic epithelium [66]. *Nkx3.1* heterozygous mice develop abnormal prostate morphology with the dysplastic epithelium [67,68]. Importantly, *Nkx3.1*-null mice show changes in prostate epithelial morphology with severe dysplasia [67]. Kim et al. demonstrated that the loss of function of *Pten* and *Nkx3.1* in mice cooperated in PCa development. Importantly, *Pten;Nkx3.1* compound mutant mice showed a higher incidence of High-grade prostatic intraepithelial neoplasia (HGPIN) [69]. In addition to the critical tumor suppressor genes described above, the *MYC* proto-oncogene is also amplified in PCa [70–72]. *MYC* encodes a transcription factor that regulates the expression of several genes involved in cell proliferation, metabolism, mitochondrial function, and stem cell renewal [73–75]. Several studies suggest that *MYC* is activated through overexpression, amplification, rearrangement, Wnt/β-catenin pathway activation, germline *MYC* promotor variation, and loss of *FOXP3* in PCa [76–79], and is a critical oncogenic event driving PCa initiation and progression [71,80].

Other than *MYC*, *TMPRSS2:ERG* gene fusion, resulting from the chromosomal rearrangement, is also reported in approximately 45% of PCa. This alteration leads to the expression of the truncated *ERG* protein under the control androgen-responsive gene promoter of *TMPRSS2* [81–85]. *ERG* belongs to the *ETS* family of transcription factors (*ERG, ETV1*, and *ETV4*), and its activation is associated with PCa progression in both early- and late-stages [82,83,86]. *MYB*, another gene encoding a transcription factor, is also reported to be amplified in PCa and exhibits an increased amplification frequency in castration resistant PCa (CRPC) [87]. Research from our laboratory has shown that *MYB* plays a vital role in PCa growth, malignant behavior, and androgen-depletion resistance [56].

3. Prostate Cancer Research Models

As discussed above, we have made appreciable progress in our understanding of PCa pathobiology over the past several years. These insights resulted from the efforts at multiple levels: (i) recording of clinicopathological data and histopathological examination of tumor sections at the microscopic levels, (ii) molecular profiling of clinical specimens to identify molecular aberrations associated with defined histopathological characteristics, and (iii) conducting laboratory assays to define the functional significance of identified molecular aberrations. The development of PCa research models by scientists played a significant role in these laboratory and preclinical efforts. Prostate cell lines (cancer and non-cancer) established from patients have been instrumental as research models to gain functional and mechanistic insight. A comprehensive list of cell lines used in PCa research is given in Table 1. Moreover, quite a few mouse models have also been developed that not only provide direct evidence for the oncogenic function of a gene or gene-set but also serve as models for furthering basic and translational cancer research. Recently, 3-D in vitro cultures and patient-derived tumor xenografts (PDXs) have been developed as well, which are mostly used for translational research. Below we describe some of these models and discuss their characteristics and potential significance.

Table 1. Prostate cancer cell line models and their characteristics.

Cell Line	Origin	Doubling Time	AR	PSA	Markers	Cyto-Keratin	Source	Refs.
Non-cancerous prostate epithelial cell lines								
RWPE-1	NPEC in peripheral zone	120 h	+	+	p53, Rb	8, 18	ATCC	[88,89]
BPH-1	Primary prostatic tissue	35 h	−	−	p53, BAX, PTEN, p21	8, 18, 19	ACCEGEN, Creative Bioarray, DSMZ	[90]
pRNS-1-1	radical prostatectomy	72 h	−	−	PTEN	5, 8	NCI and Stanford University	[91]
RC77N/E	Non-malignant tissue of a PCa patient	No report	+	−	NKX3.1, p16	8	Tuskegee University	[92]
HprEpC	Normal human prostate	No report	+	+	Cytokeratin 18	14, 18, 19	Cell applications, iXcells Biotechnologies, EZ biosystem	[93]
Hormone sensitive								
LNCaP	lymph node metastatic	28–60 h	+	+	WT p53, PTEN loss, vimentin, PAP, CBP, negative desmin	8, 18, 20	ATCC, Creative Bioarray, ACCEGEN, SIGMA	[94]
LAPC-4	lymph node metastatic from an androgen insensitive patient	72 h	+	+	p53 mutation	5, 8, 18	ATCC *	[95]
LAPC-9	bone metastasis from a patient with ADT	No report	+	+	Ki67, PTEN loss	5	ATCC *	[96]
VCaP	metastatic tumor	51 h	+	+	p53 mutation, Rb, PAP, PTEN	8, 18	ATCC, SIGMA, ACCEGEN	[97]
MDA-PCa 2a/2b	bone metastasis from an African-American male	82–93 h/42–73 h	+	+	WT p53, p21, Rb, Bcl-2	5, 8, 18	ATCC	[98]
LuCaP 23.1	lymph node and liver metastatic	11–21 days	+	+	5α-reductase type I, WT PTEN	No report	University of Washington	[99]
RC-77T/E	Radical prostatectomy from an African-American patient	No report	+	+	p16, NKX3.1, β-catenin, α-actinin-1, filamin-A	8	Tuskegee University	[92]
Castration resistant								
PC-3	lumbar vertebral metastasis	33 h	−	−	PTEN loss, no p53 expression, TGF-α, EGFR, transferrin receptor	7, 8, 18, 19	ATCC, SIGMA, ACCEGEN, Creative Bioarray	[100]
DU-145	Brain metastasis	34 h	−	−	TGF-α/β, EGFR, IGF-1, EGF	5, 7, 8, 18	ATCC, ACCEGEN	[101]

Table 1. *Cont.*

Cell Line	Origin	Doubling Time	AR	PSA	Markers	Cyto-Keratin	Source	Refs.
C4-2/ C4-2B	mouse vertebral metastasis LNCaP cell xenograft	48 h	+	+	p53, PTEN loss, marker chromosome m1	8	ATCC	[102,103]
22Rv1	CWR22R xenograft derivative	35–40 h	+	+	kallikrien-like serine protease, AR splice variant	8, 18	ATCC, SIGMA, ACCEGEN, Creative Bioarray	[104]
ARCaP	ascites fluid of a patient with advanced metastatic disease	No report	+	+	EGFR, c-erb B2/neu, c-erb B3, bombesin, serotonin	8, 18	Novicure Biotechnology	[105]

(* = Discontinued).

3.1. Cell Line Models

3.1.1. Non-Cancerous Prostate Epithelial Cell Lines

RWPE-1

This cell line model was established from the peripheral zone of a histologically normal adult human prostate from a 54-year-old man. The cells were immortalized by transduction with human papillomavirus 18 (HPV-18) to establish a stable line [88]. RWPE-1 cells exhibit the expression of AR and androgen-inducible expression of kallikrein-3 (KLK3) or PSA. These cells also express CK8 and CK18, which are the characteristic markers of the luminal prostatic epithelium [89]. Further, RWPE-1 cells exhibit heterogeneous nuclear staining for p53 and Rb proteins as well [89]. The growth of these cells is induced upon treatment with the epidermal growth factor (EGF) and fibroblast growth factor (FGF) in a dose-dependent manner, whereas TGF-β treatment inhibits their growth [89,106,107].

BPH-1

BPH-1 is an immortalized benign prostatic hyperplasia cell line model established from primary prostatic tissue obtained by transurethral resection from a 68-year-old patient [90]. Immortalization of these cells was achieved by transduction with simian virus 40 (SV40) large T antigen [90]. BPH-1 cells express wild type (WT) PTEN, WT p53 as well as CK8, CK18, and CK19 suggestive of their luminal epithelial origin [108], but are negative for AR, PSA, and prostatic acid phosphatase (PAP) [90]. Cytogenetic analysis of these cells revealed an aneuploidy karyotype with a modal chromosome number of 76 (range 71-79). EGF, TGF-β, FGF-1, and FGF-7 treatment induces the proliferation of these cells, while FGF-2, TGF-β1, and TGF-β2 are shown to have an opposite effect [90]. Due to the lack of AR expression, these cells do not respond to androgen treatment [90]. They are non-tumorigenic in nude mice [108].

pRNS-1-1

pRNS-1-1 is a human prostatic epithelial cell line model derived from a 53-year-old male who had undergone radical prostatectomy. These cells were transfected with a plasmid, pRNS-1-1, containing the SV40 genome expressing T-antigen to establish a stable line. pRNS-1-1 cells express WTPTEN, and CK5 and CK8 suggestive of their epithelial origin [91]. The pRNS-1-1 cells do not express either AR or PSA [109,110]. The growth of these cells is promoted by EGF, IGF, and bovine pituitary extract treatment, while TGF-β has an inhibitory effect. pRNS-1-1 cells do not form tumors when injected subcutaneously in nude mice [109].

RC-77N/E

The RC-77N/E prostate epithelial cell line model was derived from the non-malignant prostate tissue isolated from a 63-year-old African American (AA) man diagnosed with PCa [92]. RC-77N/E cells are immortalized by the expression of HPV-16E6/E7 and exhibit an epithelial morphology. These cells are androgen-sensitive and express CK8, AR, PSA, and p16. RC-77N/E does not form tumors in severe combined immunodeficiency (SCID) mice [92]. This line could be useful for racial disparity associated PCa studies.

HprEpC

Human prostate epithelial cells (HprEpCs) were isolated from the normal human prostate. HPrEpC model cells express both prostatic basal epithelial marker CK14 and luminal prostatic epithelium markers CK18 and CK19 suggesting that they are intermediate cells [93]. Besides their application as normal control cells for PCa research, HprEpC cells are useful tools in studying the hormonal regulation and secretory function of the prostate.

3.1.2. Prostate Cancer Cell Lines

Prostate cancer cell lines established from human patients are broadly categorized into two types (castration-sensitive and castration-resistant) depending upon their survivability under androgen-deprived conditions.

Castration-Sensitive

LNCaP

LNCaP is a widely used human PCa cell line model. This cell line was developed in 1980 from a lesion in the left supraclavicular lymph node metastasis of human prostatic adenocarcinoma from a 50-year-old Caucasian male [94]. LNCaP cells are weakly adherent and slow-growing and have a doubling time of about 60-72 h. LNCaP cells express AR and PSA and exhibit a biphasic regulation of growth following androgen treatment [111]. These cells have a point mutation in AR (T877A) and express WT p53 [112,113]. These cells also harbor one mutated and other deleted alleles of *PTEN* [114]. Additionally, these cells are CK8, CK18, CK20, and vimentin-positive [115]. LNCaP cells require androgens to sustain their growth, but several derivative androgen-depletion resistant cell lines have been developed following slow and long-term androgen-deprivation or through their selection from mouse-xenograft tumors [116,117].

LAPC-4

LAPC-4 (Los Angeles prostate cancer 4) model cell line was established from a lymph node metastasis of a hormone-refractory PCa patient through direct transfer of surgically removed tissues (2–3 mm sections) into male SCID mice. The tissue explants were subcutaneously xenografted into the mice, and later tumor cells were harvested from mouse xenografts and plated on the culture dish to generate the cell line [95]. These cells are very slow growing, with a doubling rate of around 72 h [113]. LAPC-4 cells express wild type AR and PSA [118]. The expression of both CK5 (a basal epithelial marker) and CK8 (luminal epithelium marker) is also detected in these cells suggestive of their dedifferentiation [95]. Although these cells are castration-sensitive, forced overexpression of human epidermal growth factor receptor 2 (HER-2/neu) is shown to cause ligand independence by activation of the AR pathway [119]. Further, HER2 overexpression synergizes with low levels of androgen to potentiate AR activation [119]. LAPC4 are tumorigenic and can grow subcutaneously, orthotopically, or intratibially in nude mice [120–122].

LAPC-9

The LAPC-9 (Los Angeles prostate cancer 9) cell line was derived from the bone metastasis of the prostate cancer patient that had undergone androgen-ablation therapy [96]. These cells express AR and PSA and undergo growth arrest upon androgen ablation [123]. It is shown that LAPC-9 cells can remain in a dormant state for at least six months following castration and can emerge as castration-resistant following a long period of androgen deprivation [96]. LAPC-9 cells develop tumors in nude mice upon subcutaneous injection [96,124]. They can respond rapidly to androgen replenishment and re-enter the cell cycle and resume growth [96].

RWPE-2

The RWPE-2 cell line is derived from the HPV-18 immortalized RWPE-1 cells by transformation with Ki-ras using the Kirsten murine sarcoma virus (Ki-MuSV). The overexpression of Ki-ras bestowed tumorigenicity to these cells since Ki-ras activation is implicated in prostate carcinogenesis [89]. These cells express CK8, CK18, WT p53, WT Rb, AR, and PSA and are hormone responsive. EGF and FGF promote RWPE-2 cell growth, and in contrast, TGF-β has growth inhibitory effects on these cells. RWPE-2 cells that form colonies in agar have an invasive potential [89] and form tumors when injected subcutaneously into the nude mice [125].

VCaP

The VCaP (vertebral cancer of the prostate) cell line was established in 1997 from a metastatic prostate tumor that developed in the vertebrae of a 59-year-old Caucasian patient with the hormone-refractory disease who had failed androgen deprivation therapy [97]. VCaP was passaged as xenografts in nude mice and then cultured in vitro. The VCaP cells exhibit multiple features of clinical PCa, including expression of PSA, PAP, and AR. One study has also shown the elevated expression of the AR-V7 variant in VCaP xenograft after castration by next-generation RNA-Seq [126]. Additionally, these cells express CK-8, CK-18, Rb, and p53 (with A248W mutation). As per the American Type Culture Collection, the doubling time of this cell line was about 51 h (VCaP ATCC CRL-2876TM). These cells form tumors when injected subcutaneously in SCID mice [97,127]. The presence of the *TMPRSS2:ERG* fusion gene has been shown to stimulate the growth of the VCaP orthotopic mouse model [128].

MDA-PCa 2a/2b

MDA-PCa 2a and MDA-PC 2b cell lines were established from two distinct areas of prostate tumor derived from a 63-year-old African American (AA) subject having a late-stage bone metastasis [98]. The patient was under relapse following castration therapy at the time of cell isolation. MDA-PCa 2a/2b cells express WT AR, WT p53, KLK3/PSA, WT PTEN, and p21 [129,130]. Coming from two different areas of the tumor, they have different doubling times. MDA-PCa 2a cells double in number in about 82–93 h, whereas MDA-PCa2b has a doubling time of 42–73 h [98]. These cells can form tumors in mice when injected subcutaneously [98]. Although, the MDA-PCa 2a/2b cells are derived from an androgen-independent tumor but are sensitive and responsive to androgens [98]. Among these lines, MDA-PCa 2b is androgen dependent [131]. Later, a new androgen refractory subline MDA-PCa 2b-hr was developed following 35 weeks of androgen depletion to represent clinical PCa recurrence during androgen ablation treatment [131]. These lines could also be useful for racial disparity-associated PCa studies.

LuCaP 23.1

LuCaP 23.1, Lucan 23.8, and LuCaP 23.12 cell line series were developed in 1996 from two different lymph node metastases (LNM) of a 63-year-old Caucasian PCa patient (adenocarcinoma with Gleason score 8). Cancer tissues from this subject were xenografted subcutaneously in nude mice and passaged serially to establish these xenograft lines. All three lines are AR-positive and responsive to androgen and express WT PTEN at mRNA levels [99]. Notably, androgen depletion in mice harboring these three lines prolonged tumor growth with a concomitant decrease in the PSA expression level. However, some of the tumors eventually relapsed following castration and were considered hormone-refractory. Thus, studying these models could be invaluable to unravel the sequential molecular events driving relapse and acquirement of androgen independence. Moreover, tumor progression in these models can be monitored by measuring the PSA level. The LuCaP 35 model was developed from the LNM of a 66-year-old PCa patient (Stage T4c) through subcutaneous implantation in nude mice, as described above. This line expresses PSA and AR (harbors AR amplification and C1863T mutation) and is androgen-sensitive [132]. The LuCaP 35 cells can be cultured in vitro, unlike the LuCaP 23 cells, and produce LN and pulmonary metastases when implanted orthotopically. The LuCaP 35V cells were established from recurrent LuCaP 35 cells and are androgen-independent. Collectively, these are unique in vivo and in vitro models to study the mechanism of castration resistance [133]. Later, several cell lines such as LuCaP 23.12, LuCaP 23.8, LuCaP 35, LuCaP 41, LuCaP 49, LuCaP 58, and LuCaP 73 were developed. LuCaP 23.1, LuCaP 23.12, LuCaP 23.8, LuCaP 35, LuCaP 41, LuCaP 49, LuCaP 58, and LuCaP 73 cells express AR and PSA.

RC-77T/E

The RC-77T/E cell line was developed from the radical prostatectomy specimen of a 63-year-old AA patient with a clinical-stage T3c adenocarcinoma [92]. From the same patient, anon-malignant cell line RC-77N/E was also developed (discussed above). The RC-77T/E cells express AR, PSA, NKX 3.1, CK8, and p16 [92]. RC-77T/E cells also express β-catenin, α-actinin-1, and filamin-A [134]. These cells are androgen-responsive and form tumors when injected subcutaneously in nude mice [92]. This cell line model could be useful for racial disparity-associated PCa studies.

12T-7f

12T-7f (12: 12 kb, T: Tag transgene, f: fast) is a mouse cell line developed from the probasin-large T antigen transgenic mouse (a.k.a LADY) model along with six other transgenic cell lines. These cells were split into three groups based on the stage of neoplasia and their rapid growth pattern. Inoculation of these cells in mice resulted in the development of prostate tumors. The most aggressive line from these pools was designated as 12T-7f, which could progress to late-stage adenocarcinoma [135]. Notably, tumors developed through 12T-7f xenografting regressed upon castration but progressed after androgen administration.

Castration-Resistant Cell Lines

As discussed in the earlier section, castration-resistance could develop due to AR-dependent and AR-independent mechanisms. Therefore, two types of castration-resistant cell lines (AR-positive and AR-negative) have been developed and are discussed below:

Androgen-Receptor Expressing

C4-2/C4-2B

These cell lines were derived from LNCaP mouse xenografts. C4-2 was isolated from the vertebral metastasis of the LNCaP xenograft, whereas C4-2B was derived from the bone metastasis of the C4-2 tumor-bearing mice [102,103]. Both cell lines express AR and PSA and low levels of p53 and develop tumors when subcutaneously injected in the nude mice [103].

Rv1

The 22Rv1cell line was introduced in 1999. This cell line was derived from the mouse CWR22R xenograft developed from the prostate tumor of a patient with bone metastasis [104]. The 22Rv1 cells harbor the H874Y mutation in the AR like CWR22R xenograft and express PSA and kallikrein-like serine protease [104,136]. EGF is shown to promote the growth of 22Rv1 in vitro [104]. Recently, it has been shown that 22Rv1 prostate carcinoma cells produce high-titer of the human retrovirus XMRV (xenotropic murine leukemia virus-related virus) [137].

Androgen-Receptor Non-Expressing

PC-3

The PC-3 cell line was developed from lumbar vertebral metastasis of a grade IV prostatic adenocarcinoma from a 62-year-old Caucasian man [100]. In the karyotypic analysis, these cells were found to be near triploid having 62 chromosomes. PC3 cells express CK7, CK8, CK18, and CK19 but not AR and PSA and exhibit characteristics of a poorly differentiated adenocarcinoma with a doubling time of about 33 h [138,139]. These cells respond positively to EGF while being insensitive to FGF and are tumorigenic when orthotopically injected in mice [100,140–143].

DU-145

The DU145 cell line was established from the brain metastasis of a 69-year-old prostate cancer patient [101]. These cells express CK5, CK7, CK8, CK18, and CK19 [93,144,145]. Being AR negative, DU145 cells are hormone-insensitive and do not express PSA [146]. This cell line has a doubling time of about 34 h and exhibits a growth response to EGF [147] and also a high level of EGFR expression [148]. DU-145 cells metastasize to spleen and liver when injected subcutaneously in a nude mouse [149,150].

ARCaP

ARCaP (androgen-refractory cancer of the prostate) was established from the ascites of a patient with advanced metastatic disease. Interestingly, it is shown that androgen and estrogen treatment as a dose-dependent suppressive impact on the growth of ARCaP cells [105]. ARCaP cells express low levels of AR and PSA and exhibit positive immunostaining for EGFR, HER2/neu, HER3, bombesin, serotonin, neuron-specific enolase, and the mesenchymal–epithelial transition factor (C-MET). These cells are tumorigenic and highly metastatic that preferably colonize to the lung, pancreas, liver, kidney, and bone [151–153]. These cells form ascites fluid in athymic mice [105].

3.2. Genetically Engineered Mouse Models of Prostate Cancer

The mouse models are beneficial resources to improve our understanding of the disease pathobiology and to establish the role of candidate oncogenes in the pathogenic processes. As discussed below, several genetically engineered mouse models of PCa have been developed that have provided insights into tumor initiation, progression, and metastasis and are being used in preclinical research.

3.2.1. TRAMP

The transgenic adenocarcinoma of the mouse prostate (TRAMP) mice model was generated and characterized in 1996. The chloramphenicol acetyltransferase (CAT) gene was introduced into the germ line of mice under the control of the rat probasin (PB) promoter. In TRAMP mice, expression of both the large and small SV40 T antigens (TAG) is regulated by the prostate-specific rat PB promoter [154]. The PB-SV40 T antigen (PB-Tag) transgene is spatially restricted to the dorsolateral and ventral lobes of the prostate. The gene expression is male specific and restricted to the epithelial cells of the lateral, dorsal, and ventral prostatic lobes of the murine prostate [155]. TRAMP is a very useful model for studying the pathology of PCa as the progression occurs through PIN lesions to malignant disease, like human disease, in a predictable time. Epithelial hyperplasia develops by 10 weeks of age, PIN by 18 weeks of age, and lymphatic metastases after 28 weeks of age [154,156,157].

The TRAMP model has been used for PCa prevention and treatment studies [158,159]. It is also the first genetically engineered mouse model (GEMM) that displays castration-resistant disease progression [160]. One of the limitations of the TRAMP model, however, is that these mice often develop neuroendocrine PCa [161]. A simultaneous loss of *Rb* and *p53* could be the reason for the development of neuroendocrine cancer [161,162]. Considering the higher chances of neuroendocrine disease, the TRAMP mouse model is clinically more relevant to study PCa of neuroendocrine origin.

3.2.2. LADY

The LADY PCa mouse model was developed in 1998 and is similar to the TRAMP model [163]. There are, however, a few key differences between the TRAMP and LADY. In the LADY, a larger fragment (12 kb) of the PB (a.k.a. LPB) promoter upstream of the SV40 T-antigen is used that contains additional androgen and growth factor-responsive sequences and thus allows consistently high transgene expression. Additionally, the LPB promoter is linked with a deletion mutant of the SV40 T-antigen (deleted small T-antigen) to allow the expression of large T-antigen, unlike small t-antigen in the TRAMP model. The purpose of deleting small t-antigen was to analyze the importance of neuroendocrine differences in metastatic lesions developed by LADY [164]. LADY model mice develop metastases to the liver, lymph nodes, and bones [164]. The metastases, however, primarily contain neuroendocrine cells, which is unlike the human metastasis [135,165]. Thus, the LADY mice are different from the most common type of human PCa from the perspective of rapid tumor growth and neuroendocrine tumor development. Nevertheless, the LADY model possesses the molecular changes similar to the human prostate, such as the multifocal nature of tumorigenesis, histopathologically changes from low- to high-grade dysplasia similar to PIN in humans, and the androgen-dependent growth of the primary tumors. Hence, the LADY model could be beneficial for investigating the stepwise mechanisms of PCa progression as well as therapeutic intervention [163].

3.2.3. Pten Deficient Mice

Loss of the *PTEN* tumor suppressor is a critical event in PCa initiation, as discussed above. However, homozygous knockout of *Pten* in mice embryonic stem cells through the deletion of the phosphatase domain led to embryonic lethality [166,167]. To overcome this limitation, Wang et al. generated *Pten* null mice by conditional deletion of *Pten* in the murine prostatic epithelium. They generated *Pten* $^{loxp/loxp}$: PB-Cre4 mice in order to attain the prostate-specific *Pten* biallelic deletion. They showed that *Pten* null PCa progressed with a short latency of PIN formation by 6 weeks of age compared to heterozygous *Pten* deletion mice, which developed PIN by 10 months. Moreover, homozygous *Pten* deletion mice developed invasive adenocarcinoma by 9 weeks of age and metastasis to the lymph node and lung by 12 weeks of age. The effect of hormone ablation therapy on *Pten* null mice was evaluated by performing the castration of mice at week 16. The response of *Pten* null tumors at day 3 and day 6 post-castration was analyzed. In response to androgen abolition, the AR-positive prostatic epithelium showed an increase in the apoptosis leading to the decrease of prostate volume. Hence, these homozygous *Pten* mutant mice recapitulate the PCa by mimicking the histopathological features of human disease [40]. In contrast, heterozygous mutant ($Pten^{+/-}$) mice developed neoplasia in multiple tissues, including mammary glands, lymphoid cells, small intestines, thyroid, endometrial, and adrenal glands [166,168,169], further limiting the applicability of the heterozygous mutant over *Pten* null mice.

The *Pten* knockout model has been used to demonstrate the role of the tumor microenvironment, particularly interleukin-17 (IL-17), in the growth and progression of PCa [170,171]. To test how tumor suppressor *Rb* interacts with *Pten*, Bai et al. developed mice with double mutations in both the cyclin-dependent kinase (CDK) inhibitor *p18Ink4c* and *Pten* [172]. The double mutant mice develop a broader spectrum of prostate tumors in the anterior and dorsolateral lobes at an accelerated rate [172]. Loss of function of *Nkx3.1* is crucial for PCa progression and has been associated with the development of prostatic epithelial hyperplasia, dysplasia, and PIN [30,67,173]. *Nkx3.1* and *Pten* are shown to cooperate in prostate carcinogenesis in mice. *Nkx3.1;Pten* double mutant mice demonstrated an increased incidence of HGPIN, which resembles the early stages of human PCa [69].

3.2.4. Pten$^{pc-/-}$Smad4$^{pc-/-}$

To examine a cooperative action of *Pten* and *Smad4* loss in PCa pathogenesis, De Pinho lab developed mice having prostate-specific genetic ablation of *Smad4* in Pten-null mice. These mice were highly aggressive and exhibited profound lymph node and pulmonary metastasis [45]. The importance of *Smad4* in PCa was further revealed by the development of metastatic and lethal PCa with 100% penetrance in *Smad4* and *Pten* double knockout mouse prostate [45]. *Pten*$^{pc-/-}$*Smad4*$^{pc-/-}$ has been used to analyze the efficacy of hypoxia-prodrug TH-302 and checkpoint blockade combination therapy. The combination of the hypoxia-prodrug and checkpoint blockade significantly extended the survival of *Pten*$^{pc-/-}$*Smad4*$^{pc-/-}$ mice [174]. Furthermore, Wang and colleagues utilized the *Pten*$^{pc-/-}$*Smad4*$^{pc-/-}$ mice model and identified that polymorphonuclear myeloid-derived suppressor cells (MDSCs) are one of the significant infiltrating immune cells in PCa and their depletion blocks PCa progression [175].

3.2.5. Hi/Lo-Myc

Two plasmids having a rat probasin (PB) promoter alone (PB-Mycfor lo-Myc) and PB coupled with a sequence of the ARR2 (ARR2PB for hi-Myc) were used to achieve prostate-specific overexpression of c-Myc. The ARR2PB promotor contained two additional androgen response elements that forced the development of invasive adenocarcinoma from prostatic intraepithelial neoplasia (mPIN) in about 26 weeks [27,176,177]. Hi-Myc mice also displayed a decreased expression of Nkx3.1 at both mRNA and protein levels [27]. The PB-Myc mice showed similar pathological changes, but a slower progression of 30 weeks (time to invasive PCa development from PIN lesions) [27]. The main differences between these two models are their androgen responsiveness. The Hi-Myc is androgen-responsive, while the Lo-myc model displays no such sensitivity [27]. The mice model generated by non-viral oncogene ARR2PB-Myc and PB-Myc develop invasive adenocarcinoma and offer advantages over those expressing SV40. However, they do not develop metastasis, which is a major drawback of this model. Hubbard et al. in 2016 showed that the combination of *Myc* overexpression and *Pten* loss in mice resulted in the development of lethal prostatic adenocarcinoma with distant metastases [29]. Moreover, homeobox protein Hox-B13 (HOXB13) was suggested to participate in the *MYC* activation and *Pten* loss genomic instability and aggressive prostate cancer [29,178].

3.2.6. MPAKT

The mouse prostate Akt (MPAKT) model is useful in studying the role of protein kinase B (Akt) in the transformation of prostate epithelial cells and in developing the biomarkers relevant to human PCa. This mouse model was developed by the introduction of Akt1 along with a myristoylation sequence (myr) and a hemagglutinin (HA) epitope in the form of the linearized rPb-myr-HA-Akt1. This insert was injected into the pronuclei of fertilized oocytes, and the friend leukemia virus B (FVB) mice founders were verified [179]. These mice exhibited the formation of PIN by 8 weeks. Immunohistochemistry analysis of the PIN lesions of MPAKT demonstrated numerous important findings such as Akt results in the activation of p70S6K and is associated with the development of PIN in MPAKT mice and Akt-induced PIN might be linked to neovascularization. Histological evaluation revealed that MPAKT mice had distinct phenotypic characteristics, including disorganized epithelial layers, loss of cell polarity, intraepithelial lumen formation, and nuclear atypia and apoptotic bodies. However, the MPAKT did not develop invasive carcinoma even after 78 weeks [180].

3.3. *Patient Tumor-Derived Models*

Patient-derived models are useful tools for translational research as they mimic human tumors. They are instrumental in studying the response of various therapies undergoing preclinical evaluation since they carry intrinsic tumor factors and microenvironmental presence involved in disease progression and therapy resistance.

3.3.1. Three-Dimensional (3-D) Organoid Cultures

The transition from monolayer PCa cultures to the three-dimensional (3-D) cultures is a remarkable breakthrough in cancer research. Although culturing cancer cell lines is cost-effective and easy to handle, established cell lines do not carry the heterogeneity and genetic makeup of tumors from which they were initially derived [181,182]. These limitations are mostly overridden by the establishment of 3-D organoid culture models from the patient-derived tumors [183]. Dong et al. established the first PCa 3-D organoid culture from the biopsy of a patient in 2014 [184]. This organoid culture maintained the molecular signature of PCa, including *TMPRSS2-ERG* fusion, *SPOP* mutation, Chromodomain Helicase DNA Binding Protein 1 (*CHD1)* loss, and serine protease inhibitor Kazal-type 1 (*SPINK1)* overexpression. Further, whole-exome sequencing revealed mutations in several other genes, as well as the loss of the p53 and RB tumor suppressor pathway function [184]. Puca and colleges developed patient-derived organoids from needle biopsies of metastatic lesions from patients with neuroendocrine CRPC. These organoids showed genomic, epigenomic, and transcriptomic association with corresponding patient tumors [185]. 3-D models are thus beneficial for drug discovery and preclinical evaluation of therapeutic drugs for efficacy under in vitro setting that mimics the complex in vivo environment.

3.3.2. Patient-Derived Xenografts (PDX)

Patient-derived xenografts (PDXs) are essential tools in cancer research as the results obtained from these resources more accurately predict clinical responses in patients (Table 2). The reason is that these models retain the genetic diversity of patient tumors and maintain a closely resembling tumor microenvironment [186]. PDX grown in immunocompromised mice carry essential histological and molecular features of the patient tumors, including gene expression programs, mutations, epigenetic regulators, and structural genomic events that ultimately drive their 3D growth [187,188]. Recent technical advancements, including the co-injection of PCa tissues with extracellular matrix (ECM) and transplantation into renal capsules, have increased the success rate of PDX establishment in mice [189–191]. The first androgen-dependent PCa xenograft model, designated as PC-82, was developed in 1977 by Schröder and colleagues at Erasmus University Rotterdam [192]. For this, the patient prostatic tumor tissue was grafted into the shoulder of nude mice. Later, two more androgen-independent in vivo models, designated as PC-133 and PC-135, were developed [192]. In 1996, seven other PDX models were established [193]. During 1991-2005, numerous other PDX models were developed that carried the *TMPRSS-ERG* rearrangement, *RB1* loss, AR amplification, *PTEN* deletion, *SPOP* mutation, *Tp53* deletion and mutation, and *BRCA2* loss [132,194,195]. The success rate of the localized PDX model has been increased in recent years due to the implantation of the chimeric graft with neonatal mouse mesenchyme. This method improved the survival rate and doubled the proliferation index of xenografted cancer cells [196]. The PDX models, however, have two significant limitations, i.e., the absence of functional human immunity and the lack of orthotopic modeling in the mice [197]. Further, the model takes a long time (about 8 months) for validation of detectable tumor growth in mice that limits its utility for the high-throughput drug screening [198].

Table 2. The advantages and limitations of patient-derived xenograft models.

Model	Advantages	Limitations	Sources
3D-organoid	• In vivo-like complexity • Retain 3D architecture • Maintain heterogeneity • Good for high-throughput screening • Good for drug response testing	• Low establishment rate with primary hormone-sensitive tumor • Success in only aggressive PCa specimens • Lack vasculature • Deficient microenvironment and immunity	Primary prostate cancer patient-derived tissue

Table 2. *Cont.*

Model	Advantages	Limitations	Sources
PDX	• Maintain heterogeneity • Retain 3D architecture • Intact endocrine system • Includes microenvironment	• Time-consuming and expensive • Established in a mouse with deficient immunity • Microenvironment is different from a human	Primary prostate cancer patient-derived tissue, CrownBio, The Jackson Laboratory

3.4. *Other Models*

3.4.1. Rat Models

Rat is one of the models for PCa research that was first established in the year 1937 by Moore and Melchionna after injecting the white rat prostate with benzpyrene. Following treatment, the columnar prostate epithelium underwent squamous metaplasia and also led to the induction of cancer in both the healthy and atrophic prostates [199]. These tumors spontaneously developed from a dorsal prostatic adenocarcinoma in an inbred Copenhagen rat and then were transplanted into a syngenic Copenhagen × Fischer F1 hybrid rat. These rat prostate tumors are well differentiated and slow growing [200]. The albino Lobund–Wistar (LW) rat model was first described by Pollard [201]. The LW rat developed spontaneous tumors at a mean age of 26 months. Moreover, a combination of N-methyl-N-nitrosourea (MNU) and testosterone treatments induced the development of prostate adenocarcinoma in the LW rat at a mean time of 10.5 months. The cancer of the LW rat resembles the human PCa in several aspects, including spontaneous development and progression to androgen independence and metastasis [201]. However, a major limitation of the rat models is that they have a long latency period for tumor development (2–3 years), have low tumor incidence, and lack spontaneous metastases.

3.4.2. Zebrafish Model

The zebrafish model for cancer research has been utilized by many to acquire information that is traditionally obtained by mice and cell culture systems, although there are limited studies on zebrafish in an in vivo model for PCa research. The zebrafish model is suitable for visual observation of labeled tumor cells through the imaging technique since they are transparent. Nevertheless, the limitation of orthotopic transplantation could be the hurdle owing to the anatomical difference between zebrafish and the human body such as the breast, prostate, or lung [202]. The cancer cells can be injected into a different site in the zebrafish embryos, such as the blastodisc region, the yolk sac, the hindbrain ventricle, and into the circulation via the duct of Cuvier [203,204]. Melong et al. inoculated androgen-sensitive LNCaP cells into zebrafish and observed the effect of testosterone on the growth. Administration of exogenous testosterone increased the proliferation of PCa cells [205]. Further, the growth-promoting effect of testosterone was reversed by the anti-androgen receptor drug, enzalutamide. The invasive potential of PC3 cells overexpressing the calcitonin receptor (CTR) has also been evaluated in the zebrafish model [206]. The zebrafish model has several advantages, including the fact that zebrafish are small and can generate a large number of offspring in a short time, and they are easy to maintain and observe owing to their transparency. Moreover, humans and zebrafish have 71% protein similarity, and, most importantly, zebrafish absorb molecules from water providing an additional route for drug administration.

4. Conclusions and Future Outlook

In the past years, understanding of PCa pathobiology paired with mechanistic studies has remarkably advanced the field of PCa research. This insight has only been possible because of the availability of several types of research models. These models have been extremely helpful in improving our knowledge of PCa etiology, development, and metastatic progression. The cell line models have offered an easy and inexpensive platform to study the functions of aberrantly-expressed genes and various types of genetic alterations including gene mutations, splice variants, gene rearrangements, etc. Furthermore, cell lines serve as a primary model for screening of newer drugs or drug combination and provide us data on the molecular mechanisms of therapy resistance that is crucial for drug development. Since cell lines do not completely capture the tumor heterogeneity and are not grown in a complex microenvironment that tumor cells encounter in vivo, other in vivo models play an important role in further evaluation of gene functions and drug efficacies. The 3D-tissue culture model mimics the in vivo system under in vitro settings and has proven very useful in drug screening. Further, as the field of precision medicine is developing, these models could be of great significance in patient-tailored treatment planning based on preliminary assessment. Patient-derived xenografts (PDXs) grown in mice are useful as they more closely mimic a human tumor in vivo microenvironment. Genetically engineered mouse models (GEMs) are useful as they capture the complete progression of PCa from initiation to metastatic spread under a non-immunocompromised environment. Further, these models also develop a variety of PCa tumor types although they do not have the complete molecular diversity of human tumors (Figure 3). Regardless of limitations, each model has its own importance and these models often complement each other and are often utilized in progressive sets of experiments. There is, however, a need to develop models representing PCa of different racial and ethnic groups considering racial health disparities in incidence and clinical outcomes. Our refined knowledge of tumor genetics and awareness of health disparities and technologically advances will help us make further progress and we would continue to add to our list of PCa tumor models.

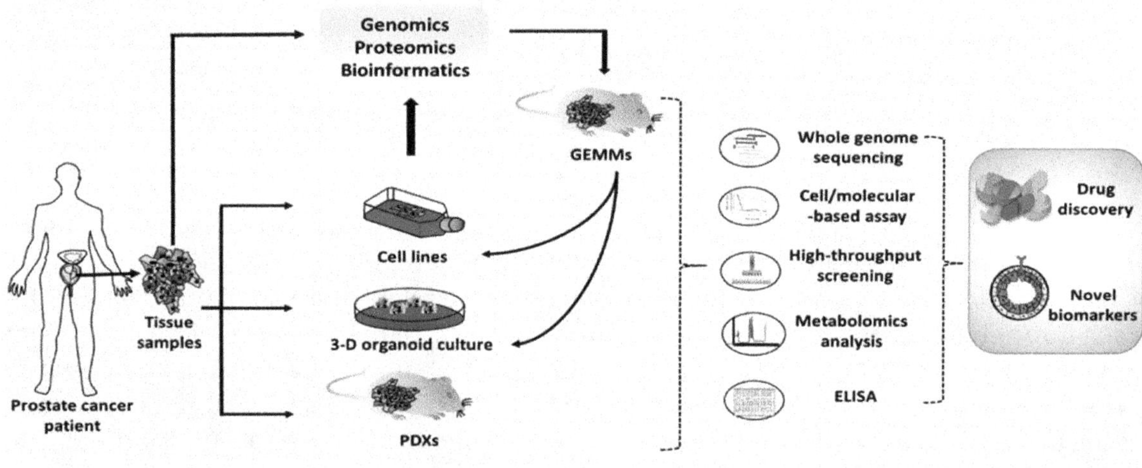

Figure 3. Application of the prostate cancer model in basic and preclinical cancer research. To develop the novel drugs or biomarkers, the prostate cancer models are required for in vitro and in vivo studies. The prostate cell lines, 3D-organiods, and patient-derived tumor xenografts (PDXs) can be generated from prostate tumor tissue from human patients. Patient tumor tissues can be also used to create genetically engineered mouse models (GEMMs). The results from research and preclinical studies are validated through several techniques such as whole genome sequencing, cell and molecular-based assays, high-throughput screening, metabolomics analysis, and ELISA. The promising drugs or biomarkers that emerge from those works will subsequently progress to preclinical and clinical studies.

Author Contributions: Conceptualization: A.P.S., S.S. (Seema Singh), S.D., S.P., S.S. (Sirin Saranyutanon), and S.K.D.; Supervision; A.P.S., S.S. (Seema Singh), and S.D.; Resources: A.P.S. and S.S. (Seema Singh); Writing, review and editing: A.P.S., S.S. (Seema Singh), S.D., S.P., S.S. (Sirin Saranyutanon), and S.K.D. All authors have read and agreed to the published version of the manuscript.

Acknowledgments: Sirin Saranyutanon would also like to acknowledge the financial support provided by the Royal Thai Government Scholarship.

References

1. Siegel, R.L.; Miller, K.D.; Jemal, A. Cancer statistics, 2020. *CA Cancer J. Clin.* **2020**, *70*, 7–30. [CrossRef]
2. Powell, I.J. Prostate cancer and African-American men. *Oncology (Williston Park)* **1997**, *11*, 599–605.
3. Fuletra, J.G.; Kamenko, A.; Ramsey, F.; Eun, D.D.; Reese, A.C. African-American men with prostate cancer have larger tumor volume than Caucasian men despite no difference in serum prostate specific antigen. *Can. J. Urol.* **2018**, *25*, 9193–9198.
4. Humphrey, P.A. Histopathology of Prostate Cancer. *Cold Spring Harb. Perspect. Med.* **2017**, *7*, a030411. [CrossRef] [PubMed]
5. Inamura, K. Prostatic cancers: Understanding their molecular pathology and the 2016 WHO classification. *Oncotarget* **2018**, *9*, 14723–14737. [CrossRef]
6. Hoffman, R.M.; Gilliland, F.D.; Adams-Cameron, M.; Hunt, W.C.; Key, C.R. Prostate-specific antigen testing accuracy in community practice. *BMC Fam. Pract.* **2002**, *3*, 19. [CrossRef]
7. Punglia, R.S.; D'Amico, A.V.; Catalona, W.J.; Roehl, K.A.; Kuntz, K.M. Effect of verification bias on screening for prostate cancer by measurement of prostate-specific antigen. *N. Engl. J. Med.* **2003**, *349*, 335–342. [CrossRef]
8. Brawley, O.W. Prostate cancer screening: Biases and the need for consensus. *J. Natl. Cancer Inst.* **2013**, *105*, 1522–1524. [CrossRef]
9. Donnelly, B.J.; Saliken, J.C.; Brasher, P.M.; Ernst, S.D.; Rewcastle, J.C.; Lau, H.; Robinson, J.; Trpkov, K. A randomized trial of external beam radiotherapy versus cryoablation in patients with localized prostate cancer. *Cancer* **2010**, *116*, 323–330. [CrossRef]
10. Hayden, A.J.; Catton, C.; Pickles, T. Radiation therapy in prostate cancer: A risk-adapted strategy. *Curr. Oncol.* **2010**, *17* (Suppl. 2), S18–S24. [CrossRef]
11. Shipley, W.U.; Verhey, L.J.; Munzenrider, J.E.; Suit, H.D.; Urie, M.M.; McManus, P.L.; Young, R.H.; Shipley, J.W.; Zietman, A.L.; Biggs, P.J.; et al. Advanced prostate cancer: The results of a randomized comparative trial of high dose irradiation boosting with conformal protons compared with conventional dose irradiation using photons alone. *Int. J. Radiat. Oncol. Biol. Phys.* **1995**, *32*, 3–12. [CrossRef]
12. Perlmutter, M.A.; Lepor, H. Androgen deprivation therapy in the treatment of advanced prostate cancer. *Rev. Urol* **2007**, *9* (Suppl. 1), S3–S8.
13. Miller, E.T.; Chamie, K.; Kwan, L.; Lewis, M.S.; Knudsen, B.S.; Garraway, I.P. Impact of treatment on progression to castration-resistance, metastases, and death in men with localized high-grade prostate cancer. *Cancer Med.* **2017**, *6*, 163–172. [CrossRef]
14. Moreira, D.M.; Howard, L.E.; Sourbeer, K.N.; Amarasekara, H.S.; Chow, L.C.; Cockrell, D.C.; Pratson, C.L.; Hanyok, B.T.; Aronson, W.J.; Kane, C.J.; et al. Predicting Time From Metastasis to Overall Survival in Castration-Resistant Prostate Cancer: Results From SEARCH. *Clin. Genitourin. Cancer* **2017**, *15*, 60–66.e2. [CrossRef]
15. Lee, C.H.; Akin-Olugbade, O.; Kirschenbaum, A. Overview of prostate anatomy, histology, and pathology. *Endocrinol. Metab. Clin. N. Am.* **2011**, *40*, 565–575. [CrossRef]
16. McNeal, J.E. The zonal anatomy of the prostate. *Prostate* **1981**, *2*, 35–49. [CrossRef]
17. Wang, G.; Zhao, D.; Spring, D.J.; DePinho, R.A. Genetics and biology of prostate cancer. *Genes Dev.* **2018**, *32*, 1105–1140. [CrossRef]
18. Zhang, D.; Zhao, S.; Li, X.; Kirk, J.S.; Tang, D.G. Prostate Luminal Progenitor Cells in Development and Cancer. *Trends Cancer* **2018**, *4*, 769–783. [CrossRef]
19. Xin, L. Cells of origin for cancer: An updated view from prostate cancer. *Oncogene* **2013**, *32*, 3655–3663. [CrossRef]
20. Wang, Z.A.; Toivanen, R.; Bergren, S.K.; Chambon, P.; Shen, M.M. Luminal cells are favored as the cell of origin for prostate cancer. *Cell Rep.* **2014**, *8*, 1339–1346. [CrossRef]

21. Stoyanova, T.; Cooper, A.R.; Drake, J.M.; Liu, X.; Armstrong, A.J.; Pienta, K.J.; Zhang, H.; Kohn, D.B.; Huang, J.; Witte, O.N.; et al. Prostate cancer originating in basal cells progresses to adenocarcinoma propagated by luminal-like cells. *Proc. Natl. Acad. Sci. USA* **2013**, *110*, 20111–20116. [CrossRef]
22. Garber, K. A tale of two cells: Discovering the origin of prostate cancer. *J. Natl. Cancer Inst.* **2010**, *102*, 1528–1529, 1535. [CrossRef]
23. Shen, M.M.; Abate-Shen, C. Molecular genetics of prostate cancer: New prospects for old challenges. *Genes Dev.* **2010**, *24*, 1967–2000. [CrossRef] [PubMed]
24. Krajewska, M.; Krajewski, S.; Epstein, J.I.; Shabaik, A.; Sauvageot, J.; Song, K.; Kitada, S.; Reed, J.C. Immunohistochemical analysis of bcl-2, bax, bcl-X, and mcl-1 expression in prostate cancers. *Am. J. Pathol.* **1996**, *148*, 1567–1576.
25. Martignano, F.; Gurioli, G.; Salvi, S.; Calistri, D.; Costantini, M.; Gunelli, R.; De Giorgi, U.; Foca, F.; Casadio, V. GSTP1 Methylation and Protein Expression in Prostate Cancer: Diagnostic Implications. *Dis. Markers* **2016**, *2016*, 4358292. [CrossRef] [PubMed]
26. Gurel, B.; Iwata, T.; Koh, C.M.; Jenkins, R.B.; Lan, F.; Van Dang, C.; Hicks, J.L.; Morgan, J.; Cornish, T.C.; Sutcliffe, S.; et al. Nuclear MYC protein overexpression is an early alteration in human prostate carcinogenesis. *Mod. Pathol.* **2008**, *21*, 1156–1167. [CrossRef]
27. Ellwood-Yen, K.; Graeber, T.G.; Wongvipat, J.; Iruela-Arispe, M.L.; Zhang, J.; Matusik, R.; Thomas, G.V.; Sawyers, C.L. Myc-driven murine prostate cancer shares molecular features with human prostate tumors. *Cancer Cell* **2003**, *4*, 223–238. [CrossRef]
28. McMenamin, M.E.; Soung, P.; Perera, S.; Kaplan, I.; Loda, M.; Sellers, W.R. Loss of PTEN expression in paraffin-embedded primary prostate cancer correlates with high Gleason score and advanced stage. *Cancer Res.* **1999**, *59*, 4291–4296.
29. Hubbard, G.K.; Mutton, L.N.; Khalili, M.; McMullin, R.P.; Hicks, J.L.; Bianchi-Frias, D.; Horn, L.A.; Kulac, I.; Moubarek, M.S.; Nelson, P.S.; et al. Combined MYC Activation and Pten Loss Are Sufficient to Create Genomic Instability and Lethal Metastatic Prostate Cancer. *Cancer Res.* **2016**, *76*, 283–292. [CrossRef]
30. Gurel, B.; Ali, T.Z.; Montgomery, E.A.; Begum, S.; Hicks, J.; Goggins, M.; Eberhart, C.G.; Clark, D.P.; Bieberich, C.J.; Epstein, J.I.; et al. NKX3.1 as a marker of prostatic origin in metastatic tumors. *Am. J. Surg. Pathol.* **2010**, *34*, 1097–1105. [CrossRef]
31. Tomlins, S.A.; Laxman, B.; Varambally, S.; Cao, X.; Yu, J.; Helgeson, B.E.; Cao, Q.; Prensner, J.R.; Rubin, M.A.; Shah, R.B.; et al. Role of the TMPRSS2-ERG gene fusion in prostate cancer. *Neoplasia* **2008**, *10*, 177–188. [CrossRef]
32. Furusato, B.; Tan, S.H.; Young, D.; Dobi, A.; Sun, C.; Mohamed, A.A.; Thangapazham, R.; Chen, Y.; McMaster, G.; Sreenath, T.; et al. ERG oncoprotein expression in prostate cancer: Clonal progression of ERG-positive tumor cells and potential for ERG-based stratification. *Prostate Cancer Prostatic Dis.* **2010**, *13*, 228–237. [CrossRef] [PubMed]
33. Blattner, M.; Liu, D.; Robinson, B.D.; Huang, D.; Poliakov, A.; Gao, D.; Nataraj, S.; Deonarine, L.D.; Augello, M.A.; Sailer, V.; et al. SPOP Mutation Drives Prostate Tumorigenesis In Vivo through Coordinate Regulation of PI3K/mTOR and AR Signaling. *Cancer Cell* **2017**, *31*, 436–451. [CrossRef]
34. Shoag, J.; Liu, D.; Blattner, M.; Sboner, A.; Park, K.; Deonarine, L.; Robinson, B.D.; Mosquera, J.M.; Chen, Y.; Rubin, M.A.; et al. SPOP mutation drives prostate neoplasia without stabilizing oncogenic transcription factor ERG. *J. Clin. Investig.* **2018**, *128*, 381–386. [CrossRef]
35. Lara, P.N., Jr.; Heilmann, A.M.; Elvin, J.A.; Parikh, M.; de Vere White, R.; Gandour-Edwards, R.; Evans, C.P.; Pan, C.X.; Schrock, A.B.; Erlich, R.; et al. TMPRSS2-ERG fusions unexpectedly identified in men initially diagnosed with nonprostatic malignancies. *JCO Precis. Oncol.* **2017**, *2017*. [CrossRef]
36. Guo, C.C.; Dancer, J.Y.; Wang, Y.; Aparicio, A.; Navone, N.M.; Troncoso, P.; Czerniak, B.A. TMPRSS2-ERG gene fusion in small cell carcinoma of the prostate. *Hum. Pathol.* **2011**, *42*, 11–17. [CrossRef] [PubMed]
37. Gerhardt, J.; Montani, M.; Wild, P.; Beer, M.; Huber, F.; Hermanns, T.; Muntener, M.; Kristiansen, G. FOXA1 promotes tumor progression in prostate cancer and represents a novel hallmark of castration-resistant prostate cancer. *Am. J. Pathol.* **2012**, *180*, 848–861. [CrossRef] [PubMed]

38. Annala, M.; Taavitsainen, S.; Vandekerkhove, G.; Bacon, J.V.W.; Beja, K.; Chi, K.N.; Nykter, M.; Wyatt, A.W. Frequent mutation of the FOXA1 untranslated region in prostate cancer. *Commun. Biol.* **2018**, *1*, 122. [CrossRef]
39. Jamaspishvili, T.; Berman, D.M.; Ross, A.E.; Scher, H.I.; De Marzo, A.M.; Squire, J.A.; Lotan, T.L. Clinical implications of PTEN loss in prostate cancer. *Nat. Rev. Urol.* **2018**, *15*, 222–234. [CrossRef]
40. Wang, S.; Gao, J.; Lei, Q.; Rozengurt, N.; Pritchard, C.; Jiao, J.; Thomas, G.V.; Li, G.; Roy-Burman, P.; Nelson, P.S.; et al. Prostate-specific deletion of the murine Pten tumor suppressor gene leads to metastatic prostate cancer. *Cancer Cell* **2003**, *4*, 209–221. [CrossRef]
41. Chen, W.S.; Alshalalfa, M.; Zhao, S.G.; Liu, Y.; Mahal, B.A.; Quigley, D.A.; Wei, T.; Davicioni, E.; Rebbeck, T.R.; Kantoff, P.W.; et al. Novel RB1-Loss Transcriptomic Signature Is Associated with Poor Clinical Outcomes across Cancer Types. *Clin. Cancer Res.* **2019**, *25*, 4290–4299. [CrossRef] [PubMed]
42. Graham, M.K.; Meeker, A. Telomeres and telomerase in prostate cancer development and therapy. *Nat. Rev. Urol.* **2017**, *14*, 607–619. [CrossRef] [PubMed]
43. Graham, M.K.; Kim, J.; Da, J.; Brosnan-Cashman, J.A.; Rizzo, A.; Baena Del Valle, J.A.; Chia, L.; Rubenstein, M.; Davis, C.; Zheng, Q.; et al. Functional Loss of ATRX and TERC Activates Alternative Lengthening of Telomeres (ALT) in LAPC4 Prostate Cancer Cells. *Mol. Cancer Res.* **2019**, *17*, 2480–2491. [CrossRef] [PubMed]
44. Schmitz, M.; Grignard, G.; Margue, C.; Dippel, W.; Capesius, C.; Mossong, J.; Nathan, M.; Giacchi, S.; Scheiden, R.; Kieffer, N. Complete loss of PTEN expression as a possible early prognostic marker for prostate cancer metastasis. *Int. J. Cancer* **2007**, *120*, 1284–1292. [CrossRef] [PubMed]
45. Ding, Z.; Wu, C.J.; Chu, G.C.; Xiao, Y.; Ho, D.; Zhang, J.; Perry, S.R.; Labrot, E.S.; Wu, X.; Lis, R.; et al. SMAD4-dependent barrier constrains prostate cancer growth and metastatic progression. *Nature* **2011**, *470*, 269–273. [CrossRef] [PubMed]
46. Zhang, D.T.; Shi, J.G.; Liu, Y.; Jiang, H.M. The prognostic value of Smad4 mRNA in patients with prostate cancer. *Tumour Biol.* **2014**, *35*, 3333–3337. [CrossRef]
47. Lakshmikanthan, V.; Zou, L.; Kim, J.I.; Michal, A.; Nie, Z.; Messias, N.C.; Benovic, J.L.; Daaka, Y. Identification of betaArrestin2 as a corepressor of androgen receptor signaling in prostate cancer. *Proc. Natl. Acad. Sci. USA* **2009**, *106*, 9379–9384. [CrossRef]
48. Taichman, R.S.; Cooper, C.; Keller, E.T.; Pienta, K.J.; Taichman, N.S.; McCauley, L.K. Use of the stromal cell-derived factor-1/CXCR4 pathway in prostate cancer metastasis to bone. *Cancer Res.* **2002**, *62*, 1832–1837.
49. Chinni, S.R.; Sivalogan, S.; Dong, Z.; Filho, J.C.; Deng, X.; Bonfil, R.D.; Cher, M.L. CXCL12/CXCR4 signaling activates Akt-1 and MMP-9 expression in prostate cancer cells: The role of bone microenvironment-associated CXCL12. *Prostate* **2006**, *66*, 32–48. [CrossRef]
50. Wu, X.; Scott, H.; Carlsson, S.V.; Sjoberg, D.D.; Cerundolo, L.; Lilja, H.; Prevo, R.; Rieunier, G.; Macaulay, V.; Higgins, G.S.; et al. Increased EZH2 expression in prostate cancer is associated with metastatic recurrence following external beam radiotherapy. *Prostate* **2019**, *79*, 1079–1089. [CrossRef]
51. Yang, Y.A.; Yu, J. EZH2, an epigenetic driver of prostate cancer. *Protein Cell* **2013**, *4*, 331–341. [CrossRef]
52. Augello, M.A.; Den, R.B.; Knudsen, K.E. AR function in promoting metastatic prostate cancer. *Cancer Metastasis Rev.* **2014**, *33*, 399–411. [CrossRef] [PubMed]
53. Jernberg, E.; Bergh, A.; Wikstrom, P. Clinical relevance of androgen receptor alterations in prostate cancer. *Endocr. Connect.* **2017**, *6*, R146–R161. [CrossRef] [PubMed]
54. Casimiro, S.; Mohammad, K.S.; Pires, R.; Tato-Costa, J.; Alho, I.; Teixeira, R.; Carvalho, A.; Ribeiro, S.; Lipton, A.; Guise, T.A.; et al. RANKL/RANK/MMP-1 molecular triad contributes to the metastatic phenotype of breast and prostate cancer cells in vitro. *PLoS ONE* **2013**, *8*, e63153. [CrossRef] [PubMed]
55. Armstrong, A.P.; Miller, R.E.; Jones, J.C.; Zhang, J.; Keller, E.T.; Dougall, W.C. RANKL acts directly on RANK-expressing prostate tumor cells and mediates migration and expression of tumor metastasis genes. *Prostate* **2008**, *68*, 92–104. [CrossRef]
56. Srivastava, S.K.; Bhardwaj, A.; Singh, S.; Arora, S.; McClellan, S.; Grizzle, W.E.; Reed, E.; Singh, A.P. Myb overexpression overrides androgen depletion-induced cell cycle arrest and apoptosis in prostate cancer cells, and confers aggressive malignant traits: Potential role in castration resistance. *Carcinogenesis* **2012**, *33*, 1149–1157. [CrossRef] [PubMed]

57. Ganaie, A.A.; Beigh, F.H.; Astone, M.; Ferrari, M.G.; Maqbool, R.; Umbreen, S.; Parray, A.S.; Siddique, H.R.; Hussain, T.; Murugan, P.; et al. BMI1 Drives Metastasis of Prostate Cancer in Caucasian and African-American Men and Is A Potential Therapeutic Target: Hypothesis Tested in Race-specific Models. *Clin. Cancer Res.* **2018**, *24*, 6421–6432. [CrossRef]
58. Deplus, R.; Delliaux, C.; Marchand, N.; Flourens, A.; Vanpouille, N.; Leroy, X.; de Launoit, Y.; Duterque-Coquillaud, M. TMPRSS2-ERG fusion promotes prostate cancer metastases in bone. *Oncotarget* **2017**, *8*, 11827–11840. [CrossRef]
59. Tian, T.V.; Tomavo, N.; Huot, L.; Flourens, A.; Bonnelye, E.; Flajollet, S.; Hot, D.; Leroy, X.; de Launoit, Y.; Duterque-Coquillaud, M. Identification of novel TMPRSS2:ERG mechanisms in prostate cancer metastasis: Involvement of MMP9 and PLXNA2. *Oncogene* **2014**, *33*, 2204–2214. [CrossRef]
60. Stambolic, V.; Suzuki, A.; de la Pompa, J.L.; Brothers, G.M.; Mirtsos, C.; Sasaki, T.; Ruland, J.; Penninger, J.M.; Siderovski, D.P.; Mak, T.W. Negative regulation of PKB/Akt-dependent cell survival by the tumor suppressor PTEN. *Cell* **1998**, *95*, 29–39. [CrossRef]
61. Berenjeno, I.M.; Guillermet-Guibert, J.; Pearce, W.; Gray, A.; Fleming, S.; Vanhaesebroeck, B. Both p110alpha and p110beta isoforms of PI3K can modulate the impact of loss-of-function of the PTEN tumour suppressor. *Biochem. J.* **2012**, *442*, 151–159. [CrossRef] [PubMed]
62. Vocke, C.D.; Pozzatti, R.O.; Bostwick, D.G.; Florence, C.D.; Jennings, S.B.; Strup, S.E.; Duray, P.H.; Liotta, L.A.; Emmert-Buck, M.R.; Linehan, W.M. Analysis of 99 microdissected prostate carcinomas reveals a high frequency of allelic loss on chromosome 8p12-21. *Cancer Res.* **1996**, *56*, 2411–2416.
63. Emmert-Buck, M.R.; Vocke, C.D.; Pozzatti, R.O.; Duray, P.H.; Jennings, S.B.; Florence, C.D.; Zhuang, Z.; Bostwick, D.G.; Liotta, L.A.; Linehan, W.M. Allelic loss on chromosome 8p12-21 in microdissected prostatic intraepithelial neoplasia. *Cancer Res.* **1995**, *55*, 2959–2962.
64. Abdulkadir, S.A.; Magee, J.A.; Peters, T.J.; Kaleem, Z.; Naughton, C.K.; Humphrey, P.A.; Milbrandt, J. Conditional loss of Nkx3.1 in adult mice induces prostatic intraepithelial neoplasia. *Mol. Cell. Biol.* **2002**, *22*, 1495–1503. [CrossRef]
65. Qian, J.; Jenkins, R.B.; Bostwick, D.G. Genetic and chromosomal alterations in prostatic intraepithelial neoplasia and carcinoma detected by fluorescence in situ hybridization. *Eur. Urol.* **1999**, *35*, 479–483. [CrossRef]
66. Abate-Shen, C.; Shen, M.M.; Gelmann, E. Integrating differentiation and cancer: The Nkx3.1 homeobox gene in prostate organogenesis and carcinogenesis. *Differentiation* **2008**, *76*, 717–727. [CrossRef]
67. Bhatia-Gaur, R.; Donjacour, A.A.; Sciavolino, P.J.; Kim, M.; Desai, N.; Young, P.; Norton, C.R.; Gridley, T.; Cardiff, R.D.; Cunha, G.R.; et al. Roles for Nkx3.1 in prostate development and cancer. *Genes Dev.* **1999**, *13*, 966–977. [CrossRef]
68. Kim, M.J.; Bhatia-Gaur, R.; Banach-Petrosky, W.A.; Desai, N.; Wang, Y.; Hayward, S.W.; Cunha, G.R.; Cardiff, R.D.; Shen, M.M.; Abate-Shen, C. Nkx3.1 mutant mice recapitulate early stages of prostate carcinogenesis. *Cancer Res.* **2002**, *62*, 2999–3004.
69. Kim, M.J.; Cardiff, R.D.; Desai, N.; Banach-Petrosky, W.A.; Parsons, R.; Shen, M.M.; Abate-Shen, C. Cooperativity of Nkx3.1 and Pten loss of function in a mouse model of prostate carcinogenesis. *Proc. Natl. Acad. Sci. USA* **2002**, *99*, 2884–2889. [CrossRef] [PubMed]
70. Chen, H.; Liu, W.; Roberts, W.; Hooker, S.; Fedor, H.; DeMarzo, A.; Isaacs, W.; Kittles, R.A. 8q24 allelic imbalance and MYC gene copy number in primary prostate cancer. *Prostate Cancer Prostatic Dis.* **2010**, *13*, 238–243. [CrossRef] [PubMed]
71. Fromont, G.; Godet, J.; Peyret, A.; Irani, J.; Celhay, O.; Rozet, F.; Cathelineau, X.; Cussenot, O. 8q24 amplification is associated with Myc expression and prostate cancer progression and is an independent predictor of recurrence after radical prostatectomy. *Hum. Pathol.* **2013**, *44*, 1617–1623. [CrossRef]
72. Qian, J.; Jenkins, R.B.; Bostwick, D.G. Detection of chromosomal anomalies and c-myc gene amplification in the cribriform pattern of prostatic intraepithelial neoplasia and carcinoma by fluorescence in situ hybridization. *Mod. Pathol.* **1997**, *10*, 1113–1119. [PubMed]
73. Dang, C.V. MYC on the path to cancer. *Cell* **2012**, *149*, 22–35. [CrossRef] [PubMed]
74. Zanet, J.; Pibre, S.; Jacquet, C.; Ramirez, A.; de Alboran, I.M.; Gandarillas, A. Endogenous Myc controls mammalian epidermal cell size, hyperproliferation, endoreplication and stem cell amplification. *J. Cell Sci.* **2005**, *118*, 1693–1704. [CrossRef] [PubMed]

75. Dang, C.V. MYC, metabolism, cell growth, and tumorigenesis. *Cold Spring Harb. Perspect. Med.* **2013**, *3*, a014217. [CrossRef]
76. Koh, C.M.; Bieberich, C.J.; Dang, C.V.; Nelson, W.G.; Yegnasubramanian, S.; De Marzo, A.M. MYC and Prostate Cancer. *Genes Cancer* **2010**, *1*, 617–628. [CrossRef]
77. He, T.C.; Sparks, A.B.; Rago, C.; Hermeking, H.; Zawel, L.; da Costa, L.T.; Morin, P.J.; Vogelstein, B.; Kinzler, K.W. Identification of c-MYC as a target of the APC pathway. *Science* **1998**, *281*, 1509–1512. [CrossRef]
78. Wang, L.; Liu, R.; Li, W.; Chen, C.; Katoh, H.; Chen, G.Y.; McNally, B.; Lin, L.; Zhou, P.; Zuo, T.; et al. Somatic single hits inactivate the X-linked tumor suppressor FOXP3 in the prostate. *Cancer Cell* **2009**, *16*, 336–346. [CrossRef]
79. Sotelo, J.; Esposito, D.; Duhagon, M.A.; Banfield, K.; Mehalko, J.; Liao, H.; Stephens, R.M.; Harris, T.J.; Munroe, D.J.; Wu, X. Long-range enhancers on 8q24 regulate c-Myc. *Proc. Natl. Acad. Sci. USA* **2010**, *107*, 3001–3005. [CrossRef]
80. Pettersson, A.; Gerke, T.; Penney, K.L.; Lis, R.T.; Stack, E.C.; Pertega-Gomes, N.; Zadra, G.; Tyekucheva, S.; Giovannucci, E.L.; Mucci, L.A.; et al. MYC Overexpression at the Protein and mRNA Level and Cancer Outcomes among Men Treated with Radical Prostatectomy for Prostate Cancer. *Cancer Epidemiol. Biomark. Prev.* **2018**, *27*, 201–207. [CrossRef]
81. Zhou, C.K.; Young, D.; Yeboah, E.D.; Coburn, S.B.; Tettey, Y.; Biritwum, R.B.; Adjei, A.A.; Tay, E.; Niwa, S.; Truelove, A.; et al. TMPRSS2:ERG Gene Fusions in Prostate Cancer of West African Men and a Meta-Analysis of Racial Differences. *Am. J. Epidemiol.* **2017**, *186*, 1352–1361. [CrossRef]
82. Tomlins, S.A.; Rhodes, D.R.; Perner, S.; Dhanasekaran, S.M.; Mehra, R.; Sun, X.W.; Varambally, S.; Cao, X.; Tchinda, J.; Kuefer, R.; et al. Recurrent fusion of TMPRSS2 and ETS transcription factor genes in prostate cancer. *Science* **2005**, *310*, 644–648. [CrossRef] [PubMed]
83. Demichelis, F.; Fall, K.; Perner, S.; Andren, O.; Schmidt, F.; Setlur, S.R.; Hoshida, Y.; Mosquera, J.M.; Pawitan, Y.; Lee, C.; et al. TMPRSS2:ERG gene fusion associated with lethal prostate cancer in a watchful waiting cohort. *Oncogene* **2007**, *26*, 4596–4599. [CrossRef]
84. Lapointe, J.; Kim, Y.H.; Miller, M.A.; Li, C.; Kaygusuz, G.; van de Rijn, M.; Huntsman, D.G.; Brooks, J.D.; Pollack, J.R. A variant TMPRSS2 isoform and ERG fusion product in prostate cancer with implications for molecular diagnosis. *Mod. Pathol.* **2007**, *20*, 467–473. [CrossRef] [PubMed]
85. Perner, S.; Mosquera, J.M.; Demichelis, F.; Hofer, M.D.; Paris, P.L.; Simko, J.; Collins, C.; Bismar, T.A.; Chinnaiyan, A.M.; De Marzo, A.M.; et al. TMPRSS2-ERG fusion prostate cancer: An early molecular event associated with invasion. *Am. J. Surg. Pathol.* **2007**, *31*, 882–888. [CrossRef]
86. Tomlins, S.A.; Palanisamy, N.; Siddiqui, J.; Chinnaiyan, A.M.; Kunju, L.P. Antibody-based detection of ERG rearrangements in prostate core biopsies, including diagnostically challenging cases: ERG staining in prostate core biopsies. *Arch. Pathol. Lab. Med.* **2012**, *136*, 935–946. [CrossRef]
87. Edwards, J.; Krishna, N.S.; Witton, C.J.; Bartlett, J.M. Gene amplifications associated with the development of hormone-resistant prostate cancer. *Clin. Cancer Res.* **2003**, *9*, 5271–5281. [PubMed]
88. Webber, M.M.; Trakul, N.; Thraves, P.S.; Bello-DeOcampo, D.; Chu, W.W.; Storto, P.D.; Huard, T.K.; Rhim, J.S.; Williams, D.E. A human prostatic stromal myofibroblast cell line WPMY-1: A model for stromal-epithelial interactions in prostatic neoplasia. *Carcinogenesis* **1999**, *20*, 1185–1192. [CrossRef]
89. Bello, D.; Webber, M.M.; Kleinman, H.K.; Wartinger, D.D.; Rhim, J.S. Androgen responsive adult human prostatic epithelial cell lines immortalized by human papillomavirus 18. *Carcinogenesis* **1997**, *18*, 1215–1223. [CrossRef]
90. Hayward, S.W.; Dahiya, R.; Cunha, G.R.; Bartek, J.; Deshpande, N.; Narayan, P. Establishment and characterization of an immortalized but non-transformed human prostate epithelial cell line: BPH-1. *Vitr. Cell. Dev. Biol. Anim.* **1995**, *31*, 14–24. [CrossRef]
91. D'Abronzo, L.S.; Bose, S.; Crapuchettes, M.E.; Beggs, R.E.; Vinall, R.L.; Tepper, C.G.; Siddiqui, S.; Mudryj, M.; Melgoza, F.U.; Durbin-Johnson, B.P.; et al. The androgen receptor is a negative regulator of eIF4E phosphorylation at S209: Implications for the use of mTOR inhibitors in advanced prostate cancer. *Oncogene* **2017**, *36*, 6359–6373. [CrossRef] [PubMed]
92. Theodore, S.; Sharp, S.; Zhou, J.; Turner, T.; Li, H.; Miki, J.; Ji, Y.; Patel, V.; Yates, C.; Rhim, J.S. Establishment and characterization of a pair of non-malignant and malignant tumor derived cell lines from an African American prostate cancer patient. *Int. J. Oncol.* **2010**, *37*, 1477–1482. [CrossRef]

93. Sherwood, E.R.; Berg, L.A.; Mitchell, N.J.; McNeal, J.E.; Kozlowski, J.M.; Lee, C. Differential cytokeratin expression in normal, hyperplastic and malignant epithelial cells from human prostate. *J. Urol.* **1990**, *143*, 167–171. [CrossRef]
94. Horoszewicz, J.S.; Leong, S.S.; Chu, T.M.; Wajsman, Z.L.; Friedman, M.; Papsidero, L.; Kim, U.; Chai, L.S.; Kakati, S.; Arya, S.K.; et al. The LNCaP cell line–a new model for studies on human prostatic carcinoma. *Prog. Clin. Biol. Res.* **1980**, *37*, 115–132.
95. Klein, K.A.; Reiter, R.E.; Redula, J.; Moradi, H.; Zhu, X.L.; Brothman, A.R.; Lamb, D.J.; Marcelli, M.; Belldegrun, A.; Witte, O.N.; et al. Progression of metastatic human prostate cancer to androgen independence in immunodeficient SCID mice. *Nat. Med.* **1997**, *3*, 402–408. [CrossRef] [PubMed]
96. Craft, N.; Chhor, C.; Tran, C.; Belldegrun, A.; DeKernion, J.; Witte, O.N.; Said, J.; Reiter, R.E.; Sawyers, C.L. Evidence for clonal outgrowth of androgen-independent prostate cancer cells from androgen-dependent tumors through a two-step process. *Cancer Res.* **1999**, *59*, 5030–5036.
97. Korenchuk, S.; Lehr, J.E.; MClean, L.; Lee, Y.G.; Whitney, S.; Vessella, R.; Lin, D.L.; Pienta, K.J. VCaP, a cell-based model system of human prostate cancer. *Vivo* **2001**, *15*, 163–168.
98. Navone, N.M.; Olive, M.; Ozen, M.; Davis, R.; Troncoso, P.; Tu, S.M.; Johnston, D.; Pollack, A.; Pathak, S.; von Eschenbach, A.C.; et al. Establishment of two human prostate cancer cell lines derived from a single bone metastasis. *Clin. Cancer Res.* **1997**, *3*, 2493–2500.
99. Whang, Y.E.; Wu, X.; Suzuki, H.; Reiter, R.E.; Tran, C.; Vessella, R.L.; Said, J.W.; Isaacs, W.B.; Sawyers, C.L. Inactivation of the tumor suppressor PTEN/MMAC1 in advanced human prostate cancer through loss of expression. *Proc. Natl. Acad. Sci. USA* **1998**, *95*, 5246–5250. [CrossRef]
100. Kaighn, M.E.; Narayan, K.S.; Ohnuki, Y.; Lechner, J.F.; Jones, L.W. Establishment and characterization of a human prostatic carcinoma cell line (PC-3). *Investig. Urol.* **1979**, *17*, 16–23.
101. Stone, K.R.; Mickey, D.D.; Wunderli, H.; Mickey, G.H.; Paulson, D.F. Isolation of a human prostate carcinoma cell line (DU 145). *Int. J. Cancer* **1978**, *21*, 274–281. [CrossRef] [PubMed]
102. Pfitzenmaier, J.; Quinn, J.E.; Odman, A.M.; Zhang, J.; Keller, E.T.; Vessella, R.L.; Corey, E. Characterization of C4-2 prostate cancer bone metastases and their response to castration. *J. Bone Miner. Res.* **2003**, *18*, 1882–1888. [CrossRef]
103. Thalmann, G.N.; Anezinis, P.E.; Chang, S.M.; Zhau, H.E.; Kim, E.E.; Hopwood, V.L.; Pathak, S.; von Eschenbach, A.C.; Chung, L.W. Androgen-independent cancer progression and bone metastasis in the LNCaP model of human prostate cancer. *Cancer Res.* **1994**, *54*, 2577–2581. [PubMed]
104. Sramkoski, R.M.; Pretlow, T.G., 2nd; Giaconia, J.M.; Pretlow, T.P.; Schwartz, S.; Sy, M.S.; Marengo, S.R.; Rhim, J.S.; Zhang, D.; Jacobberger, J.W. A new human prostate carcinoma cell line, 22Rv1. *Vitr. Cell. Dev. Biol. Anim.* **1999**, *35*, 403–409. [CrossRef] [PubMed]
105. Zhau, H.Y.; Chang, S.M.; Chen, B.Q.; Wang, Y.; Zhang, H.; Kao, C.; Sang, Q.A.; Pathak, S.J.; Chung, L.W. Androgen-repressed phenotype in human prostate cancer. *Proc. Natl. Acad. Sci. USA* **1996**, *93*, 15152–15157. [CrossRef]
106. Sun, Y.; Schaar, A.; Sukumaran, P.; Dhasarathy, A.; Singh, B.B. TGFbeta-induced epithelial-to-mesenchymal transition in prostate cancer cells is mediated via TRPM7 expression. *Mol. Carcinog.* **2018**, *57*, 752–761. [CrossRef]
107. Millena, A.C.; Vo, B.T.; Khan, S.A. JunD Is Required for Proliferation of Prostate Cancer Cells and Plays a Role in Transforming Growth Factor-beta (TGF-beta)-induced Inhibition of Cell Proliferation. *J. Biol. Chem.* **2016**, *291*, 17964–17976. [CrossRef]
108. Hayward, S.W.; Wang, Y.; Cao, M.; Hom, Y.K.; Zhang, B.; Grossfeld, G.D.; Sudilovsky, D.; Cunha, G.R. Malignant transformation in a nontumorigenic human prostatic epithelial cell line. *Cancer Res.* **2001**, *61*, 8135–8142.
109. Lee, M.; Garkovenko, E.; Yun, J.; Weijerman, P.; Peehl, D.; Chen, L.; Rhim, J. Characterization of adult human prostatic epithelial-cells immortalized by polybrene-induced DNA transfection with a plasmid containing an origin-defective sv40-genome. *Int. J. Oncol.* **1994**, *4*, 821–830. [CrossRef]
110. Shi, X.B.; Xue, L.; Tepper, C.G.; Gandour-Edwards, R.; Ghosh, P.; Kung, H.J.; DeVere White, R.W. The oncogenic potential of a prostate cancer-derived androgen receptor mutant. *Prostate* **2007**, *67*, 591–602. [CrossRef]
111. De Launoit, Y.; Veilleux, R.; Dufour, M.; Simard, J.; Labrie, F. Characteristics of the biphasic action of androgens and of the potent antiproliferative effects of the new pure antiestrogen EM-139 on cell cycle kinetic parameters in LNCaP human prostatic cancer cells. *Cancer Res.* **1991**, *51*, 5165–5170. [PubMed]

112. Nesslinger, N.J.; Shi, X.B.; deVere White, R.W. Androgen-independent growth of LNCaP prostate cancer cells is mediated by gain-of-function mutant p53. *Cancer Res.* **2003**, *63*, 2228–2233. [PubMed]
113. van Bokhoven, A.; Varella-Garcia, M.; Korch, C.; Johannes, W.U.; Smith, E.E.; Miller, H.L.; Nordeen, S.K.; Miller, G.J.; Lucia, M.S. Molecular characterization of human prostate carcinoma cell lines. *Prostate* **2003**, *57*, 205–225. [CrossRef] [PubMed]
114. Vlietstra, R.J.; van Alewijk, D.C.; Hermans, K.G.; van Steenbrugge, G.J.; Trapman, J. Frequent inactivation of PTEN in prostate cancer cell lines and xenografts. *Cancer Res.* **1998**, *58*, 2720–2723.
115. Mitchell, S.; Abel, P.; Ware, M.; Stamp, G.; Lalani, E. Phenotypic and genotypic characterization of commonly used human prostatic cell lines. *BJU Int.* **2000**, *85*, 932–944. [CrossRef]
116. Kokontis, J.M.; Hay, N.; Liao, S. Progression of LNCaP prostate tumor cells during androgen deprivation: Hormone-independent growth, repression of proliferation by androgen, and role for p27Kip1 in androgen-induced cell cycle arrest. *Mol. Endocrinol.* **1998**, *12*, 941–953. [CrossRef]
117. Hudson, T.S.; Perkins, S.N.; Hursting, S.D.; Young, H.A.; Kim, Y.S.; Wang, T.C.; Wang, T.T. Inhibition of androgen-responsive LNCaP prostate cancer cell tumor xenograft growth by dietary phenethyl isothiocyanate correlates with decreased angiogenesis and inhibition of cell attachment. *Int. J. Oncol.* **2012**, *40*, 1113–1121. [CrossRef]
118. Arnold, J.T.; Gray, N.E.; Jacobowitz, K.; Viswanathan, L.; Cheung, P.W.; McFann, K.K.; Le, H.; Blackman, M.R. Human prostate stromal cells stimulate increased PSA production in DHEA-treated prostate cancer epithelial cells. *J. Steroid Biochem. Mol. Biol.* **2008**, *111*, 240–246. [CrossRef]
119. Craft, N.; Shostak, Y.; Carey, M.; Sawyers, C.L. A mechanism for hormone-independent prostate cancer through modulation of androgen receptor signaling by the HER-2/neu tyrosine kinase. *Nat. Med.* **1999**, *5*, 280–285. [CrossRef]
120. Garcia, R.R.; Masoodi, K.Z.; Pascal, L.E.; Nelson, J.B.; Wang, Z. Growth of LAPC4 prostate cancer xenograft tumor is insensitive to 5alpha-reductase inhibitor dutasteride. *Am. J. Clin. Exp. Urol.* **2014**, *2*, 82–91.
121. Patrawala, L.; Calhoun-Davis, T.; Schneider-Broussard, R.; Tang, D.G. Hierarchical organization of prostate cancer cells in xenograft tumors: The CD44+alpha2beta1+ cell population is enriched in tumor-initiating cells. *Cancer Res.* **2007**, *67*, 6796–6805. [CrossRef] [PubMed]
122. Tsingotjidou, A.S.; Zotalis, G.; Jackson, K.R.; Sawyers, C.; Puzas, J.E.; Hicks, D.G.; Reiter, R.; Lieberman, J.R. Development of an animal model for prostate cancer cell metastasis to adult human bone. *Anticancer Res.* **2001**, *21*, 971–978. [PubMed]
123. Nickerson, T.; Chang, F.; Lorimer, D.; Smeekens, S.P.; Sawyers, C.L.; Pollak, M. In vivo progression of LAPC-9 and LNCaP prostate cancer models to androgen independence is associated with increased expression of insulin-like growth factor I (IGF-I) and IGF-I receptor (IGF-IR). *Cancer Res.* **2001**, *61*, 6276–6280. [PubMed]
124. Lee, Y.; Schwarz, E.; Davies, M.; Jo, M.; Gates, J.; Wu, J.; Zhang, X.; Lieberman, J.R. Differences in the cytokine profiles associated with prostate cancer cell induced osteoblastic and osteolytic lesions in bone. *J. Orthop. Res.* **2003**, *21*, 62–72. [CrossRef]
125. McLean, D.T.; Strand, D.W.; Ricke, W.A. Prostate cancer xenografts and hormone induced prostate carcinogenesis. *Differentiation* **2017**, *97*, 23–32. [CrossRef] [PubMed]
126. Watson, P.A.; Chen, Y.F.; Balbas, M.D.; Wongvipat, J.; Socci, N.D.; Viale, A.; Kim, K.; Sawyers, C.L. Constitutively active androgen receptor splice variants expressed in castration-resistant prostate cancer require full-length androgen receptor. *Proc. Natl. Acad. Sci. USA* **2010**, *107*, 16759–16765. [CrossRef] [PubMed]
127. Linxweiler, J.; Korbel, C.; Muller, A.; Hammer, M.; Veith, C.; Bohle, R.M.; Stockle, M.; Junker, K.; Menger, M.D.; Saar, M. A novel mouse model of human prostate cancer to study intraprostatic tumor growth and the development of lymph node metastases. *Prostate* **2018**, *78*, 664–675. [CrossRef]
128. Wang, J.; Cai, Y.; Yu, W.; Ren, C.; Spencer, D.M.; Ittmann, M. Pleiotropic biological activities of alternatively spliced TMPRSS2/ERG fusion gene transcripts. *Cancer Res.* **2008**, *68*, 8516–8524. [CrossRef]
129. Martinez, L.A.; Yang, J.; Vazquez, E.S.; Rodriguez-Vargas Mdel, C.; Olive, M.; Hsieh, J.T.; Logothetis, C.J.; Navone, N.M. p21 modulates threshold of apoptosis induced by DNA-damage and growth factor withdrawal in prostate cancer cells. *Carcinogenesis* **2002**, *23*, 1289–1296. [CrossRef]
130. Alimonti, A.; Nardella, C.; Chen, Z.; Clohessy, J.G.; Carracedo, A.; Trotman, L.C.; Cheng, K.; Varmeh, S.; Kozma, S.C.; Thomas, G.; et al. A novel type of cellular senescence that can be enhanced in mouse models and human tumor xenografts to suppress prostate tumorigenesis. *J. Clin. Investig.* **2010**, *120*, 681–693. [CrossRef]

131. Hara, T.; Nakamura, K.; Araki, H.; Kusaka, M.; Yamaoka, M. Enhanced androgen receptor signaling correlates with the androgen-refractory growth in a newly established MDA PCa 2b-hr human prostate cancer cell subline. *Cancer Res.* **2003**, *63*, 5622–5628. [PubMed]
132. Corey, E.; Quinn, J.E.; Buhler, K.R.; Nelson, P.S.; Macoska, J.A.; True, L.D.; Vessella, R.L. LuCaP 35: A new model of prostate cancer progression to androgen independence. *Prostate* **2003**, *55*, 239–246. [CrossRef] [PubMed]
133. Gaupel, A.-C.; Wang, W.-L.W.; Mordan-McCombs, S.; Lee, E.C.Y.; Tenniswood, M. Xenograft, Transgenic, and Knockout Models of Prostate Cancer. In *Animal Models for the Study of Human Disease*; Elsevier Inc.: Amsterdam, The Netherlands, 2013.
134. Myers, J.S.; Vallega, K.A.; White, J.; Yu, K.; Yates, C.C.; Sang, Q.A. Proteomic characterization of paired non-malignant and malignant African-American prostate epithelial cell lines distinguishes them by structural proteins. *BMC Cancer* **2017**, *17*, 480. [CrossRef] [PubMed]
135. Masumori, N.; Thomas, T.Z.; Chaurand, P.; Case, T.; Paul, M.; Kasper, S.; Caprioli, R.M.; Tsukamoto, T.; Shappell, S.B.; Matusik, R.J. A probasin-large T antigen transgenic mouse line develops prostate adenocarcinoma and neuroendocrine carcinoma with metastatic potential. *Cancer Res.* **2001**, *61*, 2239–2249.
136. Attardi, B.J.; Burgenson, J.; Hild, S.A.; Reel, J.R. Steroid hormonal regulation of growth, prostate specific antigen secretion, and transcription mediated by the mutated androgen receptor in CWR22Rv1 human prostate carcinoma cells. *Mol. Cell. Endocrinol.* **2004**, *222*, 121–132. [CrossRef]
137. Knouf, E.C.; Metzger, M.J.; Mitchell, P.S.; Arroyo, J.D.; Chevillet, J.R.; Tewari, M.; Miller, A.D. Multiple integrated copies and high-level production of the human retrovirus XMRV (xenotropic murine leukemia virus-related virus) from 22Rv1 prostate carcinoma cells. *J. Virol.* **2009**, *83*, 7353–7356. [CrossRef]
138. Nagle, R.B.; Ahmann, F.R.; McDaniel, K.M.; Paquin, M.L.; Clark, V.A.; Celniker, A. Cytokeratin characterization of human prostatic carcinoma and its derived cell lines. *Cancer Res.* **1987**, *47*, 281–286. [PubMed]
139. Tai, S.; Sun, Y.; Squires, J.M.; Zhang, H.; Oh, W.K.; Liang, C.Z.; Huang, J. PC3 is a cell line characteristic of prostatic small cell carcinoma. *Prostate* **2011**, *71*, 1668–1679. [CrossRef]
140. Ravenna, L.; Principessa, L.; Verdina, A.; Salvatori, L.; Russo, M.A.; Petrangeli, E. Distinct phenotypes of human prostate cancer cells associate with different adaptation to hypoxia and pro-inflammatory gene expression. *PLoS ONE* **2014**, *9*, e96250. [CrossRef]
141. Bhardwaj, A.; Singh, S.; Srivastava, S.K.; Arora, S.; Hyde, S.J.; Andrews, J.; Grizzle, W.E.; Singh, A.P. Restoration of PPP2CA expression reverses epithelial-to-mesenchymal transition and suppresses prostate tumour growth and metastasis in an orthotopic mouse model. *Br. J. Cancer* **2014**, *110*, 2000–2010. [CrossRef]
142. Puhr, M.; Hoefer, J.; Eigentler, A.; Ploner, C.; Handle, F.; Schaefer, G.; Kroon, J.; Leo, A.; Heidegger, I.; Eder, I.; et al. The Glucocorticoid Receptor Is a Key Player for Prostate Cancer Cell Survival and a Target for Improved Antiandrogen Therapy. *Clin. Cancer Res.* **2018**, *24*, 927–938. [CrossRef] [PubMed]
143. Jarrard, D.F.; Blitz, B.F.; Smith, R.C.; Patai, B.L.; Rukstalis, D.B. Effect of epidermal growth factor on prostate cancer cell line PC3 growth and invasion. *Prostate* **1994**, *24*, 46–53. [CrossRef] [PubMed]
144. Pfeiffer, M.J.; Schalken, J.A. Stem cell characteristics in prostate cancer cell lines. *Eur. Urol.* **2010**, *57*, 246–254. [CrossRef]
145. Van Leenders, G.J.; Aalders, T.W.; Hulsbergen-van de Kaa, C.A.; Ruiter, D.J.; Schalken, J.A. Expression of basal cell keratins in human prostate cancer metastases and cell lines. *J. Pathol.* **2001**, *195*, 563–570. [CrossRef]
146. Scaccianoce, E.; Festuccia, C.; Dondi, D.; Guerini, V.; Bologna, M.; Motta, M.; Poletti, A. Characterization of prostate cancer DU145 cells expressing the recombinant androgen receptor. *Oncol. Res.* **2003**, *14*, 101–112. [CrossRef]
147. Jones, H.E.; Dutkowski, C.M.; Barrow, D.; Harper, M.E.; Wakeling, A.E.; Nicholson, R.I. New EGF-R selective tyrosine kinase inhibitor reveals variable growth responses in prostate carcinoma cell lines PC-3 and DU-145. *Int. J. Cancer* **1997**, *71*, 1010–1018. [CrossRef]
148. Sherwood, E.R.; Van Dongen, J.L.; Wood, C.G.; Liao, S.; Kozlowski, J.M.; Lee, C. Epidermal growth factor receptor activation in androgen-independent but not androgen-stimulated growth of human prostatic carcinoma cells. *Br. J. Cancer* **1998**, *77*, 855–861. [CrossRef]
149. Mickey, D.D.; Stone, K.R.; Wunderli, H.; Mickey, G.H.; Vollmer, R.T.; Paulson, D.F. Heterotransplantation of a human prostatic adenocarcinoma cell line in nude mice. *Cancer Res.* **1977**, *37*, 4049–4058. [PubMed]

150. Bastide, C.; Bagnis, C.; Mannoni, P.; Hassoun, J.; Bladou, F. A Nod Scid mouse model to study human prostate cancer. *Prostate Cancer Prostatic Dis.* **2002**, *5*, 311–315. [CrossRef]
151. Zhau, H.E.; Odero-Marah, V.; Lue, H.W.; Nomura, T.; Wang, R.; Chu, G.; Liu, Z.R.; Zhou, B.P.; Huang, W.C.; Chung, L.W. Epithelial to mesenchymal transition (EMT) in human prostate cancer: Lessons learned from ARCaP model. *Clin. Exp. Metastasis* **2008**, *25*, 601–610. [CrossRef] [PubMed]
152. Wang, R.; Chu, G.C.Y.; Mrdenovic, S.; Annamalai, A.A.; Hendifar, A.E.; Nissen, N.N.; Tomlinson, J.S.; Lewis, M.; Palanisamy, N.; Tseng, H.R.; et al. Cultured circulating tumor cells and their derived xenografts for personalized oncology. *Asian J. Urol.* **2016**, *3*, 240–253. [CrossRef] [PubMed]
153. He, H.; Yang, X.; Davidson, A.J.; Wu, D.; Marshall, F.F.; Chung, L.W.; Zhau, H.E.; Wang, R. Progressive epithelial to mesenchymal transitions in ARCaP E prostate cancer cells during xenograft tumor formation and metastasis. *Prostate* **2010**, *70*, 518–528. [CrossRef]
154. Gingrich, J.R.; Barrios, R.J.; Morton, R.A.; Boyce, B.F.; DeMayo, F.J.; Finegold, M.J.; Angelopoulou, R.; Rosen, J.M.; Greenberg, N.M. Metastatic prostate cancer in a transgenic mouse. *Cancer Res.* **1996**, *56*, 4096–4102. [PubMed]
155. Greenberg, N.M.; DeMayo, F.J.; Sheppard, P.C.; Barrios, R.; Lebovitz, R.; Finegold, M.; Angelopoulou, R.; Dodd, J.G.; Duckworth, M.L.; Rosen, J.M.; et al. The rat probasin gene promoter directs hormonally and developmentally regulated expression of a heterologous gene specifically to the prostate in transgenic mice. *Mol. Endocrinol.* **1994**, *8*, 230–239. [CrossRef] [PubMed]
156. Maroulakou, I.G.; Anver, M.; Garrett, L.; Green, J.E. Prostate and mammary adenocarcinoma in transgenic mice carrying a rat C3(1) simian virus 40 large tumor antigen fusion gene. *Proc. Natl. Acad. Sci. USA* **1994**, *91*, 11236–11240. [CrossRef] [PubMed]
157. Greenberg, N.M.; DeMayo, F.; Finegold, M.J.; Medina, D.; Tilley, W.D.; Aspinall, J.O.; Cunha, G.R.; Donjacour, A.A.; Matusik, R.J.; Rosen, J.M. Prostate cancer in a transgenic mouse. *Proc. Natl. Acad. Sci. USA* **1995**, *92*, 3439–3443. [CrossRef]
158. Wang, L.; Bonorden, M.J.; Li, G.X.; Lee, H.J.; Hu, H.; Zhang, Y.; Liao, J.D.; Cleary, M.P.; Lu, J. Methyl-selenium compounds inhibit prostate carcinogenesis in the transgenic adenocarcinoma of mouse prostate model with survival benefit. *Cancer Prev. Res. (Phila)* **2009**, *2*, 484–495. [CrossRef] [PubMed]
159. Gupta, S.; Hastak, K.; Ahmad, N.; Lewin, J.S.; Mukhtar, H. Inhibition of prostate carcinogenesis in TRAMP mice by oral infusion of green tea polyphenols. *Proc. Natl. Acad. Sci. USA* **2001**, *98*, 10350–10355. [CrossRef]
160. Gingrich, J.R.; Barrios, R.J.; Kattan, M.W.; Nahm, H.S.; Finegold, M.J.; Greenberg, N.M. Androgen-independent prostate cancer progression in the TRAMP model. *Cancer Res.* **1997**, *57*, 4687–4691.
161. Chiaverotti, T.; Couto, S.S.; Donjacour, A.; Mao, J.H.; Nagase, H.; Cardiff, R.D.; Cunha, G.R.; Balmain, A. Dissociation of epithelial and neuroendocrine carcinoma lineages in the transgenic adenocarcinoma of mouse prostate model of prostate cancer. *Am. J. Pathol.* **2008**, *172*, 236–246. [CrossRef]
162. Rickman, D.S.; Beltran, H.; Demichelis, F.; Rubin, M.A. Biology and evolution of poorly differentiated neuroendocrine tumors. *Nat. Med.* **2017**, *23*, 664–673. [CrossRef]
163. Kasper, S.; Sheppard, P.C.; Yan, Y.; Pettigrew, N.; Borowsky, A.D.; Prins, G.S.; Dodd, J.G.; Duckworth, M.L.; Matusik, R.J. Development, progression, and androgen-dependence of prostate tumors in probasin-large T antigen transgenic mice: A model for prostate cancer. *Lab. Investig.* **1998**, *78*, i–xv.
164. Klezovitch, O.; Chevillet, J.; Mirosevich, J.; Roberts, R.L.; Matusik, R.J.; Vasioukhin, V. Hepsin promotes prostate cancer progression and metastasis. *Cancer Cell* **2004**, *6*, 185–195. [CrossRef]
165. Berman-Booty, L.D.; Knudsen, K.E. Models of neuroendocrine prostate cancer. *Endocr. Relat. Cancer* **2015**, *22*, R33–R49. [CrossRef] [PubMed]
166. Di Cristofano, A.; Pesce, B.; Cordon-Cardo, C.; Pandolfi, P.P. Pten is essential for embryonic development and tumour suppression. *Nat. Genet.* **1998**, *19*, 348–355. [CrossRef] [PubMed]
167. Suzuki, A.; de la Pompa, J.L.; Stambolic, V.; Elia, A.J.; Sasaki, T.; del Barco Barrantes, I.; Ho, A.; Wakeham, A.; Itie, A.; Khoo, W.; et al. High cancer susceptibility and embryonic lethality associated with mutation of the PTEN tumor suppressor gene in mice. *Curr. Biol.* **1998**, *8*, 1169–1178. [CrossRef]
168. Podsypanina, K.; Ellenson, L.H.; Nemes, A.; Gu, J.; Tamura, M.; Yamada, K.M.; Cordon-Cardo, C.; Catoretti, G.; Fisher, P.E.; Parsons, R. Mutation of Pten/Mmac1 in mice causes neoplasia in multiple organ systems. *Proc. Natl. Acad. Sci. USA* **1999**, *96*, 1563–1568. [CrossRef]

169. Stambolic, V.; Tsao, M.S.; Macpherson, D.; Suzuki, A.; Chapman, W.B.; Mak, T.W. High incidence of breast and endometrial neoplasia resembling human Cowden syndrome in pten+/− mice. *Cancer Res.* **2000**, *60*, 3605–3611. [PubMed]
170. Li, Q.; Liu, L.; Zhang, Q.; Liu, S.; Ge, D.; You, Z. Interleukin-17 Indirectly Promotes M2 Macrophage Differentiation through Stimulation of COX-2/PGE2 Pathway in the Cancer Cells. *Cancer Res. Treat.* **2014**, *46*, 297–306. [CrossRef]
171. Zhang, Q.; Liu, S.; Zhang, Q.; Xiong, Z.; Wang, A.R.; Myers, L.; Melamed, J.; Tang, W.W.; You, Z. Interleukin-17 promotes development of castration-resistant prostate cancer potentially through creating an immunotolerant and pro-angiogenic tumor microenvironment. *Prostate* **2014**, *74*, 869–879. [CrossRef]
172. Bai, F.; Pei, X.H.; Pandolfi, P.P.; Xiong, Y. p18 Ink4c and Pten constrain a positive regulatory loop between cell growth and cell cycle control. *Mol. Cell. Biol.* **2006**, *26*, 4564–4576. [CrossRef] [PubMed]
173. Bowen, C.; Bubendorf, L.; Voeller, H.J.; Slack, R.; Willi, N.; Sauter, G.; Gasser, T.C.; Koivisto, P.; Lack, E.E.; Kononen, J.; et al. Loss of NKX3.1 expression in human prostate cancers correlates with tumor progression. *Cancer Res.* **2000**, *60*, 6111–6115. [PubMed]
174. Jayaprakash, P.; Ai, M.; Liu, A.; Budhani, P.; Bartkowiak, T.; Sheng, J.; Ager, C.; Nicholas, C.; Jaiswal, A.R.; Sun, Y.; et al. Targeted hypoxia reduction restores T cell infiltration and sensitizes prostate cancer to immunotherapy. *J. Clin. Investig.* **2018**, *128*, 5137–5149. [CrossRef] [PubMed]
175. Wang, G.; Lu, X.; Dey, P.; Deng, P.; Wu, C.C.; Jiang, S.; Fang, Z.; Zhao, K.; Konaparthi, R.; Hua, S.; et al. Targeting YAP-Dependent MDSC Infiltration Impairs Tumor Progression. *Cancer Discov.* **2016**, *6*, 80–95. [CrossRef] [PubMed]
176. Wu, X.; Wu, J.; Huang, J.; Powell, W.C.; Zhang, J.; Matusik, R.J.; Sangiorgi, F.O.; Maxson, R.E.; Sucov, H.M.; Roy-Burman, P. Generation of a prostate epithelial cell-specific Cre transgenic mouse model for tissue-specific gene ablation. *Mech. Dev.* **2001**, *101*, 61–69. [CrossRef]
177. Zhang, J.; Thomas, T.Z.; Kasper, S.; Matusik, R.J. A small composite probasin promoter confers high levels of prostate-specific gene expression through regulation by androgens and glucocorticoids in vitro and in vivo. *Endocrinology* **2000**, *141*, 4698–4710. [CrossRef]
178. McMullin, R.P.; Mutton, L.N.; Bieberich, C.J. Hoxb13 regulatory elements mediate transgene expression during prostate organogenesis and carcinogenesis. *Dev. Dyn.* **2009**, *238*, 664–672. [CrossRef]
179. Majumder, P.K.; Yeh, J.J.; George, D.J.; Febbo, P.G.; Kum, J.; Xue, Q.; Bikoff, R.; Ma, H.; Kantoff, P.W.; Golub, T.R.; et al. Prostate intraepithelial neoplasia induced by prostate restricted Akt activation: The MPAKT model. *Proc. Natl. Acad. Sci. USA* **2003**, *100*, 7841–7846. [CrossRef]
180. Ramaswamy, S.; Nakamura, N.; Vazquez, F.; Batt, D.B.; Perera, S.; Roberts, T.M.; Sellers, W.R. Regulation of G1 progression by the PTEN tumor suppressor protein is linked to inhibition of the phosphatidylinositol 3-kinase/Akt pathway. *Proc. Natl. Acad. Sci. USA* **1999**, *96*, 2110–2115. [CrossRef]
181. Gao, D.; Chen, Y. Organoid development in cancer genome discovery. *Curr. Opin. Genet. Dev.* **2015**, *30*, 42–48. [CrossRef]
182. Ben-David, U.; Beroukhim, R.; Golub, T.R. Genomic evolution of cancer models: Perils and opportunities. *Nat. Rev. Cancer* **2019**, *19*, 97–109. [CrossRef]
183. Wang, S.; Gao, D.; Chen, Y. The potential of organoids in urological cancer research. *Nat. Rev. Urol.* **2017**, *14*, 401–414. [CrossRef] [PubMed]
184. Gao, D.; Vela, I.; Sboner, A.; Iaquinta, P.J.; Karthaus, W.R.; Gopalan, A.; Dowling, C.; Wanjala, J.N.; Undvall, E.A.; Arora, V.K.; et al. Organoid cultures derived from patients with advanced prostate cancer. *Cell* **2014**, *159*, 176–187. [CrossRef] [PubMed]
185. Puca, L.; Bareja, R.; Prandi, D.; Shaw, R.; Benelli, M.; Karthaus, W.R.; Hess, J.; Sigouros, M.; Donoghue, A.; Kossai, M.; et al. Patient derived organoids to model rare prostate cancer phenotypes. *Nat. Commun.* **2018**, *9*, 2404. [CrossRef] [PubMed]
186. Choi, S.Y.; Lin, D.; Gout, P.W.; Collins, C.C.; Xu, Y.; Wang, Y. Lessons from patient-derived xenografts for better in vitro modeling of human cancer. *Adv. Drug Deliv. Rev.* **2014**, *79–80*, 222–237. [CrossRef]
187. Nguyen, H.M.; Vessella, R.L.; Morrissey, C.; Brown, L.G.; Coleman, I.M.; Higano, C.S.; Mostaghel, E.A.; Zhang, X.; True, L.D.; Lam, H.M.; et al. LuCaP Prostate Cancer Patient-Derived Xenografts Reflect the Molecular Heterogeneity of Advanced Disease and Serve as Models for Evaluating Cancer Therapeutics. *Prostate* **2017**, *77*, 654–671. [CrossRef]

188. Li, Z.G.; Mathew, P.; Yang, J.; Starbuck, M.W.; Zurita, A.J.; Liu, J.; Sikes, C.; Multani, A.S.; Efstathiou, E.; Lopez, A.; et al. Androgen receptor-negative human prostate cancer cells induce osteogenesis in mice through FGF9-mediated mechanisms. *J. Clin. Investig.* **2008**, *118*, 2697–2710. [CrossRef]
189. Lee, C.H.; Xue, H.; Sutcliffe, M.; Gout, P.W.; Huntsman, D.G.; Miller, D.M.; Gilks, C.B.; Wang, Y.Z. Establishment of subrenal capsule xenografts of primary human ovarian tumors in SCID mice: Potential models. *Gynecol. Oncol.* **2005**, *96*, 48–55. [CrossRef]
190. Okada, S.; Vaeteewoottacharn, K.; Kariya, R. Establishment of a Patient-Derived Tumor Xenograft Model and Application for Precision Cancer Medicine. *Chem. Pharm. Bull. (Tokyo)* **2018**, *66*, 225–230. [CrossRef]
191. Kopetz, S.; Lemos, R.; Powis, G. The promise of patient-derived xenografts: The best laid plans of mice and men. *Clin. Cancer Res.* **2012**, *18*, 5160–5162. [CrossRef]
192. Hoehn, W.; Schroeder, F.H.; Reimann, J.F.; Joebsis, A.C.; Hermanek, P. Human prostatic adenocarcinoma: Some characteristics of a serially transplantable line in nude mice (PC 82). *Prostate* **1980**, *1*, 95–104. [CrossRef] [PubMed]
193. Van Weerden, W.M.; de Ridder, C.M.; Verdaasdonk, C.L.; Romijn, J.C.; van der Kwast, T.H.; Schroder, F.H.; van Steenbrugge, G.J. Development of seven new human prostate tumor xenograft models and their histopathological characterization. *Am. J. Pathol.* **1996**, *149*, 1055–1062. [PubMed]
194. Kiefer, J.A.; Vessella, R.L.; Quinn, J.E.; Odman, A.M.; Zhang, J.; Keller, E.T.; Kostenuik, P.J.; Dunstan, C.R.; Corey, E. The effect of osteoprotegerin administration on the intra-tibial growth of the osteoblastic LuCaP 23.1 prostate cancer xenograft. *Clin. Exp. Metastasis* **2004**, *21*, 381–387. [CrossRef]
195. Corey, E.; Quinn, J.E.; Bladou, F.; Brown, L.G.; Roudier, M.P.; Brown, J.M.; Buhler, K.R.; Vessella, R.L. Establishment and characterization of osseous prostate cancer models: Intra-tibial injection of human prostate cancer cells. *Prostate* **2002**, *52*, 20–33. [CrossRef] [PubMed]
196. Toivanen, R.; Berman, D.M.; Wang, H.; Pedersen, J.; Frydenberg, M.; Meeker, A.K.; Ellem, S.J.; Risbridger, G.P.; Taylor, R.A. Brief report: A bioassay to identify primary human prostate cancer repopulating cells. *Stem Cells* **2011**, *29*, 1310–1314. [CrossRef]
197. Morton, C.L.; Houghton, P.J. Establishment of human tumor xenografts in immunodeficient mice. *Nat. Protoc.* **2007**, *2*, 247–250. [CrossRef]
198. Yada, E.; Wada, S.; Yoshida, S.; Sasada, T. Use of patient-derived xenograft mouse models in cancer research and treatment. *Future Sci. OA* **2018**, *4*, FSO271. [CrossRef]
199. Dunning, W.F.; Curtis, M.R.; Segaloff, A. Methylcholanthrene squamous cell carcinoma of the rat prostate with skeletal metastases, and failure of the rat liver to respond to the carcinogen. *Cancer Res.* **1946**, *6*, 256–262.
200. Tennant, T.R.; Kim, H.; Sokoloff, M.; Rinker-Schaeffer, C.W. The Dunning model. *Prostate* **2000**, *43*, 295–302. [CrossRef]
201. Pollard, M. The Lobund-Wistar rat model of prostate cancer. *J. Cell. Biochem. Suppl.* **1992**, *16H*, 84–88. [CrossRef]
202. Wertman, J.; Veinotte, C.J.; Dellaire, G.; Berman, J.N. The Zebrafish Xenograft Platform: Evolution of a Novel Cancer Model and Preclinical Screening Tool. *Adv. Exp. Med. Biol.* **2016**, *916*, 289–314. [CrossRef] [PubMed]
203. Herbomel, P.; Thisse, B.; Thisse, C. Ontogeny and behaviour of early macrophages in the zebrafish embryo. *Development* **1999**, *126*, 3735–3745.
204. Le Guyader, D.; Redd, M.J.; Colucci-Guyon, E.; Murayama, E.; Kissa, K.; Briolat, V.; Mordelet, E.; Zapata, A.; Shinomiya, H.; Herbomel, P. Origins and unconventional behavior of neutrophils in developing zebrafish. *Blood* **2008**, *111*, 132–141. [CrossRef] [PubMed]
205. Melong, N.; Steele, S.; MacDonald, M.; Holly, A.; Collins, C.C.; Zoubeidi, A.; Berman, J.N.; Dellaire, G. Enzalutamide inhibits testosterone-induced growth of human prostate cancer xenografts in zebrafish and can induce bradycardia. *Sci. Rep.* **2017**, *7*, 14698. [CrossRef] [PubMed]
206. Xu, W.; Foster, B.A.; Richards, M.; Bondioli, K.R.; Shah, G.; Green, C.C. Characterization of prostate cancer cell progression in zebrafish xenograft model. *Int. J. Oncol.* **2018**, *52*, 252–260. [CrossRef]

Permissions

All chapters in this book were first published by MDPI; hereby published with permission under the Creative Commons Attribution License or equivalent. Every chapter published in this book has been scrutinized by our experts. Their significance has been extensively debated. The topics covered herein carry significant findings which will fuel the growth of the discipline. They may even be implemented as practical applications or may be referred to as a beginning point for another development.

The contributors of this book come from diverse backgrounds, making this book a truly international effort. This book will bring forth new frontiers with its revolutionizing research information and detailed analysis of the nascent developments around the world.

We would like to thank all the contributing authors for lending their expertise to make the book truly unique. They have played a crucial role in the development of this book. Without their invaluable contributions this book wouldn't have been possible. They have made vital efforts to compile up to date information on the varied aspects of this subject to make this book a valuable addition to the collection of many professionals and students.

This book was conceptualized with the vision of imparting up-to-date information and advanced data in this field. To ensure the same, a matchless editorial board was set up. Every individual on the board went through rigorous rounds of assessment to prove their worth. After which they invested a large part of their time researching and compiling the most relevant data for our readers.

The editorial board has been involved in producing this book since its inception. They have spent rigorous hours researching and exploring the diverse topics which have resulted in the successful publishing of this book. They have passed on their knowledge of decades through this book. To expedite this challenging task, the publisher supported the team at every step. A small team of assistant editors was also appointed to further simplify the editing procedure and attain best results for the readers.

Apart from the editorial board, the designing team has also invested a significant amount of their time in understanding the subject and creating the most relevant covers. They scrutinized every image to scout for the most suitable representation of the subject and create an appropriate cover for the book.

The publishing team has been an ardent support to the editorial, designing and production team. Their endless efforts to recruit the best for this project, has resulted in the accomplishment of this book. They are a veteran in the field of academics and their pool of knowledge is as vast as their experience in printing. Their expertise and guidance has proved useful at every step. Their uncompromising quality standards have made this book an exceptional effort. Their encouragement from time to time has been an inspiration for everyone.

The publisher and the editorial board hope that this book will prove to be a valuable piece of knowledge for researchers, students, practitioners and scholars across the globe.

List of Contributors

Yasuyoshi Miyata, Tomohiro Matsuo, Yuji Sagara, Kojiro Ohba and Hideki Sakai
Department of Urology, Nagasaki University Graduate School of Biomedical Sciences, 1-7-1 Sakamoto, Nagasaki 852-8501, Japan

Kaname Ohyama
Department of Pharmaceutical Science, Nagasaki University Graduate School of Biomedical Sciences, 1-7-1 Sakamoto, Nagasaki 852-8501, Japan

Manuela A. Hoffmann
Department of Occupational Health & Safety, Federal Ministry of Defense, 53123 Bonn, Germany
Clinic of Nuclear Medicine, Johannes Gutenberg-University, 55101 Mainz, Germany

Hans-Georg Buchholz, Matthias Miederer and Mathias Schreckenberger
Clinic of Nuclear Medicine, Johannes Gutenberg-University, 55101 Mainz, Germany

Helmut J Wieler
Clinic of Nuclear Medicine, Bundeswehr Central Hospital, 56072 Koblenz, Germany

Florian Rosar
Clinic of Nuclear Medicine, Johannes Gutenberg-University, 55101 Mainz, Germany
Department of Nuclear Medicine, Saarland University Medical Center, 66421 Homburg, Germany

Nicolas Fischer
Department of Urology, University of Cologne, 50937 Cologne, Germany

Marco Moschini
Department of Urology, Comprehensive Cancer Center, Medical University of Vienna, Vienna General Hospital, A-1090 Vienna, Austria
Department of Urology, Urological Research Institute, San Raffaele Scientific Institute, 20132 Milan, Italy
Department of Urology, Luzerner Kantonsspital, Spitalstrasse, 6000 Luzern, Switzerland

Francesco Montorsi, Alberto Briganti, Andrea Gallina and Armando Stabile
Department of Urology, Urological Research Institute, San Raffaele Scientific Institute, 20132 Milan, Italy

Stefania Zamboni, Agostino Mattei, Philipp Baumeister and Livio Mordasini
Department of Urology, Luzerner Kantonsspital, Spitalstrasse, 6000 Luzern, Switzerland

Francesco Soria
Department of Urology, Comprehensive Cancer Center, Medical University of Vienna, Vienna General Hospital, A-1090 Vienna, Austria
Division of Urology, Department of Surgical Sciences, University of Studies of Torino, 10124 Turin, Italy

Romain Mathieu
Department of Urology, Comprehensive Cancer Center, Medical University of Vienna, Vienna General Hospital, A-1090 Vienna, Austria
Department of Urology, Rennes University Hospital, 35000 Rennes, France

Evanguelos Xylinas
Department of Urology Bichat Hospital, Paris Descartes University, 75877 Paris, France
Department of Urology, Hôpital Cochin, APHP, 75014 Paris, France

Wei Shen Tan and John D Kelly
Division of Surgery and Intervention Science, University College London, London WC1E 6BT, UK
Department of Uro-Oncology, University College London Hospital NHS Foundation Trust, London W1T 4EU, UK

Giuseppe Simone
Department of Urology, "Regina Elena" National Cancer Institute, 00128 Rome, Italy
Department of Urology, IRCCS Regina Elena National Cancer Institute, 00144 Rome, Italy

Anoop Meraney
Urology Division, Hartford Healthcare Medical Group, Hartford, CT 06106, USA

Suprita Krishna and Badrinath Konety
Department of Urology, University of Minnesota, Minneapolis, MN 55455, USA

Rafael Sanchez-Salas and Xavier Cathelineau
Department of Urology, L'Institut Mutualiste Montsouris, Université Paris Descartes, 75014 Paris, France

Michael Rink
Department of Urology, University Medical Center Hamburg-Eppendorf, 20251 Hamburg, Germany
Department of Urology, Medical University of Hamburg, Martinistraße 52, 20246 Hamburg, Germany

Andrea Necchi
Fondazione IRCCS Istituto Nazionale dei Tumori, 20133 Milan, Italy

Pierre I. Karakiewicz
Cancer Prognostics and Health Outcomes Unit, University of Montreal Health Centre, Montreal, QC H4A 3J1, Canada

Morgan Rouprêt
Sorbonne Université, GRC no. 5, ONCOTYPE-URO, AP-HP, Hôpital Pitié-Salpêtrière, F-75013 Paris, France

Anthony Koupparis
Bristol Urological Institute, North Bristol NHS Trust, Southmead Hospital, Bristol BS10 5NB, UK

Wassim Kassouf
Department of Urology, McGill University Health Center, Montreal, QC H4A3J1, Canada

Douglas S Scherr
Department of Urology, Weill Cornell Medical College, New York-Presbyterian Hospital, New York, NY 10038, USA

Guillaume Ploussard
Department of Urology, La Croix du sud Hospital, 314000 Toulouse, France

Stephen A. Boorjian
Department of Urology, Mayo Clinic, 200 First Street Southwest, Rochester, MN 55905, USA

Yair Lotan
Department of Urology, University of Texas Southwestern Medical Center, Dallas, TX 75390, USA

Prasanna Sooriakumaran
Department of Uro-Oncology, University College London Hospital NHS Foundation Trust, London W1T 4EU, UK
Department of Molecular Medicine and Surgery, Karolinska Institutet, 17177 Stockholm, Sweden

Douglas S. Scherr
Department of Urology, Weill Cornell Medical College, New York-Presbyterian Hospital, New York, NY 10038, USA

Mathieu Roumiguié and Bernard Malavaud
Department of Urology, Institut Universitaire du Cancer, 31059 Toulouse CEDEX 9, France

Antonin Brisuda and Marek Babjuk
Department of Urology, 2nd Faculty of Medicine, Charles University, Teaching Hospital Motol, 15006 Prague, Czech Republic

Maximillian Burger
St. Josef, Klinik für Urologie, Caritas-Krankenhaus, 93053 Regensburg, Germany

Hugh Mostafid
Department of Urology, Royal Surrey County Hospital, Surrey, Guildford GU2 7RF, UK

Marc Colombel
Department of Urology, Hôpital Edouard Herriot, 69437 Lyon, France

Joan Palou Redorta
Department of Urology, Fundacio Puigvert, 08025 Barcelona, Spain

Fred Witjes
Department of Urology, Radboud UMC, 6525 GA Nijmegen, The Netherlands

Florian Janisch
Department of Urology, Medical University of Hamburg, Martinistraße 52, 20246 Hamburg, Germany
Department of Urology, Medical University of Vienna, Währinger Gürtel 18-20, 1090 Vienna, Austria

Hang Yu, Malte W. Vetterlein, Roland Dahlem, Oliver Engel, Margit Fisch and Armin Soave
Department of Urology, Medical University of Hamburg, Martinistraße 52, 20246 Hamburg, Germany

Shahrokh F. Shariat
Department of Urology, Medical University of Vienna, Währinger Gürtel 18-20, 1090 Vienna, Austria
Institute for Urology and Reproductive Health, Sechenov University, Bolshaya Pirogovskaya str. 2-4, 119991 Moscow, Russia
Department of Urology, University of Texas Southwestern Medical Center, 5323 Harry Hines Blvd, Dallas, TX 75390, USA
Karl Landsteiner Institute of Urology and Andrology, Franziskanergasse 4, a 3100 St. Poelten, Austria
Department of Urology, Second Faculty of Medicine, Charles University, Ovocný trh 5, Prague 1-116 36, Czech Republic
Department of Urology, Comprehensive Cancer Center, Medical University of Vienna, Vienna General Hospital, A-1090 Vienna, Austria
Department of Urology, Weill Cornell Medical College, New York Presbyterian Hospital, New York, NY 10021, USA
Department of Urology, The University of Texas M.D. Anderson Cancer Center, Houston, TX 77030, USA

lNiklas Klümper
Department of Urology, University Hospital Bonn, 53127 Bonn, Germany
Center for Integrated Oncology, University Hospital Bonn, 53127 Bonn, Germany
Institute of Experimental Oncology, University Hospital Bonn, 53127 Bonn, Germany

Marthe von Danwitz, Johannes Stein, Doris Schmidt, Anja Schmidt, Manuel Ritter, Abdullah Alajati and Jörg Ellinger
Department of Urology, University Hospital Bonn, 53127 Bonn, Germany
Center for Integrated Oncology, University Hospital Bonn, 53127 Bonn, Germany

Glen Kristiansen and Michael Muders
Center for Integrated Oncology, University Hospital Bonn, 53127 Bonn, Germany
Institute of Pathology, University Hospital Bonn, 53127 Bonn, Germany

Michael Hölzel
Center for Integrated Oncology, University Hospital Bonn, 53127 Bonn, Germany
Institute of Experimental Oncology, University Hospital Bonn, 53127 Bonn, Germany

Donghyun Kim and Jin Man Kim
Department of Pathology, Chungnam National University School of Medicine, 266 Munhwa Street, Daejeon 35015, Korea
Department of Pathology, Chungnam National University Hospital, 282 Munwha-ro, Daejeon 35015, Korea

Jun-Sang Kim
Department of Radiation Oncology, Chungnam National University School of Medicine, 288 Munhwa Street, Daejeon 35015, Korea
Department of Radiation Oncology, Chungnam National University Hospital, 282 Munwha-ro, Daejeon 35015, Korea

Sup Kim
Department of Radiation Oncology, Chungnam National University Hospital, 282 Munwha-ro, Daejeon 35015, Korea

Kyung-Hee Kim
Department of Pathology, Chungnam National University School of Medicine, 266 Munhwa Street, Daejeon 35015, Korea
Department of Pathology, Chungnam National University Hospital, 282 Munwha-ro, Daejeon 35015, Korea
Department of Pathology, Chungnam National University Sejong Hospital, 20 Bodeum 7-ro, Sejongsi 30099, Korea

Carlo Cattrini
Department of Internal Medicine and Medical Specialties (DIMI), School of Medicine, University of Genoa, 16132 Genoa, Italy
Prostate Cancer Clinical Research Unit, Spanish National Cancer Research Centre (CNIO), 28029 Madrid, Spain

Davide Soldato, Elisa Zanardi, Paola Barboro and Francesco Boccardo
Department of Internal Medicine and Medical Specialties (DIMI), School of Medicine, University of Genoa, 16132 Genoa, Italy
Academic Unit of Medical Oncology, IRCCS Ospedale Policlinico San Martino, 16132 Genoa, Italy

David Olmos
Prostate Cancer Clinical Research Unit, Spanish National Cancer Research Centre (CNIO), 28029 Madrid, Spain

Alessandra Rubagotti
Academic Unit of Medical Oncology, IRCCS Ospedale Policlinico San Martino, 16132 Genoa, Italy
Department of Health Sciences (DISSAL), School of Medicine, University of Genoa, 16132 Genoa, Italy

Linda Zinoli
Academic Unit of Medical Oncology, IRCCS Ospedale Policlinico San Martino, 16132 Genoa, Italy

Carlo Messina
Department of Medical Oncology, Santa Chiara Hospital, 38122 Trento, Italy

Elena Castro
CNIO-IBIMA Genitourinary Cancer Unit, Hospitales Universitarios Virgen de la Victoria y Regional de Málaga, Instituto de Investigación Biomédica de Málaga, 29010 Malaga, Spain

Zhengqiu Zhou
Department of Molecular and Cellular Biochemistry, University of Kentucky College of Medicine, Lexington, KY 40536, USA

Connor J. Kinslow
Department of Radiation Oncology, Vagelos College of Physicians and Surgeons, Columbia University Irving Medical Center, New York, NY 10032, USA

Peng Wang
Division of Medical Oncology, Department of Internal Medicine, College of Medicine, University of Kentucky, Lexington, KY 40536, USA

Bin Huang
Department of Biostatistics, College of Public Health, University of Kentucky, Lexington, KY 40536, USA

Simon K. Cheng and Israel Deutsch
Department of Radiation Oncology, Vagelos College of Physicians and Surgeons, Columbia University Irving Medical Center, New York, NY 10032, USA
Division of Medical Oncology, Department of Internal Medicine, College of Medicine, University of Kentucky, Lexington, KY 40536, USA
Department of Biostatistics, College of Public Health, University of Kentucky, Lexington, KY 40536, USA
Herbert Irving Comprehensive Cancer Center, Vagelos College of Physicians and Surgeons, Columbia University Irving Medical Center, New York, NY 10032, USA

Matthew S. Gentry
Department of Molecular and Cellular Biochemistry, University of Kentucky College of Medicine, Lexington, KY 40536, USA
Markey Cancer Center, University of Kentucky, Lexington, KY 40536, USA

Ramon C. Sun
Markey Cancer Center, University of Kentucky, Lexington, KY 40536, USA
Department of Neuroscience, University of Kentucky College of Medicine, Lexington, KY 40536, USA

Claudia Manini
Department of Pathology, San Giovanni Bosco Hospital, 10154 Turin, Italy

José I. López
Department of Pathology, Biocruces-Bizkaia Health Research Institute, Cruces University Hospital, Barakaldo, 48903 Bizkaia, Spain

Shyama U. Tetar, Omar Bohoudi, Suresh Senan, Miguel A. Palacios, Swie S. Oei, Antoinet M. van der Wel, Berend J. Slotman, Frank J. Lagerwaard and Anna M. E. Bruynzeel
Department of Radiation Oncology, Amsterdam University Medical Centers, 1081 HZ Amsterdam, The Netherlands

R. Jeroen A. van Moorselaar
Department of Urology, Amsterdam University Medical Centers, 1081 HV Amsterdam, The Netherlands

Claudia Claroni, Marco Covotta, Giulia Torregiani, Maria Elena Marcelli and Ester Forastiere
Department of Anaesthesiology, IRCCS Regina Elena National Cancer Institute, 00144 Rome, Italy

Gabriele Tuderti
Department of Urology, IRCCS Regina Elena National Cancer Institute, 00144 Rome, Italy

Alessandra Scotto di Uccio
School of Medicine, University Hospital Center "Tor Vergata", 00133 Rome, Italy

Antonio Zinilli
IRCrES, Research Institute on Sustainable Economic Growth of the National Research Council of Italy, 00185 Rome, Italy

Sofia Karkampouna, Maria R. De Filippo, Irena Klima and Eugenio Zoni
Urology Research Laboratory, Department for BioMedical Research, University of Bern, Murtenstrasse 35, 3008 Bern, Switzerland

Charlotte K. Y. Ng
Oncogenomics Laboratory, Department for BioMedical Research, University of Bern, Murtenstrasse 40, 3008 Bern, Switzerland

Martin Spahn
Lindenhofspital Bern, Prostate Center Bern, 3012 Bern, Switzerland

Frank Stein and Per Haberkant
Proteomics Core Facility, EMBL Heidelberg, Meyerhofstraße 1, 69117 Heidelberg, Germany

George N. Thalmann and Marianna Kruithof-de Julio
Urology Research Laboratory, Department for BioMedical Research, University of Bern, Murtenstrasse 35, 3008 Bern, Switzerland
Department of Urology, Inselspital, Anna Seiler Haus, Bern University Hospital, 3010 Bern, Switzerland

Jennifer Kubon, Danijel Sikic, Angela Neumann, Bastian Keck, Bernd Wullich, Helge Taubert and Sven Wach
Department of Urology and Pediatric Urology, University Hospital Erlangen, Friedrich-Alexander Universität Erlangen-Nürnberg, 91054 Erlangen, Germany

Markus Eckstein, Veronika Weyerer, Robert Stöhr and Arndt Hartmann
Institute of Pathology, University Hospital Erlangen, Friedrich-Alexander Universität Erlangen-Nürnberg, 91054 Erlangen, Germany

Ralph M. Wirtz
STRATIFYER Molecular Pathology GmbH, 50935 Cologne, Germany

Sirin Saranyutanon, Sachin Kumar Deshmukh and Santanu Dasgupta
Cancer Biology Program, Mitchell Cancer Institute, University of South Alabama, Mobile, AL 36604, USA
Department of Medical Oncology, Mitchell Cancer Institute, University of South Alabama, Mobile, AL 36604, USA

Sachin Pai
Department of Pathology, College of Medicine, University of South Alabama, Mobile, AL 36617, USA

Seema Singh and Ajay Pratap Singh
Cancer Biology Program, Mitchell Cancer Institute, University of South Alabama, Mobile, AL 36604, USA
Department of Medical Oncology, Mitchell Cancer Institute, University of South Alabama, Mobile, AL 36604, USA
Department of Biochemistry and Molecular Biology, University of South Alabama, Mobile, AL 36688, USA

Index

Printed in the USA
CPSIA information can be obtained
at www.ICGtesting.com
JSHW051400091023
49903JS00006B/214